The Karma of Love

Books by Geshe Michael Roach

THE GARDEN

THE DIAMOND CUTTER: THE BUDDHA ON STRATEGIES
FOR MANAGING YOUR BUSINESS AND YOUR LIFE

HOW YOGA WORKS

KARMIC MANAGEMENT: WHAT GOES AROUND COMES AROUND,
IN YOUR BUSINESS AND YOUR LIFE

THE ESSENTIAL YOGA SUTRA

THE TIBETAN BOOK OF YOGA

KING OF THE DHARMA: THE ILLUSTRATED LIFE OF
JE TSONGKAPA, TEACHER OF THE FIRST DALAI LAMA

THE EASTERN PATH TO HEAVEN
A GUIDE TO HAPPINESS FROM THE TEACHINGS
OF JESUS IN TIBET

THE PRINCIPAL TEACHINGS OF BUDDHISM

KING UDRAYANA AND THE WHEEL OF LIFE

THE LOGIC AND DEBATE TRADITION
 OF INDIA, TIBET, AND MONGOLIA

PREPARING FOR TANTRA

THE 18 BOOKS OF THE FOUNDATION COURSE IN BUDDHISM,
ASIAN CLASSICS INSTITUTE (ACI)

THE 10 BUDDHIST MEDITATION AND PRACTICE MODULES, ACI

THE 18 BOOKS OF THE DIAMOND WAY COURSE IN BUDDHISM, ACI

The Karma of Love

100 Answers for Your Relationship,

from the Ancient Wisdom of Tibet

Geshe Michael Roach

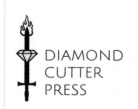

DIAMOND
CUTTER
PRESS

Published in 2013 by
Diamond Cutter Press
55 Powderhorn Drive
Wayne, New Jersey 07470

Cover design by:
        Geshe Michael Roach & Georgina Rivera

Interior design by:
        Geshe Michael Roach & Robert Ruisinger

Library of Congress Cataloging-in-Publication Data
available upon request.

ISBN 978-1-937114-06-0

www.diamondcutterpress.com
www.KarmaOfLove.com

TABLE OF CONTENTS

FOREWORD

I grew up in Arizona, had a normal American youth and the normal encounters with girls, and then after high school went east to attend Princeton University. I excelled in my schooling, and was even awarded a medal for scholarship from the President, at the White House. It seemed like my life was charmed, that I was headed for great things.

And then one night all of that changed. I was in a meeting at the university chapel for volunteers who wanted to help do something about world hunger. The priest took a telephone call, and then came and touched my arm and asked me to come with him to his office. There he told me that my mother had just died. My charmed world was shattered.

In the time that followed, I received two more phone calls—one that my younger brother had died, and another that my father had passed as well. In this sea of grief it seemed that staying in college, and in the life I had expected, held little meaning. I left school and journeyed to India, searching for answers.

I had the good fortune to meet some Tibetan monks, and gradually became a monk myself. I stayed in Tibetan monasteries for more than 25 years, and was the first westerner in six centuries to receive the degree of *Geshe,* or Master of Buddhism, from the great monastery of Sera Mey.

To finish this degree I had to undergo many tests—such as a 3-week public examination by hundreds of the monks, all in the Tibetan language. My main lama in the monastery, Khen Rinpoche, proposed for me an additional test: Could I go to New York, start a diamond company, and make a million dollars, to prove that I understood the principles of karma which I had been taught in the monastery? We would then give the money to Tibetan refugees to help with their food and other needs.

Re-entering the world, especially the world of New York City and a business as potentially dirty as the diamond business, was the last thing I wanted to do—so I avoided his advice for many months. In the end, though, the Lama's word prevails, and I had to go.

I did help to start a company, called Andin International Diamond, and helped bring it towards its $200 million in annual sales. The company was recently purchased by Warren Buffett, one of the world's wealthiest people. With the money I earned at the company, I was able to help refugees and many other people.

Our firm was one of the fastest-growing companies in the history of New

York, and naturally that drew some attention. I was approached by Doubleday Publishers and asked to write a book about how we achieved our success
by using the principles of karma—the principles of helping others.

And so I wrote a book called *The Diamond Cutter,* named after a famous
sutra which explains karma and its flipside, the Buddhist idea of emptiness.
This book has become a business bestseller around the world, translated into
some 25 languages, and is used by millions of people; it is especially popular
in the Chinese edition, and has helped many people achieve financial independence.

Inevitably, people began to ask me to come and give talks about the book.
In the years since it was written, I and my colleagues at the Diamond Cutter Institute have conducted business seminars and retreats for thousands of
people in many countries. During these programs we often hold small breakout groups called "Wisdom for Daily Life," where participants have a chance
to ask questions about their own companies and careers.

One day, during a program in China, a woman in one of these groups
asked if I would answer a question not about business, but about her relationship with her husband. Did the Diamond Cutter Principles—the principles of
karmic seeds—also apply to her family life? I answered that of course they
did; that karmic seeds in our mind are responsible for everything and everybody around us.

Suddenly a dam broke and everyone in the group began asking pent-
up questions about the most intimate issues of their relationship with their
spouse or partner. In that moment I realized that taking care of people's spiritual needs—and needs like housing and money and food—was not enough.
Our intimate relationships are the source of perhaps the greatest happiness
in life; and they can also be the source of our greatest pain. If we want to be
happy, and if we want the world to be happy, then we have to get this relationship thing right!

The ancient tradition of the Buddhist monks, surprisingly, has much wisdom to offer us about our relationship with our partner. First of all there is an
open tradition of tens of thousands of peerless books of knowledge—books
which inform us of where everything in our life is coming from, including
everything about our partner. These are the teachings on karmic seeds.

There is also a secret tradition, called the Diamond Way, thousands of
years old, which offers us new and extraordinary ways of relating to our partner—of reaching high and incomparably beautiful places with them. These
teachings even say that the Buddha himself attained his enlightenment only
with the help of Tilottama, a lady who came to be his partner at the bidding

of the highest beings of the universe. The description of how they attained spiritual perfection in each other's arms, as the sun dawned in a new day, is one of the most moving passages in the literature of the world.

As for my own qualifications in composing a book about the Karma of Love, I feel that I was most fortunate among all my fellow monks in that I had been through relationships before becoming a monk (most Tibetans enter the monastery between the ages of say 7 to 12). I knew what women were about—I knew the joys of a relationship, and I knew the very painful problems. My own parents had gone through a heart-wrenching divorce, that terrible combination of loving each other and not being able to stay with each other.

And I think most importantly, I had had a relationship which I considered divine—where I had some glimpse of what had passed between Lord Buddha and Lady Tilottama, between Dante and Beatrice, between Jesus and Mary Magdalene, in the Garden.

In the years since, I have strengthened this experience, and gained an ever-deeper understanding of it, through thousands of hours of teachings received at the feet of twelve of Tibet's greatest masters. I have been granted secret initiations into the practices of working with a partner, and I have spent many years in translating and studying thousands of pages of the ancient texts on these practices.

I have made a sincere attempt to follow these practices, sometimes attracting unwanted attention of the press and the ire of the monastic authorities, some of whom feel that this knowledge cannot be shared with the mass of people. But I do believe in a perfect world, I believe that together we can create it, and I believe that it begins and ends with a perfect relationship—with understanding the Karma of Love.

And so I would like to share with you what I have learned, to help you with your own relationship. Over many years' time, thousands of people from almost every corner of the globe have asked me questions about their relationships. I have tried to select the 100 most common questions, and to answer them here from the ancient wisdom of Tibet, through the dear blessings of my own Heart Lama. I pray that it helps you and that perfect person in your life.

Geshe Michael Roach

Rainbow House
Thanksgiving Day 2012

THE MOST IMPORTANT
QUESTION OF ALL

Question 1

I had my first girlfriend in the sixth grade, when I was 12 years old. I can't count how many relationships I've been in since then—it must be dozens, and almost all of them ended very unhappily, after a start where I had much hope, where I thought this one would be different. I've tried all kinds of advice, I've read all kinds 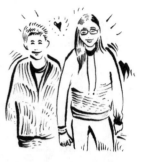 **of books, but I have this sad feeling that nothing's going to work. So in a few words, here at the beginning, can you tell me why this Karma of Love technique is going to work, when so many other things have failed?**

I know you've tried everything, or at least tried a lot of things, to find a relationship that works—and what you haven't tried you've watched others try, and seen how it didn't work. I think we can agree then that if the Karma of Love approach works, it's going to have to be something very different than anything you've ever heard of before. And it is.

First of all, the Karma of Love works, and it works every time. You see, almost everything we ever do in life we do with the understanding that it might work, or it might not work. Even just taking an aspirin for a headache, we swallow the pill; we sit and hope it will work; and then maybe it does or maybe it doesn't. Sadly, every one of us has gotten used to things working out only some of the time: nobody would ever think of taking the empty aspirin bottle back to the pharmacy and asking for half their money back, because half of the pills didn't work when they had a headache. We've become accustomed to failure; we expect it, at least some of the time, and deep down we

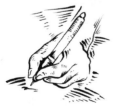 believe that this is a fact of life—something we cannot change.

Karma though works all of the time, if you really understand how to use it. Gaining that understanding takes some real effort. This book is not going to work for you if you're not ready for some new ideas, to think

about them and to act upon them. You're going to learn, for the first time, where the world around you is really coming from. And then you're going to use what you've learned to create the relationship you've always dreamed of.

So let's jump in right now, to the most basic new idea that you need to know: emptiness.

I hold a pen up in my hand, and I ask you, "What is this thing?"

"A pen," you quickly answer.

"And if a puppy dog walked into this room right now, and I waved this object in front of his nose, what would he do?"

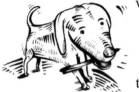

"Well I don't know, I suppose he might very well chew on it."

"So how does the puppy see the pen?"

"Well, we can say that he sees it as a chew-toy."

So that's step one in your understanding of emptiness. Now let's go a little further.

"Okay then, who's right—the person or the dog? Is this thing a pen, or is it a chew-toy?"

"Well I suppose they're both right: to me, the thing is a pen; and to the dog, it's a chew-toy."

"Good, good; animal rights and all that! So you're both correct. This object is, to different observers, both a pen and a chew-toy. Now another question. If I take this object and set it on the table here, and you and the puppy both leave the room, which one is it then—a pen, or a chew-toy?"

"Well if neither of them were here to see it one way or another, then I think we'd have to say it was neither—right then it wouldn't be a pen or a chew-toy. But it would have the potential to be either one, depending on whether a human or a dog walked back into the room."

Okay, so now you've got it; you already understand the very difficult idea of emptiness, an idea which is absolutely necessary if you're going to create your perfect partner. Try to see what "emptiness" means here. It's not like everything is black, or nothing is nothing, or nothing matters.

The object lying on the table after the human and the dog leave the room is "empty" because it's blank—like a blank white movie screen before they start the movie. Everything around us, and everybody in our life, is the same: empty, blank, available. You may feel pretty bad about the last person you shared a relationship with, but there are probably lots of other people who think they're pretty nice. They're the same as the pen: it just depends on what you see—it depends on who's looking.

"So now hold up a pen in one hand, hold it in front of your face, and show me with your other hand whether the pen is coming from its side, or from yours. Wave your hand from the pen to your eyes, if you think the pen is coming from its own side. Or wave your hand from your eyes to the pen, if you think it's coming from your side."

Almost everybody will point their finger from themselves to the pen: "It's coming from me, it must be coming from me. And the chew-toy is coming from the puppy."

"That's right. If the pen were coming from the pen's side, well then the dog would have to see it as a pen...and then they would try to grab it in their paw, and try to write a poem maybe—a poem to their dog girlfriend saying, 'You've got a great tail!'"

So there we've got it: the pen is coming from me. By itself it's not a pen or a chew-toy; it's just blank, it's just available. And so when I see a pen it's got to be coming from my own mind.

Can we just close our eyes then, and wish that the pen was a big diamond ring? Try it right now and see—you know it doesn't work. A great new boyfriend may be coming from your own mind, but that doesn't mean you can just close your eyes and wish him into existence. We can want or wish or pray all we want, but that's not going to make it happen—every lonely person in the world *wishes* they had someone, but the wishing doesn't make someone appear.

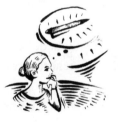

So why do we see a pen? How does it come from our mind?

There are seeds in our mind, karmic seeds. They lay deep in our subconscious, deep down in the mind, and when the time is ready they crack open, like a seed for a tree. I hold a black stick up in front of your face and in that microsecond a karmic seed splits open in your mind, and out pops a luminous image of a pen. This tiny picture of a pen jumps out between you and the black stick in a thousandth of a second—so fast that you've never in your life noticed that it was happening—and then you see a pen.

And it's a *real* pen. Mental pictures are that good. You can pick it up and write with it.

Do you see where this is going? If you're a woman looking for a partner and a good-looking man walks in the door at Starbucks Coffee and heads towards your table, he's the same as the pen. He's coming from a seed in your mind. Ah! Now all we need to know is how to plant the seed!

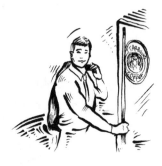

To put it briefly, we can only plant a seed with another person. Whatever we want, we need to see that somebody else gets it first. When we help someone else get what they want, it plants a seed in our mind to get the same thing ourselves later on, as the seed ripens and splits open.

What this means is that you can *plant* your future partner, or change anything you want about the partner you have now—because it's all coming from you. You just need to know how to do it: to be a good farmer, you need to learn how to plant seeds right, and take care of them right. Then you can have everything.

And so the answer to your first question, the most important question of all, is *Yes, you can have any partner you want, any relationship you want,* if you just learn how to plant the right karmic seeds. And that's what we're going to cover with the 100 questions you find in this book. Every time we answer somebody's question, it will teach you one more thing about the technique of karmic farming. So what I want you to do is sit down first and read this whole book through from beginning to end—even the parts where we're talking about a question that you may not have right now.

In the process, you'll learn everything there is to know about the Karma of Love. Then go back to the questions which relate to your own life, and you'll be ready to carry out the answers that you find there. It's a new system, a completely new system, from ancient Tibet. But if you really understand this system, then it works all the time—and that's why it's different from everything you've ever tried before.

And by the way, almost all the questions you find here relate to traditional partnerships—girlfriends & boyfriends, husbands & wives—because this is mostly how the questions came to me, all over the world. The principles you learn here though have been successfully applied by a great many people to other relationships: family, friends, business associates, co-workers, and relationships with those of the same sex. So feel free to use the Karma of Love in all of your connections with other people.

FINDING THEM

Question 2

Where should I look for my partner?

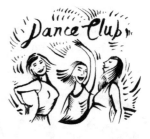

Ann came to me a few years ago with a strange request. (As with everything else in this book, this is a true story, or several true stories glued together, with the names changed to respect the privacy of my friends.)

Ann is from Asia, and so she uses my traditional title: "Geshe La, you're a monk. Buddhist monks are *fa li wu bian,* as we say in China—they have special spiritual powers. I know lots of monks who can do *mo,* who can tell the future, for people who need to know something. And I need to know something."

"Like what?" I ask.

Ann looks a little sheepish. "Well," she says, "I need a boyfriend, but I'm not sure where to look for him. I figure it would save me a lot of time and trouble if you could just peek into the future and tell me where I'm going to meet him."

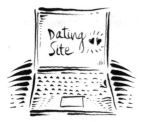

I'm a little taken aback; I expected a question like "What kind of meditation should I be doing this week?" I stall for time.

"So…where do you *think* you might meet him?"

"I'm thinking either to try the internet, or go to a dance club. Problem is, I'm thinking that any boy I meet on the internet is going to be a nerd—the kind who spends more time with his laptop than he does with his girlfriend. Then again, any boy I meet in a dance club is going to be…well, the kind of boy who *goes* to a club. He might not be the type to stay in a long-term relationship."

Now I don't usually do this fortune-telling thing, but in one of the Tibetan monasteries where I lived—this one smack dab in the middle of New Jersey—there were a lot of ancient monks from Mongolia who were really good at it. I watched them for years, and so I know how to put on a good show if it will help someone.

Fortunetelling by Tibetan monks is done with a pair of dice, but the Mongols do them one better. They take the knuckle bones of a sheep, which are pretty much cube-shaped, and boil them down to pure white. You toss the bones on the table and see how they land and then tell the 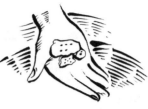 person what's going to happen. And so I throw the sheep knuckles and bend over them, looking *very* serious.

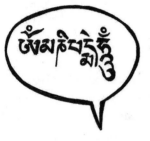

"Hmm!" I say, and "hum!" And then I throw in a few mantras for good measure: *"Om mani padme hung, Om mani padme hung!"*

After that you should yell "Ah! There it is!"

Ann leans over the knuckle bones. "So Geshe La, will I find him on the internet?"

"No, no!" I say gravely. "Not the internet! It cannot be the internet!"

"Oh," she cries, "then it must be at a dance club!"

I bend very slowly over the bones and scrutinize them. "No, nor there; you will not meet him in a club!"

"So where?" she asks.

I pause, stoop over the bones and stare at them some more, then slowly straighten up and look her in the eyes. "You will need to go…to a nursing home!"

"A nursing home?" Ann's eyes widen and she looks at me incredulous. A long pause and then, "But Geshe La, you don't understand."

"Don't understand what?" I growl.

"I mean," she blushes, "I mean…Geshe La, I want a *young* boy!"

I laugh and tell her, "No, it's you who don't understand. Tell me, *why* do you want a boy?"

"Well," she replies immediately, "look at how I live my life. I have a good job, in an office here in Manhattan. I work a good long day, I enjoy my work, and then I come home. I cook myself a little dinner, which takes like 45 minutes. Then I sit down alone to eat it, which takes about 5 minutes. And then I wash the dishes, which takes another half an hour. So you see, I spend over an hour on dinner, just to sit down and eat it by myself, with no one sitting across the table to eat it with me, to enjoy my cooking, to ask me how my day went."

"So you're lonely," I say. "And what you want is someone to be with: you want companionship, from someone you love."

"Exactly," she sighs, relieved.

"Exactly," I repeat back, "which is why you need to go to the nursing home. What you want is companionship. So first you need to plant a karmic seed in your mind for companionship, and that seed will crack open and you will meet the boy, wherever it may be. The way to plant a seed for companionship is to provide companionship to someone else, first. And one of the best ways to provide companionship is to go to a nursing home.

"Go to a nursing home, go visit an elderly woman, someone who's old, someone that nobody wants to visit, somebody with bad breath from their bad teeth, someone wrinkled and forgotten, someone who will sit there and say to you over and over, every time you visit, 'Did I tell you about the boyfriend I had in high school? Now *he* was a handsome one!'

"You don't need to be with her all the time—just visit once in a while, say once a week, or every two weeks. Bring her some flowers, take her out to dinner sometimes, help her fill out her pension forms or fix up her room. But most of all give her companionship: listen to the stories of her life, even if it's the hundredth time she's told them to you, and share your own stories too. You will learn much from her life, and she will have some good advice for your own.

"This will plant a seed of companionship, and when that seed opens, you will meet your boy. If the seed is there it doesn't matter where you look for him—on the internet, at a club, or just sitting in your own apartment—he will come, he has to come. And if you don't make this new seed and you go on the internet or to a club, you might find him and you might not, because there might be an old seed sitting there in your mind, and there might not."

So Ann, you see, she is completely different from almost everybody I've ever given advice to. Because she actually goes out and does exactly what I've told her to do.

A few months later she gives me a call.

"Geshe La! Great news!"

"What?"

"Well, I did what you said with the old lady. And then I was visiting San Francisco, teaching a yoga class there. And the whole class came into the room, one by one, and I was watching for him, you see..."

"Yes?"

"And, well…you know, most yoga classes are mostly girls anyway, and he didn't show up!"

I'm getting confused. "And?"

"And then well the door opens, 5 minutes after the class has already started, and there's this boy standing there in the doorway, because he got there late."

"Yes?"

"And well, he looks across the room at me, and you know…it's just like in the movies—like, totally, love at first sight—him for me, and me for him. Like we're just sitting there and the whole class is waiting for me to say something, and all I can do is look at this delicious boy."

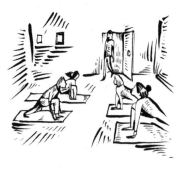

Six months later I get another call. "Geshe La, this is Ann. So…you're a monk right, a Buddhist monk?"

"That I am," I concur.

"Well…do Buddhist monks like…do they ever do marriage ceremonies?" Yes, they do, and I did. And it was beautiful, all white lace and black suits, there in Manhattan.

You get the point. Ann didn't *find* a partner. Ann *created* a partner. When you follow the principles of the Karma of Love—that is, the Diamond Cutter Principles— nothing is an accident. We decide what we want, clearly, and then we help someone else get the same thing first, to plant a karmic seed. After that, things just take care of themselves—no worrying, no wondering. He comes, and he gives us companionship, because we have given companionship to someone else.

So don't sit there trying to decide about clubs or the internet or yoga classes. Seek out those who are lonely—and when you do seek, you'll begin to find them everywhere: not just lonely old people, but lonely children whose parents are too busy, and lonely peers sitting right next to you at work, or on the bus. Offer to be their friend, give them companionship, and keep it up—make it your mission. The seed will be planted, and your partner will come; it doesn't matter where you go.

Question 3

What should I look for in a partner?

Karen, a veteran of many of my talks, collars me on the way to the parking lot after a long night's presentation to a largish group in the Southwest; I'm really exhausted, but my assistants have told her that she can "buy" the walk out to the car. We call it "walk and talk," and thankfully they keep the two of us moving through the crowd.

I pretty much know what she wants to talk about. Karen had a pretty good relationship going with a pretty good guy—good job, friendly personality—but it seems like he wants to move on.

So she looks up at me with not a little pain in her face and says, "Geshe La, it didn't work out; I think you've heard all the gory details. He's gone. And now I've got to start looking again, but first I want to ask what you think about…about what I should look for in a partner this time. To make it work better…" Her voice trails off, and I feel for her.

"Look Karen," I reply. "I'm a monk, and you know that, and I know you know that, and so I know what you're expecting me to say. 'Find someone who has a good heart—go for a nice person. Don't worry about what he looks like, or what kind of job he has, or how smart he is'."

She nods, as if that's assumed. And maybe that's part of her whole problem.

"Well, you can forget about that," I begin. "That's okay if you don't know what you're doing—if you've been *looking* for Mr. Right, and you don't know anything about *creating* Mr. Right.

"If Mr. Right is somebody you *find,* then you're definitely going to have to make some compromises. If you have to *find* a partner, then sure you'll either find somebody who is handsome and smart, but not so stable and nice; or else stable and nice, but not so handsome and smart.

"And then you're going to have to sweat over it and decide whether you want to spend the rest of your life with someone who's only like 75% of everything you really want in a partner."

She doesn't say anything, but I can feel that Karen's getting a little uncomfortable…that her whole life, she's been playing exactly this kind of odds game.

"So what's the alternative?"

"You've got to see that this isn't how it works with the Diamond Cutter system. Here, you're *creating* your partner—you're *making* them by planting the right karmic seeds.

"Before you create anything else in this life—a painting, a cake, whatever—you have to sit down first and decide what you want it to be like. You think carefully and make a list of everything you want the thing to be, and then you create each part of it the way you want it.

"It's the same with creating Mr. Right. Make a list of what you want, and be careful! You'll get exactly everything that you try to get, so make sure you know what you want. Oh, you can change him later if you decide to, but why go through the trouble?"

I stop dead, right there in the parking lot, and turn to look into Karen's eyes. "Get someone who is *everything,*" I say. "*Make* someone who is everything. *Use the seeds!* Whadda you think I've been teaching you all this time!"

"Okay, okay!" she yelps. "Tell me where to start."

"Alright then. Let's say you want somebody who's everything I just mentioned: somebody who has a good heart, and who is smart, who has a good job, and…why not?…who looks exactly like what you always dreamed of.

Make your list of what you want

"Make your list, and then plant the karmic seed in your mind for each of the qualities you want him to have. Each of these qualities will require a *different* seed, because each quality is *different* from the other."

In the course of this book, we'll cover just about all the qualities you'd ever want your partner to have. But for a start, why don't we cover the ones that Karen wants?

"Alright, first," I say. "If you want to have smart people around you, you need to plant the seeds for smart. That's easy, because the smartest thing in the world is figuring out exactly how the world works. And the world works through these little seeds in your mind—it pops out of these seeds, just like we saw with the pen.

"Keep this in mind; think about it often; bring it to mind as you walk down the street, as you drive your car. And talk about it with others whenever it seems they might be interested, or need some help. All this plants smart seeds, and as they open you'll find that you're surrounded by smarter and smarter people—including your partner.

"Got that?" I ask. We're already standing next to my car, and I'm looking longingly at the front seat.

"Got it," Karen smiles. "Next?" She's actually got a little journal out, and she's taking notes. When I see people do that, I know there's a good chance they're going to actually *do* what I suggest. That spurs me on.

"Okay, if you also want a partner with a good job then you're obviously going to have to help other people find the job they're looking for—that's a no-brainer. How many people do you have to help? As many as it takes. You'll know it's enough when you meet the boy, and he has a good job." She nods, writing furiously.

Now about the good looks? We'll talk about it more here later on, at Question 8. But to Karen, I say: "Let's just put it briefly. The trick here is that the more calm you can stay in tense or upsetting situations—the more cool you can stay—then the more seeds you plant to be beautiful, and to meet a beautiful partner."

"As for the good heart—well that really is the most important thing in a partner, for one good reason. Someone with a good heart is helping everybody around them, all the time. And that means they're planting good karmic seeds in their mind, all the time. If you're living with someone who is constantly planting good seeds, it's going to rub off on you."

"The best kind of good heart is one that *understands* why to be good—otherwise, if things get tough, the good heart under pressure might stop being good. To meet people who understand why they *must* be kind, you're going to have to try as hard as you can to understand this yourself."

"Can you be a little more specific?" she asks.

"It means, just think about the seeds, as often as you can. Think about how everything comes from being kind to others. On the day that you really understand where things are coming from, you will understand that what's holding up the walls of the very room you're sitting in right now is kindness—not wood, not iron, not cement. Kindness makes the world go round, because everything we do comes round."

She finishes writing that last sentence with a flourish and snaps shut her journal. "Will do!" And she opens the door of the car and sends me off without another word.

That little exchange in the parking lot has a really happy ending. Karen got on it with the seeds, and created quite an extraordinary hunk: taller than the original, much more gentle and considerate, much more devoted. I feel really happy when people get *everything* they want. To me it feels like we deserve it, all of us. Sort of a human right.

TIME PRESSURE

Question 4

My husband and I really love each other, but we both have such hectic schedules that on many days the only time we cross paths is when we're running in or out the door. How can we get more time together?

Now this time thing is an important issue for most of us, but it's not really important enough to come up here at the start of the book. Except that we're going to use it to explain the *technique* of seed planting: we call this technique the "Four Starbucks Steps," and you're going to have to use them with every one of the 100 questions that you find in this book. So let's get to these four, right away.

I didn't actually get asked this "time" question myself. It was my friend, Viet Duong. He and his wife Elisha were heading up a DCI tour to Vietnam, including stops in Hanoi and Ho Chi Minh. About seven of us were sitting up on the stage in a semicircle, fielding questions from the audience.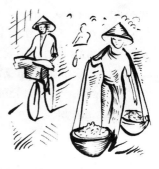

Viet doesn't even blink. He grabs the mike and launches right in. Luckily our translator is sitting next to me, and he fills me in on what Viet is saying. I mean, Vietnamese has got to be one of the toughest languages in the world. I've tried but I can't even learn to say "Hi!"

"So if you want more money," says Viet to the audience, leaning forward like an old-time preacher, "what do you have to do?"

"Help somebody else make money," the audience chants back.

"And if you want more time," smiles Viet, "what do you have to do then?"

Mouths open, and promptly close. People look around to see if anybody else has the answer. One brave young man does.

"Help somebody else get more time?" he yells.

Give what you want

"Right!" beams Viet, with his usual sunshine smile. "Which means that you're going to have to give somebody else some of your time."

The lady who asked the question scowls a bit. I don't need a translator to understand what she says next: "But I don't have any time to give; that's why I'm asking you the question in the first place!"

Viet doesn't back down.

"It's exactly the same thing as money, don't you see? We give other people money, with the proper technique, and that plants seeds to see money come back to us; a lot more money. When we don't have time—enough time to spend quality time with our partner—then we have to *give* time."

Ms. Scowl still doesn't look happy.

"Look," says Viet. "If you want to work on your problem in a new way, in the Diamond Cutter way, then you're going to have to think about planting seeds, no matter what it is you want in your life. Now how can you plant some seeds for more time? Who can you give some of your time to?"

Ms. Scowl does that looking-at-the-ceiling-while-I'm-thinking thing. Then she comes back to Viet.

"Maybe help my sister."

"Your sister? What kind of help does she need?"

"She's got like, two kids, you see, and between that and cleaning and cooking for her family—and holding down a full-time job—she's always frazzled. She never has enough time."

"Great!" beams Viet. "So just give her some time! Maybe offer to watch her kids for the evening while she and her husband go out for once!"

Ms. Scowl scowls even more, if that's possible. "I come to you asking how my husband and I can get more time, and you tell me to take what little time I have and watch my sister's kids?"

"Right!" smiles Viet. It's like he's matching her, smile for scowl. "Just for a few hours!"

Now the lady starts to look confused. "Give my sister a few hours, so I can get a few hours back? What's the point? Why don't I just keep my few hours?"

"Ah," intones Viet. "Now I see your problem. Look, you have to understand one thing about the seeds. You give your sister a few hours of the precious little time that you have, and it comes back ten times more!" Then he pauses and looks at the ceiling himself. "That is, if you do it with *technique...*" he adds.

"Technique?" says Ms. Scowl, but like many people who ask tough questions about the Diamond Cutter Principles, you can see that she's actually very intelligent and really wants to know. These are the best kind of people for learning this new system. They want to know exactly how it's going to work, before they try it. And then when they do try it, they're superstars, because they've already worked out all their questions.

"Okay," says Viet, putting on his thinking cap. "Suppose you take a watermelon seed, a good one. Is it going to make a watermelon?"

"Well sure," says Ms. Interested, "if you plant it."

Viet gestures towards the floor of the stage. "Even if I plant it here?"

"Well no," she says. "I mean, you have to plant it in the right place—you have to know what you're doing. And if you want it to grow well there's a lot of other stuff you're going to have to know: how much water is too much or too little for this particular plant; how much sunlight; what kind of fertilizer, in what quantities."

Viet nods in that sunny way of his. "Right. In the Diamond Cutter system, we call this 'technique.' If you know the right farming technique, then a watermelon seed will make you a big bunch of nice watermelons. And it will grow faster. Spend a few hours watching you sister's kids *with technique,* and you get back whole days of free time that you and your partner can spend together."

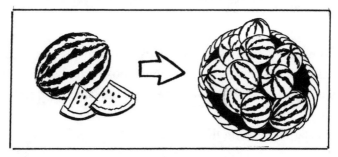

Ms. Scowl is starting to look a little more like Ms. Intrigued. She pulls out a pen and pad and looks up at Viet expectantly. I'm starting to feel very proud of him, as I often do when I watch our DCI teachers at work around the world.

"Okay look," he says. "The technique for planting karmic seeds is called the Four Starbucks Steps."

Ms. Intrigued looks confused.

"Uh, we'll talk later about the Starbucks thing," says Viet.

"Okay, Starbucks Step Number One. We call it **A Single Sentence.** Say what it is that you want, in a single, short sentence."

"I want more time, to be with my partner," she answers.

"Good. Now Starbucks Step Number Two. We call it **The Plan.** The plan has two parts. First you have to plan where you're going to plant your seed. When you plant a seed for a flower or tree, you need to choose your soil.

"For a karmic seed, you need another person: other people are the earth in which you plant your seeds. It's almost impossible to plant a seed just in yourself—you need someplace else to plant it, another person. So part of step two, part of the planning, is to choose this person.

"It should be someone who wants the same thing that you want."

"But we did that already," she breaks in. "We chose my sister, who also desperately needs some time."

"Right," says Viet. "And now the second half of the planning is to decide *where* you're going to help her."

"Well, at *her* house," she replies. "It's not like I'm going to have those little monsters running around *my* house, tearing it up."

"Of course!" he smiles. "But what I'm talking about is where you're going to sit down with her and talk about the whole idea of helping her get some more time for herself. And that's where Starbucks comes in!

"Give your sister a call, ask her if she can meet you at Starbucks for a few minutes over coffee—tell her you need her help with something. Tell her she can bring the kids."

Ms. Scowl looks dubious. "Those kids—okay, but I don't think they can stay long. Last time I took them out with their mom to Starbucks so she and I could talk, they went over and pulled down all the bags of coffee for sale and started stacking them in the middle of the floor."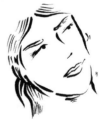

"Right!" says Viet, as if that were the plan all along. "So Starbucks Step Two is covered: we've made a plan, we've chosen a person and a place where we'll help them.

"And by the way that's why we say 'go to Starbucks,' and not just 'go to a coffee shop.' If you want your seed to grow big and to grow fast, then the plan has to be as specific as possible: you want hours watching her kids to turn into days spent at your partner's side, within the next month or two.

"So don't just say, 'I choose to help my sister, and I'll try to get in touch with her sometime and talk about it.' Instead I want to hear you say, 'I choose to help my sister, and I'll call her and take her out to the Starbucks on 4ᵗʰ Street at 2pm this Friday afternoon."

"Got it," says Ms. Hopeful. She's been writing furiously, which is very typical when smart people hear about the Four Starbucks Steps. They already see how this whole approach makes a lot of sense: it explains almost everything in the world immediately, and it also *feels right* that the solution to all our problems should also be a win/win for everybody else around us. "Step Three?" she asks.

Viet frowns for a second and then asks simply, "What do you think comes next?"

She's ready. "I take her to the Starbucks! I talk to her about helping her with her kids! And then I actually *help* her with her kids!"

"Right on!" gushes Viet. "I mean, you can plant some seeds just by planning to help somebody, but they won't be very strong. You have to **actually carry your plan out,** to get the result you want. And simply, that's all there is to Starbucks Step Three. Call her, meet and talk about how you can help her get some time to herself, and then actually help her get that time."

"As for the last one, Starbucks Step Four, I think…" Viet glances across the stage to me mischievously. "I think Geshe Michael can help us with that one!" The crowd gives him a big hand of appreciation, and then they quiet down and look to me. The microphone makes its way down the line of chairs.

"Uh, okay then. Starbucks Step Number Four," I begin. "That's easy: **Coffee Meditation!**"

I watch the crowd as the translator translates this last part. Vietnam has gone through a lot of changes, but people are still pretty sharp when it comes to Buddhism. They've never heard of Coffee Meditation, and it doesn't sound like something that's going to get them more time with their partner. Lots of quizzical looks.

"Alright," I settle into my chair. "Here's how my Tibetan teacher taught me Coffee Meditation.

"He was a super-tough lama, one of the last of the grand lamas who finished all their training in Old Tibet. In my teacher's day, Tibet was completely isolated from the outside world. It's not enough to say he had never seen a car—he had never even ridden on a bicycle. I mean, it was over a mile from his monastery to the nearest town, and if people needed something they just set aside a big part of the day and walked there and back.

"Then he had to run away from his country, and spent years in a refugee camp in India, and eventually ended up in the United States. When he got there, he spent many years teaching the people who came to him for help, all for free. But he also knew how to relax, which is an important skill for all of us to learn.

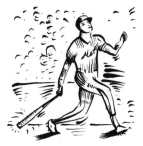

"And so my Lama discovered TV. And he discovered baseball. And for some reason he fell in love with the New York Mets, who for years had one of the worst records in baseball history." I mean, I'm not going to lay this on an audience in Vietnam, but it was my Lama furiously doing mantras that miraculously lifted Darryl Strawberry's line drive over the home run fence in the fifth game of the championship series against the Astros, back in 1986.

"And I would come home, exhausted, after like 12 hours working at my office in New York, and two hours on subways and buses to get back home to the monastery, and I'd hear him upstairs, watching a game.

"Now I'm not that interested in TV, or in baseball, but probably a lot of you know that when you come home from work really wiped out, there's a certain comfort in sitting in front of a television with your mind turned off. Am I right?"

Lots of nods and smiles—Vietnam is full of smiles.

"And so I trudge in the front door and throw down my coat and my briefcase and I can hear him up in his room enjoying a game. And I'm thinking to myself, How am I gonna get up there and watch it with him? 'Cause us young monks aren't supposed to watch TV, you see.

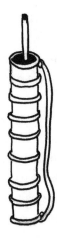

"But I had an old trick that I would use to get into his room. Tibetans like butter tea, lots of butter tea—sometimes 15 or 20 cups a day. And it's always appropriate for a student to whip up a cup and take it to their lama's room.

"So I pour and boil the water, break a corner off a brick of black Chinese tea, throw it in, and add salt, cream, butter, and milk. Ladle it high and drop it back like 50 times to mix the tea and butter—or just throw it into one of those ancient Tibetan tea churns and *swoosh* it up—then throw it all into a cup. Run upstairs and knock on the door. I can already hear the comforting voice of Tim McCarver, my favorite Mets announcer.

When he hears the knock, Lama yells *"Sho!"* Which is sort of like "Get your rear end in here!"

I step in and—following the traditional etiquette—kneel down and set the butter tea down on the little table in front of his easy chair. I glance up to make sure he's really focused on the game: he is, with his right hand whipping out mantras on his rosary, like a washing machine spinning at full speed. I stay crouched low, quietly move to the side of his chair and back a bit, and sit on the floor where he can't see me. Sometimes Lama doesn't notice me for a half hour or more—or at least it seems like he's not noticing me.

But tonight Lama says immediately, in that gruff low voice of his, "Did you meditate today?"

"Uh, no, Lama. You know, I had to get up at 5:30 this morning, and jump in the shower, and run down to catch the bus—it's been non-stop since then, and I just got home."

"You have to meditate," he growls, without taking his eyes off the baseball game.

"Now?" I whine.

"Now."

I get up to go downstairs to my tiny little room. He grabs my hand and waves towards his golden sofa. "Over there," he growls again, pointedly pushing me past so I don't block his view of the next play. "Sit over there."

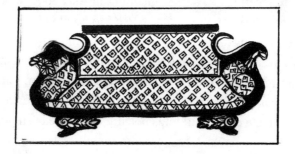

Now you have to understand one thing about Lama's sofa. It was presented to him by a wealthy sponsor. It's handmade, and it took like a year to finish it. All dark, polished hardwood on the arms and legs; and the fabric is this expensive pale-yellow silk-like stuff, with gold threads woven through it.

The sofa's been there on the side of his room for years, and *no one has ever sat on it,* not even Lama. Except once the Dalai Lama made a few hours' visit to our temple, and *he* got to sit on it.

Sometimes a lama will ask you to do something wrong, just to see if you're dumb enough to do it. And then when you do do it, they yell at you, or—in the monastery, if it's a really big thing—they might give you the Prayer Beads Treatment.

You think those Buddhist prayer beads are only for prayers? Walk around our monastery some time and listen to the Tibetan version of "Spare the rod, spoil the child." You hear this *whoosh whoosh* of a prayer beads being swung at full force, and then a young monk walks out of a doorway rubbing his head ruefully.

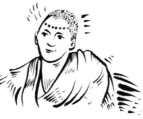

The idea is that your teacher whacks you on the head a few times with the beads when you've been really naughty. It leaves a little row of rosy-colored dots across your forehead, and all your friends make fun of you for a few hours—"Ha ha ha! Look who got the Prayer Beads Treatment!"

I cover my head casually with my hand, like I'm just scratching or something. "That's okay Lama, I can meditate downstairs in my room."

"Sit on the couch," he growls again. And now no choice but to sit; if a lama has to ask three times, then you get The Treatment anyway.

I sit down on the couch and wait while Lama concentrates on a particularly important play in the baseball game. Then, "Lie down on the couch!"

This is getting serious. There's this thing in Asia about a person's feet. In a lot of those countries, you're not supposed to point your feet at anything: I can remember in Bangkok visiting the Temple of the Emerald Buddha, and seeing signs all over the place that say "Don't point your feet at the Buddha!" Lying down on the couch means I have to put my feet on one of Lama's things, which is another great way to get the Prayer Bead Treatment.

"Uh, Lama, I can do the full lotus posture now, I've been practicing."

"Lie down!" I lie down.

Lama rings his bell, and the other attendant, a young Tibetan monk, runs up the stairs.

"Fix Mike a cup of coffee," growls Lama. The cup comes promptly.

"Drink the coffee."

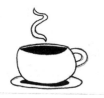

My hands are shaking. I'm trying to drink coffee lying down, and I know if I spill a drop on the Golden Sofa I'm going to get something worse than a rosary.

"Now meditate."

I start to sit up and Lama shakes his head, eyes still glued to the TV. "Lie down. Meditate lying down."

I've never heard of such a thing—the lamas are always demanding that we have to sit up to meditate, and keep a super-straight back.

"Meditate about what?" I ask, lying back. I tuck an arm under my head and stare at the ceiling. Hey, I could get used to this. It feels really comfortable and calm.

"Starbucks," grumbles Lama. "Think about Starbucks. Who did you take to Starbucks today?"

I know what he means—who did I take out for a cup of tea or coffee (or better of course, a fruit smoothie)? Whose problems have I listened to today? Who have I tried to help?

The point is that you make a lot of karmic seeds in your mind just by doing the first three Starbucks Steps. Deciding what you want in your life plants some seeds. Planning to help somebody else plants a lot more. And then actually helping them piles more seeds on top of these. But the most important is this last step, Coffee Meditation.

Just leaning back on your bed at night and thinking about all the things you've done today to help someone else is absolutely the most powerful way to plant seeds. If you want to know the secret weapon that I used to help build a zillion-dollar company, it's Coffee Meditation—just that. It seems too easy; we feel like we need to suffer bigger to get bigger goals in our life, but maybe the truth is just the opposite.

Maybe the most powerful karmic seeds are the ones we plant just by relaxing and being contented about the small goodnesses that we've been doing for others. It's not a matter of pride, just enjoying whatever we've been able to do.

None of us is perfectly good, but none of us is perfectly bad either. We have a choice, as we go to sleep at night, to think about the problems of our life, or to think about the bright spots. When we're tired, we tend to exaggerate our problems. The very word *meditation* means that we take the normal flow of our thoughts—in this case, worrying about our problems while we fall off to sleep—and muscle the mind over to some good thoughts: Who did I try to help today? This is exactly the goal of meditation: to control the direction in which the mind flows.

So come home from work, and cook your dinner. Clean up the dishes, and watch a bit of TV if you really have to—or do a bit of emailing or Facebook. Then take your bath, and get into your nightclothes.

Sit down on your bed, or just lie halfway down on some pillows and prop your chin up on your hand, and stare at the ceiling. Get that dreamy look on your face that you used to have in high school when you were thinking about your boyfriend or girlfriend, wondering when your next date would be.

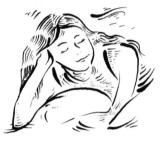

It may seem strange to say it, but that day-dreaming was pretty close to real meditation. Don't feel like you have to tie your legs up in a pretzel to get to this same deep place in your mind.

And then just go into your Coffee Meditation: the last of the Four Starbucks Steps, the true technique for farming mental seeds. Plant your seeds with these four, and the things you want to happen in your life will come to you, fast and strong. Remember them for the rest of this book, and for the rest of your life:

The Four Starbucks Steps

1) Say what it is you want in your life, <u>in a single short sentence.</u>

2) <u>Plan</u> who it is you're going to help get the same thing, and which Starbucks you're going to take them to, to talk about it.

3) <u>Actually do something</u> to help them.

4) Do your <u>Coffee Meditation</u>: as you go to sleep, think of the good things you're doing to help them.

COMMITMENT

Question 5

I don't have any trouble finding men to go out on dates with me, but they never want to take the next step, into a long-term relationship. What seed do I need to plant to see some commitment?

It does seem that a lot of the advice I give people is yelled over my shoulder as we move through a crowd after a talk…this time it was in Paris, leaving a dinner meeting with a group of businesspeople who had flown in from all over—Hong Kong, the Middle East, and Germany.

Cathy walks toward me with that purposeful stride of someone who's on a mission. I remember her from a talk in America the year before, and wonder what's pressing enough to bring her halfway around the world for some follow-up. She had been completely alone for some time and was pretty desperate for a boyfriend, any boyfriend. I took her through Ann's nursing-home thing, and I knew she would try it. She's a pretty determined person.

"Okay Geshe La, so…hey, this stuff really works! But it works too well! I didn't get the boy, I got a whole bunch of boys! Cute boys and" (she blushes) "hot boys!"

I'm a little surprised at this complaint, and I arch my eyebrows. "So Cathy, I don't get it. What's the problem?"

"Lots of boys," she whines, "but none of them willing to *commit*. I mean, we go out on a couple of dates, and then when I start to talk about anything long-term they get nervous and start to back off. What kind of seeds do I need to plant for one of them to get excited about something more permanent?"

As usual, we need to think about the essence of what you want. We need to think about the idea of commitment. What is the essence of commitment? Let's ask Maitreya.

We all know that the Buddha lived a long time ago in India—about 2,500 years ago, to be exact—but what many people don't know is that this Buddha was just one of many who are supposed to be on their way to this world. The Tibetans say that the next Buddha to appear here will be someone named

Maitreya, and that he has already sent some messages on ahead of him, in the form of scriptures revealed to a sage more than 16 centuries ago.

One of these teachings is a description of something that the Tibetans call *hlaksam namdak*. This means taking total responsibility for things—sort of a "buck stops here" attitude, but on a very big level. It means taking responsibility, during every situation we find ourselves in, all day long, for seeing

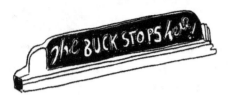

that other people around us get the things they do want, and don't run into the things they don't want. It means taking responsibility for others even when we know nobody's going to help us.

"Look Cathy," I explain, as we stroll past some beautiful old manses on the riverfront, gaslights flickering in the dark. "You've got to get into this kind of thinking—you've got to get into taking personal responsibility for what other people need. Sort of 'I will be the one to make it happen,' for lots of people around you. That plants the karmic seed to meet a young man who's willing to make a long-term commitment."

Now it's fine to think that we're going to take care of others, but we need a little help here. First of all, it's not easy to keep up this kind of long-term commitment. We all know that it's nice and good to help others but—as many people have pointed out to me many times—most of us are struggling just to get by with our own needs: covering the bills, keeping the house or apartment clean, getting the laundry done before work.

It may be true that I'm not going to get commitment from the boy until I take responsibility for what the people around me need, but I don't see how that's going to happen if I'm already overwhelmed just taking care of what *I* need.

The answer to this problem is really amazing. There's a place where taking care of our own needs connects with taking care of other people's needs. There's a place where they become the same thing.

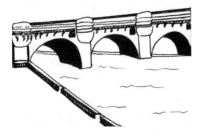

Think about it. The discussion we had about the pen changes the way we think about everything. If I want to see a pen in my world (and not a chew-toy), then I need to provide pens to others, first. If I want companionship for myself, then I have to provide companionship to others, first.

Cathy and I stop at a lovely spot above the Left Bank, overlooking the Seine and people strolling along the other path, down near the water.

"Suppose," I explain, "that all I want is to get my favorite kind of donut, a maple-covered donut. It may look like I get a donut by going to the donut shop and paying the money; it may look like the donut was baked in the back of the shop, from flour and milk and sugar. But now we know that none of these things is the real cause of the donut. You can have money and you can go to a donut shop, but they might be out of donuts. On the other hand, a friend can hand you a donut without you paying for it.

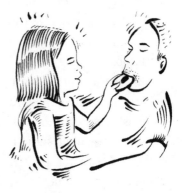

"The real cause of the donut, as we saw with the pen, is that I provided someone else with something like a donut in the past. Which is to say, if I want to eat a donut, then I need to help someone else eat a donut first. That is, I have to cause a donut to pass through another person's lips, before I can see a donut pass through my own lips. If I don't get a donut going into your mouth, I don't get one coming into mine.

"All of us are used to seeing a difference between 'my' mouth and 'your' mouth, because when you get a donut into your mouth it doesn't mean that I get a donut into mine. But now we understand what's really happening: that getting a donut into one is how you get a donut into the other. *Visually,* your mouth looks different than mine; *functionally,* there's no difference between them. And so there's no longer any point to discriminating between the two. Your mouth *is* my mouth, because my mouth can't get a donut unless your mouth does.

Your mouth is my mouth

"What this means as far as getting commitment out of a boy is that it's *a lot easier* to plant the necessary karmic seed if you know what's going on. The karmic seed for commitment from your partner is to take personal responsibility for others around you all the time, all day long. Someone is in a rush and needs that parking space; you make sure they have it. Someone at the table didn't get the olives they wanted on their pizza; you're the one who stands up to go find some. A box falls off a truck on the highway; you pick up your cell to let the police know about the obstruction in the road.

"You need to take responsibility for others if you want the boy to show some commitment. And now it's totally easy to take responsibility, because you've figured out the karmic seed story: you know that taking care of others is actually the same thing as taking care of yourself. You can't take care of yourself without taking care of others, and you can't take care of others without taking care of yourself.

"Because you *are* others."

Cathy pauses for a long moment to digest all this. I know it will take some time, so I stay quiet (which for me is sometimes a challenge). Then I see it register in her eyes, and I know she's got it. I know she's ready to ask the most important question; I can see it coming.

"Okay Geshe La, I get it...but...*on a practical level,* what exactly are you suggesting that I do?"

Okay then, let's get practical. You won't get anything done if we don't make it something specific. For one or two weeks, take responsibility for the happiness of everyone you eat together with. Make sure everybody gets exactly what they want, and if something at the table's not right for somebody, make sure it gets fixed for them. Just take responsibility for everybody, and get used to the idea that you are actually taking responsibility for yourself as well. Make this kind of commitment at dinner a habit...and then watch, as he commits to you.

And yes, Cathy now has one of the most beautiful relationships I've ever seen. It's been quite a few years now, and the boy is quietly and steadily devoted to her, in a constant daily flow of small kindnesses and consideration for what she needs and wants. And she keeps planting the same seeds, so he keeps flowing with the same deep commitment to her.

Question 6

My partner is always getting emails from old flames, some of whom she seems a little too chummy with. What's the karma to see her more devoted to me?

A young man named Carl, whom I had known for quite a few years, popped this question on me one night. We were sitting in front of the fireplace in a faculty house at our university, in a quiet corner of southeast Arizona. I was sadly surprised, because (as is often the case) I had thought his relationship with Joanna was going pretty well.

"Well," I begin, "I can see where you're coming from. I mean, the karma for loyalty is perhaps one of the most basic karmas in any relationship—you don't need any other advice about your relationship if there isn't any real relationship in the first place: if there's no unique bond between the two of you."

He nods expectantly; you can see he's been thinking exactly the same thing.

"Alright then," I nod back. "The Tibetan tradition has an extremely simple and effective method for making sure that your partner stays loyal. You're going to have to be extremely loyal yourself, regardless of what your partner is doing right now.

"The way they're acting has been created by negative karmic seeds which you yourself planted, at some point in the past. To get rid of those seeds, you're going to have to maintain a high degree of integrity yourself—a very conscious and *unilateral* degree of integrity."

Carl looks a little confused. "What do you mean exactly when you say 'unilateral'?"

"Right. Well, this is a really exciting thing about the Diamond Cutter system. If we run into a problem with our partner getting emails from old flames, then normally we feel like we need to talk to the partner, to find out how serious this thing is, to let them know how concerned we feel about it."

Carl nods. "Exactly. In fact I was going to ask Joanna that tonight."

I put up my hand. "Hold off for a bit. You and I both know that talking to her might work, and it might not work. What I want is for you to start being skeptical of these things that might work, or might not work. Because if they might work and they might not work, then the fact is that *they don't work.* Stop knocking your head against the wall. *Find a way that works every time.*

Find a way that works every time

"Look, the great thing is that you don't need to talk to your partner at all, because *that's not going to fix the problem every time.* No more negotiation, no more circular discussions that stretch late into the night. That doesn't fix the karmic seed.

"We have to do something which does fix the seed, and you don't need your partner to do it—because the seed's inside of you, and you're the one who put it there. We need to change this questionable emailing or texting into a seed for perfect loyalty, and the place we need to grow the seed is inside of us, not them. That will fix what Joanna's doing, without getting her involved at all. Make sense?" He nods; you can see he's taking notes in his head.

"So here's what the Tibetans say we have to do. Throughout the day, every day, everywhere you go, no matter who you're with, just remember one thing.

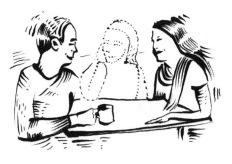

"Never say, or do, or even think something to another person that you wouldn't say or do or think if Joanna were sitting there right next to you, watching and listening—listening even to your innermost thoughts.

"A woman comes up to you at work, or walks by you in the grocery store, and she looks at you in a certain way. And you just don't return the look at all: you are perfectly loyal, the same as you would be if Joanna were there right next to you, carefully watching your eyes."

Carl nods, but slow—and I can see the problem that's coming up in his mind. He thinks he's headed for some kind of psychic jail for the rest of his life.

"It's not like that," I assure him. "If you really get into this kind of loyalty you'll find that it's extremely happy and refreshing, not any burden or feeling of being controlled or restricted.

"The women around you will feel happy, because they know there's a man in the room who will respect them and treat them with dignity. The men in your life will come to feel completely comfortable and trusting of you, because deep down they register how much you honor their relationship.

"And of course all the same applies from a woman's point of view. You build a whole community of trust, and plant deep seeds. Without you really noticing it, Joanna suddenly changes—and she only wants to hear from you."

Carl did plant these seeds, and—as you will come to expect—they came back in a rather unexpected way. Joanna lost her interest in email and texting, and switched over to Facebook, posting pictures and news to her friends in an open way that Carl could not only see for himself, but could actually participate in, several times a day. He became a partner in her messages, instead of a slightly nervous bystander.

Question 7

My partner wants to get married, but I'm not sure if I want to make a lifelong commitment like that. What should we do?

I got this question one night from an old friend named Herb, standing together on a dirt road in rural Arizona, outside a rambling country farmhouse where he and his partner Irene were about to do a short retreat together.

I really like them both and I would really like to see them together for forever. But I have a personal rule against making people's decisions for them. I prefer to give them some cool ideas to chew on, and then let them apply the ideas in their own way. Let them plant their own seeds, and I know it's going to be a happy ending for them—one that I can enjoy watching.

"Look Herb," I start. "We don't get a lot of opportunities in our life to make a decision like this—a decision about whether we really want to spend the rest of our life with another person that we really care about. We all know, we all sense, that there's a time when we should jump. Not to jump might be the mistake of a lifetime. And to leave Irene hanging for a long time, while you agonize over whether to jump or not, might ruin the magic between you two forever.

"On the other hand, we don't want to enter a commitment like this without a lot of thought and care; it's very serious bad karma to make a formal long-term commitment and then break this commitment later on. It may well mean that we'll never find another person in our entire life who makes a true commitment to us."

Herb is a thoughtful guy, and I can see that he gets it. He nods and stays quiet for a while, looking off into the horizon, into the deep desert darkness. "Exactly," he agrees then. "That puts it all in a nutshell. So where do I go from here?"

Now Buddhist monks are really into vows—they take a lot of vows, and they study carefully what the vows involve before they take them. Then they're trained how to keep these vows well, for the rest of their life. I myself have committed to no less than 518 vows: 22 basic ones when I first got to the monastery; another 253 when I became a monk; 120 extra ones that relate to taking care of other people; and another 123 which require special permission from ones lama.

I guess the first thing my lama ever told me about taking vows is that a well-kept vow is a very, very powerful karmic seed. At the time, we were talking about whether I wanted to make a commitment not to eat meat. When I first visited a monastery, I had a very strange dream one night. I was out in the countryside, on a farm, and there was a cow who was going to be slaughtered and made into meat.

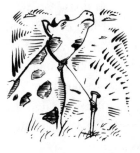

The cow's neck was tied tightly with a rope, and the other end of the rope was fixed to a thick wooden stake pounded into the ground. Nobody had come yet with the knife to cut the cow's throat, but somehow the cow knew what was about to happen. The cow was screaming, screaming loud, and the scream was the scream of a human, not the scream of a cow. Even in the dream it was really creepy, and the hair on the back of my neck was standing up straight.

I woke up with a start, there in the darkness of the monastery, surrounded by monks spread sleeping on the floor. I could never forget the dream, and every time I ate a piece of meat, I found myself asking myself if I would still eat it if I had to kill the animal with my own hands just before the meal. That's when I decided to stop eating meat.

Now my lama told me that if I were going to do this, I should consider making a promise not to eat meat—to take a vow. He said that the karmic seed would be a lot stronger than if I just decided not to take meat. The seed that this particular vow plants, by the way, is one to see your own life protected and strong—and in the 30 years since I took this vow not to eat meat, I've almost always enjoyed excellent health.

Bodily strength doesn't lie inside of protein, any more than a pen lies inside of a pen. We ourselves put the strength into the protein, by protecting life all around us. There's a reason why there's so much cholesterol in meat, and why the cholesterol kills so many people.

And so if you and your partner do intend to stay together, then making a formal commitment to do so will make the relationship infinitely more powerful and joyful, over the years to come.

The lamas say that before we take any vow like this—especially one as serious as a marriage vow—we have to know, first of all, exactly what it is we're promising. And so the first thing about deciding whether to make a marriage commitment is to decide, with your partner, exactly what this commitment entails. Is it really "till death do us part"? Are you really going to stick with each other both "in sickness and in health"? Is this an exclusive commitment, or are exceptions allowed down the line? Countless marriages have failed because the two partners ended up having different ideas about exactly what they had committed to, back in the beginning. Maybe it would be useful to write down a list which you both agree upon, ahead of time.

Keeping vows is considered an art form of in Tibet. It does start with understanding the vows in detail, but then we need to get lots of help and support in keeping them. A Tibetan monk most often takes their vows from the one lama in their life who has always been closest to them: from one who knows their history, who knows their strengths and their weaknesses, and who makes a commitment to stay in their life and guide them through the day-to-day, especially when problems come up with keeping one of the vows.

Tradition says that if you take a vow from someone you already have a close relationship with, then you will be more careful to keep the vow, simply because it would be so embarrassing for us to have them find out that we've broken it—and because they from their side would be so hurt and disappointed. So rather than finding a random priest or minister or similar vow-giver out of a phone book, you might want to seek out someone that you can both forge a more lasting relationship with—someone to whom you can go to for help when challenges come up between you; a person who was there at the very start. Take your time—check this person out carefully for integrity, and for wisdom.

It's also easier to keep a vow if you both share friends and relatives who respect the vow. With Buddhist monks this is considered very important; for over two thousand years we've been encouraged to live in the company of friends who share similar values, and we are required to meet with them twice a month, to discuss together privately any problems we might be having with keeping our vows.

All this began in the days long before the invention calendars or clocks—and so if you go outside at night and see that the moon is either full, or black, then you know you're supposed to be at the vow meeting tonight. If you are contemplating getting married, then seek out the support of friends who respect this kind of commitment—friends that you can talk to whenever things get hard.

But I think what will help you the most to make your decision is something that the Tibetans call *penyun sampa.*

"Herb, look," I add. "Before you make any longtime commitment to Irene, I want you to look into your own heart and ask yourself *why* you're taking these vows, and what you expect them to do for you both, and for others.

"Maybe you want to do what we do in the monastery. Before we take our real monk's vows, the lamas make us take 'baby' monk's vows."

Herb has this way of squishing his whole face up in a fist when he's got a really serious question about something. So he does the squish thing and asks me, "What are baby vows?"

"Okay, so when we first get to the monastery the older monks give us a couple of months to try on just a few of the more basic vows, to see how they fit. Once we feel comfortable with those, then we're allowed to take on the full vows later. During this waiting period we're encouraged to sit down quietly by ourselves every day and make lists in our mind about why we want to take these vows: we make lists about all the good things that we expect to happen to us if we do accept the full vows.

"Look Herb," I admit. "My own lama wasn't sure how well a westerner living in the modern world was going to do with hundreds of ancient commitments, and he actually had me keep baby vows for eight years before he agreed to make me a full monk.

"So take your time, sit down and make a list of what you think marriage would do for you both, for your life and for the people around you. Wait until you know you're ready to keep, and keep well, any commitment that you decide to make."

Herb pauses and nods in that thoughtful way of his, and then looks up to see if there's anything more.

"And don't forget" I add (here comes the punchline). "Everything we've talked about here is just good advice; but you've got to work on the seeds too. This is the crucial thing—it's always the most important thing of all.

"If you think about it, the question doesn't boil down to whether you two guys should get married or not. The big question is how to plant the seeds to make the right decision.

"What you want is that a decision, a good decision, dawns on you clearly, and easily. We know enough now to understand that the karma of being able to make a quick, clear, and *right* decision is to look around us and find friends, family, and coworkers who are themselves faced with a difficult decision.

"Make opportunities for them to sit down with you, give them some quality time to talk about the serious choices they are facing. If you plant these seeds, then your own decision will come clear, without any other work at all.

"No anxiety, no gut-wrenching wavering between the yes or no of asking Irene to marry you," I promise. "Just plant the seeds, and sit back and relax. The right decision will come clear, like a plant that pops up out of a seed in the ground, without you worrying about it at all."

And yes, Herb and Irene did decide to tie the knot. I won't say it happened the next day, or even the next month, because it takes time for a seed to ripen, even if you plant it well. But I knew it was going to be a happy ending, because they did everything right to get there. And it makes me really happy every time I see them together, to know that I was able to help out—and to know that they both really understand *why* it worked out. I love to see those rings on their fingers.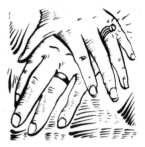

Question 8

Whenever we walk down the street, my husband gawks at every cute girl who passes by, and it really irritates me. What seed do I need to plant for him to be satisfied with looking just at me?

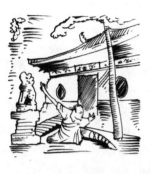

I got this question at a Diamond Cutter Institute seminar in Zhengzhou, central China. It's been an exciting trip, since the whole program was held right next to the Shaolin Temple, where Kung Fu was born. At the crack of dawn you can hear about 20,000 young men and women yelling as they go through their forms. I don't like being woken up, but I do really appreciate the passion they show.

Anyway, the person asking the question is Aiping, whose name means "love." Her husband Huanzhi is a successful businessman who's across the room schmoozing and exchanging business cards with some others during the break. Luckily, I have a really good translator and, like many Chinese, Aiping already has really good instincts into the wisdom of the Diamond Cutter, a beloved Chinese classic.

"This gets into two different kinds of karmic seeds," I begin. "The seeds to look beautiful to yourself, and seeds to look beautiful to Huanzhi." Aiping smiles and takes quick notes, the Chinese characters flying off her fingers.

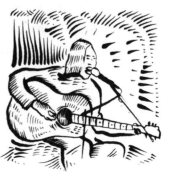

"Because it's all different, you see. You can say you just want to be beautiful, but there's no such thing. My favorite song of all time is one by Neil Young..." here the translator goes off for a while, trying to describe the rocker. I wait until she's finished and carry on.

"Well, you see, one of my best friends used

to call him 'that screaming eunuch'.." Another pause in the translation. "I see the song as epic; he sees the song as chaos. And we're both right, you see: the dog is right that the stick is a chew-toy, and the human is right that it's a pen. By itself, it's neither—no such thing."

I check to see if Aiping is still with me; she nods sharply. Right with me.

"And you're just the same, Aiping. We want to plant a seed for you to see yourself as beautiful, and a seed for Huanzhi to see you as beautiful too. Take away the two of you, and there *is* no other beautiful—and that's just one more kind of emptiness."

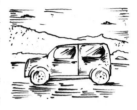

I hear the translator hit *kong shing*—the Chinese have a perfect word for this *blank-white-screen* idea—and smile.

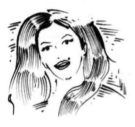

"Which means, if you think about it, that anything and anyone could be beautiful, because beauty is only in the eye of the beholder. The proof of this is all around us: supermodels with big moles on their cheeks, or cars shaped like bread boxes; and the public goes wild over both of them. If he *sees* you as beautiful, by the way, you really *are* beautiful—because you never have been more or less than what you were both seeing anyway."

"So what's the seed to see beauty?" asks Aiping.

Beauty comes from not getting angry

I nod. "It's simply to avoid getting angry in situations where you easily could get angry. Your boss at work comes into the room and starts yelling at you for something that's not your fault: You're 'The most stupid employee I've ever had' for something that somebody else did, and *he's* so stupid that he won't even give you a chance to explain it."

Ai looks up, and it registers. "Yes, yes, that's what I've always heard: that anger has a very special power to burn our good karmic seeds. The ancient scriptures say that just a few minutes of intense anger is enough to incinerate thousands of good seeds."

"Just so. Anger has a special effect on the seeds which make us see ourselves beautiful: hold a sustained anger towards someone—resentment, or bitterness—and you can literally watch over the weeks as wrinkles form on your face, and your hair turns to gray.

"The wrinkles, and the gray, are coming from us, same as the pen. And the process is completely reversible. If we can learn how *not* to get angry in situations that would make just about anyone angry, then gradually beauty will return to our face and form. And then Huanzhi will forget to look at other people walking down the street."

Sounds easy, but you and I know it's not. Not getting angry in a very tough situation is almost impossible. We're going to need some serious help.

The seeds themselves provide this help. Once you understand the seeds— once you understand where things are really coming from—then it's almost impossible to get mad at someone else. I like to a call it the "Water on the Bathroom Floor Syndrome."

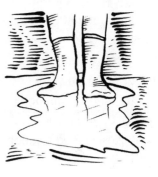

It's winter, the floors of your home are freezing cold, and you've only got one good pair of thick wool socks for puttering around the house; that is, one pair which doesn't have holes in them. You crawl sleepy out of bed and walk half conscious into the bathroom to brush your teeth. You stand in front of the mirror, and suddenly your feet are soaked with freezing water. Someone has taken a shower again without closing the shower curtain all the way, and there's water covering the floor. It's like the tenth time this month.

You hear the family having breakfast downstairs around the kitchen table, and you head down seeking some justice. Your husband and the kids are there enjoying some Cheerios; all talk stops when they see the look on your face.

"Okay, who did it?"

"Did what, dear?"

"Left the shower curtain open and spilled water all over the floor." You hold that last good pair of socks up in front of their faces; maybe even let them drip a bit on the Cheerios.

Your husband looks you straight in the eye. "Wasn't me, hon. I haven't had my shower yet this morning."

Your boy looks up with an innocent face, and before he even opens his mouth you know he's innocent. "Not me, Mom."

All eyes focus on your daughter, who stares at the ground—not a good sign. "Mommy…somebody got up really early this morning and took a shower. Wasn't it…you?"

Who spilled the water on the floor?

And then you remember—you forgot it was Saturday and you got up early for work, took your shower, forgot to close the curtain, got water all over the floor, then realized it was the weekend and dropped back into bed.

You give the three of them a sheepish look and retreat to your room.

It's the same with your yelling boss. It's not that he decided to start yelling at you, and it's not that if you get mad at him he's going to decide to stop yelling, or else yell some more. He's coming from you as surely as the pen is coming from you. You spilled the water earlier today, and now you're stepping in it.

Once we really grasp how this works, it's 100% impossible to get angry at your boss. You don't go into the bathroom and yell at yourself in the mirror (the way you might have yelled at your daughter, had she been the guilty party), because it doesn't do any good. You know you spilled the water. You just make a calm resolution not to do it again, and you hang your socks up to dry. End of story.

In the case of your boss, you watch him rant for a while and then decide that you're going to be really careful not to get angry in the small daily ways (maybe with the kids) which must have planted the seed for him. That will shut the boss's yelling down by next week; like turning off a shower faucet and watching the last of the water drip out the shower head.

And then the new seeds will change how you look. Again, please understand that it's not that you "really" look a certain way, and if you're in a good mood you'll look better. You look exactly how the seeds force you to look, and noway else. Be ready for the beauty in the mirror, and the beauty that your husband sees.

By the way, going back to what we said at the beginning of this question, it's easy to see how being beautiful in the way you respond to challenges all day is going to plant a seed for you to see yourself as beautiful. But this seed also decides how you see your husband seeing you—as beautiful. It's not that you are planting a seed in his mind, because each of us can only plant our own seeds. Rather, the same seed that makes you see yourself beautiful makes you see him seeing you as beautiful.

And so you are!

LOVE

Question 9

Sometimes when I'm with my partner, it feels like sitting in heaven next to a true Angel. I just want to know how I plant the seeds to keep that feeling going all the time.

The glimpses of heaven which we are sometimes granted are real, because they're coming from karmic seeds in our mind, just like everything else is. If we figure out the exact seeds that they come from, then we can plant those seeds and make these moments happen more often—maybe all the time. The seeds we need for this are good wishes for the whole world, and they're not so hard to come by.

The ancient Tibetans say that these powerful seeds begin with a disaster at home. If we're lucky, it comes early on in our life. Your mother dies of breast cancer, your brother takes his life.

Tragedies like this force us to face up to what's happening in the world. If everything goes really well in our time here (which is really unusual), then we can get a good job, a good partner, a good house, a good family. And then one by one, the world takes them away from us—that's just the way it is. You get old, you both get old, you weaken, you come closer to the end, with every passing day.

Deep down, we all know—even from our childhood—that this is how things will go. It gives us a sad feeling for ourselves and the world, but there's also a kind of sweetness.

I was on a flight once, when I was still a teenager—from Phoenix to Washington DC. We were scheduled to change planes in Chicago.

It was a normal flight: a pretty bad movie that people were grumbling about, a few tiny packs of peanuts that they grumbled about even more. Approaching Chicago we were surrounded by thick clouds. It seemed like it was taking us a long time to get on the ground.

Suddenly the plane shot straight up like a bullet. It peaked and then came down sharp as a roller coaster, then hit bottom and shot up again. This happened three or four times. A flight attendant stepped out of the cockpit door, looking a little sick. The captain came on the intercom.

"Uh folks, we have a little problem here. We tried to put the landing gear down, but the light in the cockpit that tells us whether or not the wheels are down isn't coming on. This could be just a bad light, or it could be that the landing gear is stuck, we don't know.

"We flew a few times by the tower to see if they could check visually whether the wheels are down, but the cloud coverage is too thick for them to tell for sure. We've just tried a couple of steep dives to see if we could knock the gear down, but the light's still not coming on. So it looks like we're just going to have to attempt a landing, and see if the wheels hold up."

Another nerve-wracking pause...

"Uh, we're going to circle the field for a bit here and give them time to get the runway ready for us. We'll keep you up to date on what's happening. Until then, please just follow the instructions you get from our flight crew."

They shut off the movie—no one's worried about it anymore, or about the peanuts. People look around a little dazed, wondering what to do. The guy next to me pulls out a piece of paper, writes for a few minutes, then folds the paper up carefully and slips it into the seat pocket in front of him.

He catches me looking. "I read about this plane that went down some-place," he explains. "Only one or two survivors, but some of the people who died wrote notes to their families that were found later."

The feeling of tension in the plane rises; the flight attendant goes to the cockpit again, comes back looking even worse. She picks up the microphone and makes an announcement.

"Well ladies and gentlemen, as you can see, we're in a holding pattern over Chicago. This will give our staff on the ground time to put foam out on the runway, just in case our wheels aren't down, or they don't hold. We... we're also trying to use up all the extra fuel on board, just in case there is a small problem on the ground..." and then she breaks down sobbing. The second attendant leads her to an empty seat and helps her down. All the rest of us are left with a very clear picture of jet fuel splashed across the runway, burning what's left of the plane.

There's a moment of silence, and then a strange thing happens. A lady in the row in front of me, across the aisle to the left, turns and hugs the lady next to her. Somebody else gets up and goes to hug the crying flight attendant. Hands reach out to clasp the hands of strangers, more hugs in every row, and suddenly comfort is flowing like electricity through the entire plane. Human

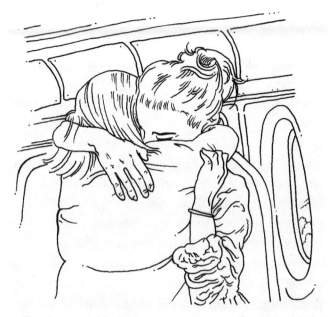

kindness, overflowing—and it dawns on every one of us that this is the original condition of the human soul, the way we were always meant to be.

Because the plane is always going down, every day of our lives, and we don't know how many minutes or hours any of us has left before it hits.

At the end they tell us take off jewelry—if there's a fire, it will burn through flesh and bone. Shoes that aren't good for jumping from the plane, or running away from it as fast as we can, should come off too.

And then just before the final approach, the worst thing of all. Cover your head with your hands, bend forward, get your face down. Think in silence about your life, and think about your death.

The wheels touched the runway, and they held. We floated like a skier through the foam on the tarmac, between two rows of vehicles parked to either side. On the left stood a line of ambulances, drawn up to transport the survivors. On the right was a line of black hearses, for the dead. We coasted to the gate, and the seatbelt sign went off with a *ding*.

People jump up from their seats. "Gotta catch my connection!" exclaims a man as he jams me in the ribs with his elbow. The love goes back to its usual place, deep down inside, to wait for another clear moment.

The plane is always falling

But I have never forgotten the sweetness in our hearts on the plane, the wave of human kindness which passed among us, and I don't think anyone else there ever forgot it either. It is a feeling that we are all mortal, that we will all pass away, and that we are in this together, regardless of what else is happening between us.

And that feeling spawns another feeling, an even deeper feeling, that we would like to take care of each other. Very deep down, we would all like to have a chance to help all the rest of us, somehow—especially against this one great enemy that all of us share: the merciless decline of human life into death. There is, deep within the heart of every living creature, a burning desire to help every other living thing live.

Every time we feel this sweet desire, this hunger to help the world, it plants within us a very special seed. This is the hunger that an angel feels all the time, and it plants inside of us the seed to be with the angels, and to become as them. This is the seed for those special moments when it feels as though you are sitting next to an angel, in heaven itself.

It is not so difficult a seed to find. Just look around on this airplane we call the world, and love those whose lives are sometimes as touching as our own.

Question 10

My husband never shows me any affection; I come home ready for a big hug but he just says "Hi" and sits down to check his email. What's the karma to see him be more warm to me?

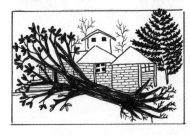

To understand the seed you have to plant to see your husband be more affectionate, you need to appreciate oak trees.

A lot of my training I did in a small, traditional Buddhist temple that was started by Mongolian refugees from World War II, right down in the middle of New Jersey. It was built in the old Mongol style, with a high roof leading up to a steeple topped by the traditional golden rafters. All around the temple stood very old oak trees, thick and tall.

One night we had a tremendous windstorm, which toppled a tree next to the temple. It fell leaning against the roof, about 30 feet off the ground, and the next morning all our little team of monks was out on the sidewalk, looking up.

"We will need to cut off the top of the tree," declares the Abbot. "And then ease the trunk down slowly so it doesn't break through the windows and walls."

The monks nod in unison. They are a strange bunch, almost all of them older than 75, straight out of the steppes of Central Asia, and the 15th century. Zungru, a hermit that we rarely see outside of his monk's cell, says quietly: "Of course, the tree must be cut by the monk with the least seniority."

I sigh. "Monk with the least seniority" is practically my middle name: I am 50 years younger than the youngest of them, and it's not like Mongolian teenagers in the community are lining up to take monk's vows, when they can hop in the car on a Saturday afternoon and be up in the dance clubs on New York's lower East Side in less than two hours.

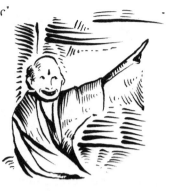

"I'll do it," I say, and reach down for the c'strous. I work my way up a very high ladder with one hand, perch myself on the edge of the temple roof, and pull on the starter rope, trying not to eject myself into space. Then I wend up towards the higher branches, jam my feet between one limb and the trunk, stand up, and cut. In about 3 minutes my legs are shaking from exhaustion and fear. I hate heights.

"Ha ha," says Zungru, way down below. "Look at Mr. Pic-Pic."

I shoot him a dirty look. *Pic-pic* is the Tibetan word for "jello," and he's calling me "Mr. Jello Legs."

Three hours later I'm done; we slide the tree safely off the temple, and I climb down the ladder. At the bottom, on the sidewalk, I see a single tiny acorn. I pick it up, let it roll around in the palm of my hand, and then suddenly I see it as it will be fully grown, maybe a hundred years from now: a huge, towering oak tree.

And I see another windstorm there in the future, and I see this new tree falling against the temple, and I see myself, a century later, still the monk with least seniority—climbing up the ladder to cut it. With a growl I take the acorn and throw it out in the middle of the street, where it can never take root.

Try to feel the difference between the weight of the acorn and the weight of the tree which it has the power to produce: half a gram, versus a few hundred tons of finished tree. The result, many thousands of times heavier than the seed that caused it.

This is the way of all seeds, outside us or inside us. Our own bodies are composed of trillions upon trillions of cells, which reproduce themselves day after day for 50, 60, or 70 years. And they came from only the one egg of your mother, and the one sperm of your father.

Mental seeds are no different; in fact, a few tiny mental seeds produce much greater results than any physical seed can. Which is good news if you want your husband to show you more affection.

Because we want him to be affectionate not for a night, or for a few days, but for the rest of your life. We want a hug—a real hug, a rib-crushing several minutes of contented silence hug—every time you leave for work, and every time you come home, and a couple more hugs scattered here and there throughout the day, every day.

The point is that all we need are some small, carefully planted seeds. Again, learn to look at the essence of what you want, and craft your seeds accordingly. What we want here boils down to genuine warmth, and to get it we first have to give it.

As you go through your day, try to be much more consciously friendly to all the people who cross your path. This doesn't need some huge effort, just more care on our part. Pat people at work on the shoulder when they're doing a good job; thank the person at the grocery check-out counter for their help; hold the door open for someone coming into the building behind you.

Most important, shower random smiles on people who walk by you on the street, or in the store. Especially if you are being careful to do the Coffee Meditation that we described back in Question 4, these small seeds will grow into a mighty tree, a lifetime of affection. Because unexpected warmth is the sweetest warmth, and your husband will be finding new ways to show it to you.

LIVING TOGETHER

Question 11

I do most of the cooking in our house, but when it comes time to clear the table and wash the dishes, my husband suddenly disappears like magic, and pops up in the living room in front of the television. What's the karma to get him to help with the chores?

This gets into another important question about karmic seeds. When my lama challenged me to go to New York and start a successful company to prove that I understood how the seeds work, I first went to get some advice from one of the older monks—this was in the Tibetan monastery, overseas.

"When you start up your company," he said, "you're going to have to start up a charity at the same time. The charity will drive your business—it will be the engine for the profits of your business."

I nodded and made a note; he gave me some more tips, and then I popped the big question.

"So, how long is this gonna take? I mean, if I plant the seeds you're describing, how long will it take me to see some real results?"

He looks at me, smiles cheerfully, and announces, *"Tse chima la.* Next life!"

I shake my head ruefully. "Next life isn't gonna cut it, Rinpoche. Look, you know, I'm American. We like *invented* fast food. We *are* McDonald's, all over the world. If an employee at McDonald's takes more than two and a half minutes whipping up a batch of French fries, they get *fired.* I gotta get these seeds going like in a few months, or even a few weeks."

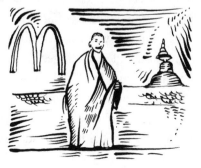

And that's important for you too, you see. I've got to show you how to plant a seed and see some results fast. If you go to a nursing home to help somebody and it takes three years for the boy to show up, there's going to be a very basic problem.

If it takes too long, you won't be sure whether going to the nursing home was what caused the boy. And then you won't buy into the system, and it won't help you for the rest of your life.

Which brings us back to your husband disappearing when it comes time to do the dishes. It's not enough just to plant seeds, because if you don't plant them in the right place, they're not going to grow properly. We all know people who are generous and help lots of other people, but the more they give away the more broke they seem to get. In many cases the seeds they're planting are the right seeds, but they've planted them in the wrong place.

The karmic seed for getting your husband to be more helpful around the house is to concentrate for a few weeks on being much more helpful to others, very consciously helpful. An example of a helpful seed planted in a bad place—in stony soil— would be to help somebody at work because you're afraid your boss will fire you if you don't. It's true that you've helped the

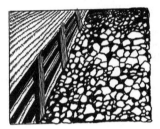

person sitting at the desk next to yours, and it's true that a seed was planted...but the person is really just someone that you're paid to help anyway. Better if you pick a heavy karmic object: fertile soil for a fast seed.

So what are some great places to plant your helpful seeds?

Choose good places to plant your seeds

The ancients of Tibet say there are three very fertile places. The first of them is anyone who's really in the middle of an emergency, especially if you're the only person they have to rely on right now. It could be someone on the street who just fell down, and you're the nearest person to help them up; or a friend who's going to lose their apartment tomorrow morning if they can't come up with another hundred dollars of rent money tonight; or people you hear about in a refugee camp somewhere on the other side of the world, who need some food, right now.

The second fertile soil for your seed is someone who has been of great help to you in the past. If I ask you who is the one person in your life who has helped you the most, it shouldn't take more than an instant for a picture of your mother to come to mind. Whatever your relationship with her is right now, the simple fact is that she taught you how to walk, taught you how to talk, how to dress yourself, how to act in the world. In modern times she usually had a choice to have you or not, and she chose to risk her life to give you yours. Nearly the same with your father. And then there are all the other teachers and mentors and family and friends who have guided you through life so far. Any help that you give them, any kindness repaid, is a seed planted in the best of soil.

Third are those who are helping many other people. I remember once I was given a donation of $10,000 from a friend who asked that I distribute it to sick people at one of our Tibetan refugee camps. I travelled to India, got to the camp, and found a small room which I could use as an office. We spread the word that the next day we would be handing out grants for people's medicine and medical care. You just had to bring a receipt for either that was dated in the last month.

We set it up carefully, of course. We didn't give people enough time to find a local doctor who was crooked and would hand out receipts for a kick-back. We prepared a stamp, and some red ink, to smear all over a receipt once we had paid it. We even stamped the left hand of each person who received a payment.

And it was a line! Two hours before we opened our door there was an orderly queue of refugees stretching down the dusty road of the camp for a mile or more. We handed out money for the next seven hours, with a few heated debates about whether a receipt for a purchased donkey was a medical expense. By the time the sun was low on the horizon, we had used up the ten thousand, and the line seemed just as long as when we had started.

I flew back to the States with the feeling that there must be a better way. In time we found a French nurse who was willing to come to the refugee camp and run a free clinic with donated Western medicine which was still usable, but had passed its expiration date.

The lesson then is to help one person who is helping many other people, rather than trying to cover each individual in need: wear shoes, say the Tibetans, rather than trying to coat the world in leather.

We're going to come back to this theme again and again. Pick your seeds carefully, plant them in a way that's going to come back thick, strong, and quick—use the Four Starbucks Steps that we saw back in Question 4. Help others in way that's smart and effective, and your husband will suddenly decide that he loves the feel of warm soapy water on his hands.

Question 12

When we moved in together, my partner (without any warning) showed up with a cat. I like pets, but I don't keep one myself, because I feel that if I do then I won't be able to go anywhere. Sure enough, now I'm stuck feeding the cat whenever my better half needs to visit her family. *And* I've discovered that I'm allergic to the cat hair. What can I do?

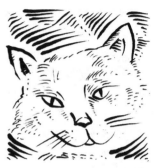

One of the companies that inspired us as we built Andin International Diamond was the Sony Corporation, and its co-founder Akio Morita. We pored over his bestselling book *Made in Japan,* the story of Sony's success. The most important idea in this book is one that you can use to fix your cat dilemma, and any other problem you might be having with a roommate.

Mr. Morita says that one of Sony's founding principles was to supply the customer with a product or feature that they really wanted, but didn't yet *know* that they wanted. Watch people, and observe their needs so carefully that you can give them something which will really help them, even if they haven't thought of it yet. I call it the Jampa Principle.

For many years with my main Tibetan teacher, Khen Rinpoche Geshe Lobsang Tharchin, I played the role of cook, dishwasher, chauffer, laundry-

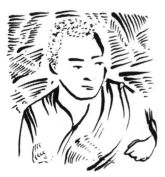

man, housemaid and gardener. After I helped start the diamond company I was gone much of the day, and had to seek a replacement for many of these tasks. I was lucky enough to find Jampa Lungrik.

Jampa was a cheerful, quiet, and extreme-ly devoted young Tibetan monk who stepped right into all these roles with perfect grace. One of our most important tasks was to manage the lines of people who would show up asking for time to talk to Lama. Make sure that everyone who wants to see him does, but at the same time assure that he's not overtaxed. The temple kitchen served as our waiting room, and it was usually filled with people wanting to see the Master. We had to make tea for them and keep them entertained for what could sometimes be a pretty long wait.

It was during this time that Jampa taught me how monks in the monastery are trained in providing hospitality for a guest—something which is considered an extremely important skill in Tibet. In the Land of Snows, the guest really is king, and my house really is your house.

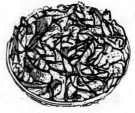

Jampa said, "Before the people get here, set plates full of goodies out on the kitchen table. Put the cookies up there on one end. Over here, a bowl of fruit. Off towards the other end of the table, maybe a pile of *kaptse:* Tibetan donuts.

"A pitcher of water goes here, a carafe of juice goes there, a tea thermos here, a pot of coffee there—with lots of cups and glasses spread around.

"The knock on the door is a crucial moment. Open the door, greet your guest, and step back, inviting them into the kitchen. As they walk in, watch their eyes carefully.

"The guest will make some eye contact with you as you greet them, but then their gaze will pass around the room, and down the kitchen table. This is where you really have to pay attention.

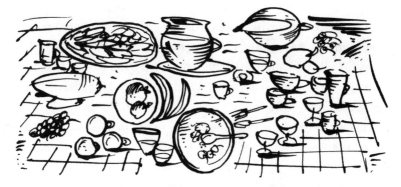

"The reason we've spread the snacks around different parts of the table is so we can tell where their eyes pause. When the guest sees something they really enjoy—maybe the Tibetan donuts—their eyes will linger there, just for a second.

Watch people's eyes to see what they need

"What you do then is ask them to be seated, and you go straight for the Tibetan donuts, pick up the plate, and hold it out to them—'Would you like one of these while you're waiting?' Then pour them a cup of whatever beverage their eyes went to.

"Watch their donut, watch their cup, and keep watching their eyes as you talk to them to learn a bit about them, and why they've come to see Rinpoche. When the cup is two-thirds empty, offer them some more.

"Keep watching their eyes; anticipate their needs. This is the essence of hospitality."

It's the same with your partner, you see. The essence of your problem with them is that they're not being sensitive to your needs. Maybe they've stuck you with a shedding cat; maybe they have noisy friends over in the middle of the night; maybe they leave stacks of dirty dishes in the sink. The point is that—if you want them to be sensitive to your needs—then you're going to have to crank up your own sensitivity to the needs of others in your life.

So start watching people's eyes; try to guess what they might want, or need. Get practical with this and, as we said before, pick some fertile soil in which to plant these seeds. Choose someone like your parents, or someone else who has really helped you in your life, and spend just a tiny bit of time every day thinking about their needs, about what you can do for them.

It doesn't have to be something big, just something which is carefully thought out, because this will produce more seeds. Select a time of the day when you regularly have some quiet moments to yourself—I like to make these plans for others while I'm eating breakfast. And having made plans is another thing you can do your Coffee Meditation on at the end of the day, to make the seeds grow super-fast.

Rather than confronting our housemate, rather than discussions or arguments or reminders, we are working on the real seeds which created them in the first place: the seeds that make us see a pen, or a pile of dirty dishes. As you learn to observe and tend to the small needs of others in your life (which is already a very pleasant task for you and for them), you will find that your roommate is suddenly becoming a much more considerate person.

The cat might one day go to a cousin who has children that love pets, without your even asking.

Question 13

My husband doesn't have a clue as far as personal hygiene—he always walks around the house with half a beard, in stinky clothes. What's the seed I need to plant to see him take a little more care of himself?

This question comes up with an older American couple from the Midwest. They've come to a talk that I'm doing in Detroit, aimed at autoworkers whose jobs are being threatened by plant closures. I identify with Jack and Kris, who are also products of the 1960's, but as in many cases some of the good parts of the counterculture got lost, while the hippie hygiene part stuck.

"You know the exercise by now," I say to Kris. "First you have to identify the essence of the problem. What would you say that is?"

She thinks for a moment. "Well, I guess the real crux of the issue is that Jack's just not thinking about how his appearance impacts on others. He's caught up in himself—which happens to just about all of us, really—and he's not thinking about how I feel."

"Alright then, sounds right. So the karmic seed you need to plant in this particular case is kind of cool. If we're seeing someone close to us ignore their personal hygiene to the point that it makes our day unpleasant, then we have to plant some seeds of the opposite kind, and things will change—no discussion, no argument. Which gets us into watermelons, and groundhogs."

Kris gives me a confused look, one that I was hoping for. It means she'll be listening to what comes next.

"Look, we counteract a negative seed by planting a positive seed of the same type. That is, if we feel lonely then we offer someone else companionship; if we want to get out of credit-card debt, then we seek others who need financial help, and offer it to them in a wise and well-considered way." She nods.

"But I want you to be aware that there's some leeway here. Just last night somebody asked me what the karmic seed was to get more chocolate-chip ice cream in their life: they wanted to know if they would have to go around handing out this specific flavor to get more of it back later.

"Makes sense," says Kris. "Everyone has their favorite flavor, and sometimes we just can't get it."

"Exactly. So generally speaking, one of the four great laws of karmic seed-planting says that you have to give something similar to what you want yourself: like creates like.

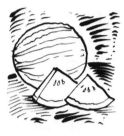

"If you think about it, this is one of the small unappreciated miracles of life. If you want watermelons in your garden this summer, you just go to a watermelon that's already around and pull some seeds out of it.

"These particular seeds will always grow into a watermelon, and never a mango or a cactus. Just think how life would be if it weren't this way—can you see farmers sitting around together at the local restaurant, discussing what might happen this year? 'I planted corn seeds this spring, and I'm hoping that I don't get bamboo sprouts coming up from them, like I did last year!'

"So a seed to see Jack be a little more attentive to his appearance is going to involve being more attentive to your own—but there is some leeway. There's a book called the *Treasure House of Wisdom,* written by a master named Vasubandhu about 17 centuries ago, and here he discusses the chocolate-chip ice cream question.

"Somebody says, look, Vasubandhu. Suppose I'm supposed to be reborn as a bear, but I happen to die just before summer, when bears aren't having babies. No problem, says the Master, you just detour into a groundhog." That gets a smile out of Kris—I suddenly suspect that she feels that the groundhog and Jack are somehow connected.

"And there's a debate about this answer, but you get the idea. You decide what result you want, and then you go for the closest seed you can; but it doesn't have to be *exactly* the same thing that you're looking for. In your mind though it's important to *dedicate* the seed to a particular purpose—to something like cleaning up your man."

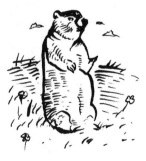

"So what would be a seed which is close?" she asks.

"Well, let's think about it. You want your husband to shine, and the reason he's not shining now is there, deep inside of you. So I'd suggest that you do the flower thing."

"Which is?"

"Which is this. Three times in the next week, when you go out, I want you to spend some time to look especially nice. Like a flower, that people love to look at.

"And you have to think of it this way; it's not for you, not for your ego. You're going to look especially beautiful so there's one more beautiful thing that the people of the world can enjoy as they walk down the street.

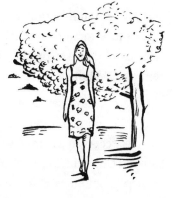

"The idea is that you do something which you might want to do anyway, for yourself— looking good as you walk down the street— but you change the motivation for it. Can you consciously try to look special for others, to make them happy?

"This is a new concept of personal beauty: doing your part to make the world a beautiful place for others. Beauty becomes a beautiful thing, and not something selfish—it becomes a visual smile for those who cross your path. Beauty becomes clean, and pure; a flower walking down the street.

Keep offering flowers

"Keep offering flowers to the world—make it a habit not just to dress this way, but to think this way for others, for the pleasure of others. To speed the seeds up, remember to do your Coffee Meditation just before bed. And then one day the seeds will crack open, and your husband will emerge from the bathroom, clean-shaven, in a crisp white shirt."

"I like it," smiles Kris. "And that's something I like about the whole seed-planting thing. It's just *fun.*"

Question 14

I have a demanding job; when I get home I'm exhausted, and I feel like I need to talk to someone about the problems at work. But my husband really doesn't want to hear about these issues, much less help me work them out. What seed do I need to plant to see some empathy?

This question came in China too. Except it wasn't quite as fun as the Kung Fu Temple. DCI has received an invitation to present the Diamond Cutter ideas in a conference of professional psychologists at a university in Harbin, China.

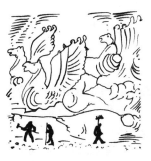

We said sure, we'd love to come, but nobody bothered to check on a map. Harbin turns out to be right next to Siberia, and it's 15 below zero when we walk out of the airport. People at midnight are running around in the snow, and their idea of a good time is constructing 3-story ice sculptures on the sidewalks that last all winter without melting. I honestly think the water inside my eyeballs is going to freeze.

But the people are warm, and their questions sincere. The one that Jiali asks me is, sadly, one that I've heard all across the world.

"So first, tell me what you think the very essence of this problem is," I begin.

Jiali thinks for a moment. "I guess the main thing is that Yongqian just isn't listening to me."

"In that case, the seed we need to plant is loud and clear: you need to start listening more carefully to others."

"And what's the best way to do that?"

"According to the ancient books, this is really just an extension of a good meditation practice: the ability to listen to your own mind—to keep your attention glued to one thing.

"When you get good at it, it feels like the mind is sliding against whatever you're trying to concentrate on, like an ice skate that travels across a mile of ice but never loses contact with it.

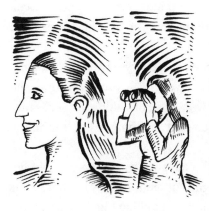

"At the beginning, it's a chore. You sit across the table from someone and try to listen to what they're saying; but instead of letting your mind wander off in between their words, you try to hold your thoughts up tight against every single syllable.

"Your mind wanders off to the cell phone in your pocket, or to what you're going to make for dinner, or to what's going on outside the window behind the person who's talking to you."

"But that seems pretty natural," Jiali replies. "Is there some trick to stopping it?"

I nod. "There is. You set a little piece of your mind to sit behind your main mind and watch how well it's listening; when the main mind wanders off, the little mind rings an alarm, and you bring your attention back. This can be exhausting, like trying to control a big uncooperative dog on a leash.

"In time though you learn to listen, and listen closely; your concentration on the words of the other person is so good that you can almost feel the thoughts in their head behind the words, as they choose which words to use. You start to get a little feeling of what it's like to be them, which is a sign that you're becoming a really good listener—better than you ever were before."

"And how, exactly, is that going to change how Yongqian listens to me?"

Send your seeds where you want them

"While you're listening, or afterwards, pause and 'send' the seeds you're planting off towards him. When you consciously direct seeds, it reinforces them inside your own mind; and it guarantees that the result will come back where you want it to.

"Keep this up until the day comes when you open the front door and—

without any prompting at all—Yongqian asks you how your day went at work."

By the way, there's another thing about the art of listening. One step further up the listening ladder, some wonderful things start to happen. If you keep up the kind of work we've been describing so far in this book, the whole story of your life is going to change.

This is because we're always making seeds—every day, every thought, every moment. Up to now we haven't been aware of this seed planting, and so it's been a little random, like somebody with a bag of wildflower seeds running through a field, spilling them out by accident and living with a mishmash of results.

And the results are mostly bad—not because we're evil people, but because we tend to have little negative thoughts all the time: It's too hot in this room; I don't like the dress she's wearing today. Nothing big, but the simple fact is that it's the small seeds that run our lives. Try to appreciate the difference in scale between an apple seed and an apple tree, and then it's no stretch to believe that our life is full of ups and downs for a very good reason.

When we do start planting some good seeds consciously for the first time, we're immediately making a huge change in our percentage of good seeds, just because we don't usually plant very many. In the case of listening, this means that we immediately begin to hear people saying a lot of amazing things that we've never had the seeds to hear before.

Keep listening, keep listening closely, and you may tune into frequencies that you've never even been aware of before—the way that animals hear things that humans can't. Maybe you'll learn things from people that you never expected; maybe one day you will talk to an angel.

Question 15

My wife is really messy—just walking through a room she leaves a trail of wreckage behind her: a sweater, a coffee cup, her laptop, and her cell phone (which later on she runs around trying to find). What's the karma to see her be a bit more tidy?

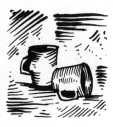

Tidiness is not exactly popular in the world right now; you almost never read that a famous movie star has been rated high on their tidiness. In the Tibetan tradition though tidiness is considered a big deal, because of the effect it has upon your mind.

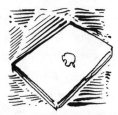

On the practical side, it just doesn't take much time at all to be tidy. We avoid washing dishes and making the bed, but it's nothing more than sheer laziness. I mean, recently I timed how long it took me to make the bed as soon as I got out of it, and we're talking well under a minute. Same with the dishes, even a big sinkful of them after executing a major Julia Child recipe: no more than 5 or 6 minutes.

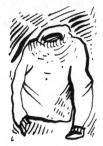

Get into the habit of putting things away while they're still in your hand; why come home, pull your coat off, throw it on the couch, and then have to come back later to pick the coat up and put it away? Just take it off and hang it straight up.

This has another big benefit, which is that you can find things when you need them. Don't set your cell phone on the counter, and then run around later trying to find it when you really need to make a call. Let it have a regular place, in your purse right next to your wallet, and when you finish a call just put it back there.

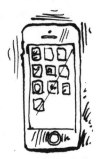

Tibetan monks have a traditional practice of walking around the house after they get up in the morning, putting things away and tidying up. This

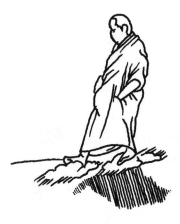

gets your body warmed up in a pleasant way for the day; monks might even throw a couple of soft rags on the floor and then skate around the room on them, polishing up the floor and getting a bit of exercise at the same time.

We're not talking about a sterile or a spotless living room here, just one that is sleek and elegant, uncluttered. When you walk through a room like this, it has a calming effect on your mind: you can think more clearly, especially about the important things in life. This idea about where your whole life is coming from—

the idea of the seeds—isn't an easy one to get your head around. It requires a certain clarity of mind, and keeping our life tidy helps us keep that clarity.

Understand that when you do follow this practice of tidiness, just a little bit each morning, you're actually doing the most effective thing you can do to make your wife more tidy. You'll find that it *works* to make her a tidy person; rather than, for example, having a long talk with her about being a tidy person—which *doesn't* work. And that calls for some explanation.

Suppose you're getting on a plane, with an airline you've never flown before. A perky flight attendant meets you at the door and holds out a clipboard.

"Excuse me sir, could you just sign this form before getting on the plane today?"

If you're like me—if you've spent any part of your life around business contracts—then you lean down and try to read the paper she's holding out to you. She pulls it back ever so slightly.

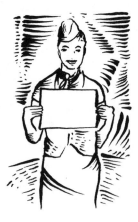

"No big deal," she says. "It's just a little form."

"What kind of form?"

"Well, a waiver—an insurance waiver."

"Insurance waiver? Why are you asking me to sign an insurance waiver?"

"Well," she says, with a condescending smile. "As you know, we're a new airline, and a lot of our staff are new too. They're getting very good at flying these planes, and most of the time we get right to where we're going, without any problem at all."

"Most of the time?" you ask.

"Well, you know, we have had a few little incidents from time to time and…well, you know, the relatives of the victims can be so…demanding!"

She holds out the waiver again, but you're already headed back to the ticket counters, to find a company that knows how to fly their planes, *all of the time.*

So get this—we talked about it a bit at the beginning. In the case of a plane that you're going to trust your life to, **working sometimes is the same as not working at all.** Only a fool would risk their life on a plane that only works sometimes. But all of us risk our lives in the very same way, every hour of the day. We do things that might work, or might not work—which means that *we don't really know how things work.* If we did, we'd just do what works, no problem.

Now how does all this relate to your wife's tidiness?

Talking to your wife about her lack of tidiness, trying to convince her how much it bothers you when she strews her things all over the house, is like the airline we were talking about—and you know it. You know very well, from much past experience, that talking to your wife might work, and it might *not* work. And that means it *doesn't* work.

Planting seeds is different. Do this little monk practice of tidying up your own place every morning, and it plants a seed to see her start tidying up—especially if you're topping it off with Coffee Meditation before bed. There's no discussion, no tension, and it never doesn't work. Which means it works. All the time.

That's the great thing about the karmic seed method, what we call the Diamond Cutter system, all throughout this book. Once you get good at it, it takes all the guesswork out of your life. There's no reason why you can't have all the things you've always wanted. There's no reason why you have to keep putting up with disappointment.

**When something works
sometimes it doesn't
work at all**

SEX, PART ONE

Question 16

Is there any way, karmically, to get my boyfriend to be a little more tender during sex? Half the things he does to turn me on just hurt.

Again we first have to look at the essence of what your boyfriend is doing to you, and I think we can agree on calling it unintended hurt.

And once again, we could sit him down and talk to him, and there's a chance that he'll get it; but there's a (good) chance that he won't understand what you're trying to say, and either he'll get offended (because all men like to think that their romantic skills are already unprecedented) or he'll get tentative in bed, which is maybe even worse.

So let's stop doing things that might not work. Let's go straight to seeds, because they work every time.

The most common type of unintended hurt that we ever inflict upon others is with the things that we say. In general, karmic seeds can be planted in three different ways: by doing, by saying, or by thinking, anything—good or bad. In almost every case (there are a few exceptions), we need someone else to rebound the karma off of in order to plant a seed—sort of like how you need a wall to get an echo, or a floor to bounce a basketball.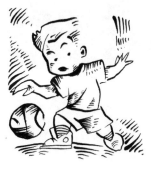

Physical and verbal actions are considered byproducts of mental actions—we think before we do or say, and so thoughts are "raw" karma, karma at its most basic level. Fully intentional words that hurt someone else are called a "path of karma," or a "full" karma—they include both the mental trigger, and the words that come out a moment later and hurt the other person. Words that hurt unintentionally do create some negative seeds, although they are less powerful than the intentional kind. And these are the kinds of seeds that create a boyfriend who hurts us trying to please us.

In the next few weeks you're going to need to be very careful to watch what you say to others. Try to be very sensitive about how your words affect people; watch their faces closely as you speak to them, to see how they react to your words. It's very difficult to really control everything we say to others, but with practice and awareness we can make a lot of improvement.

What I'm guessing is that sometimes you say slightly sarcastic things to others which you consider cute or funny, and perhaps you'll find that some people are hurt by this. Ask your closest friends—the ones who you know will be honest with you—whether some of the things you say end up hurting other people. I have this problem myself; I'm often struck by the irony of situations and make some slightly acid comment, more to the world than to the individual in front of me. But I've been told by good friends that I often hurt people's feelings this way.

So watch, and try to speak more gently. Consciously send the seeds to your boyfriend, and he'll become more gentle too.

Question 17

My wife has lost her interest in sex, but I haven't! What's the karma to get the heat back into our relationship?

It is said that the Buddha, two and a half thousand years ago, spoke no less than 84,000 massive collections of wisdom, each later written down using the amount of ink that could be carried on the back of a mythical elephant who was the size of modern-day 18-wheeler truck.

Each one of these collections is thousands of pages long, and each of them was meant to address a single one of the 84,000 different negative thoughts that a normal person has deep inside their head.

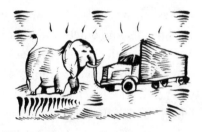

Lord Buddha of course realized that most of us would be so busy entertaining all these negative emotions that we would never have enough mental space to watch out for all 84,000. So he narrowed the list down a bit for us. He created a Top 10—very similar to the Ten Commandments of the Jewish and Christian traditions.

Now if a bad thought makes it into the Top 10, you've got to appreciate that most of us are having it every day—if not every hour, or every few minutes.

One of the most insidious of the Top Ten is our strange human habit of being happy when something bad happens to someone else. Witness our fascination with the troubles of movie stars and politicians; or our tendency to stop and stare at a bad car accident.

This is one of the seeds that you can work on in order to see your wife's interest in intimacy return. The idea is that you are being denied something that you would very much like to have; and that means you have seeds ripening in your mind from wishing this kind of thing on others.

Now you may say that you're not having these kinds of negative thoughts towards others—that actually you do not take any particular interest in the misfortunes of others. If though you are being denied some happiness, the fact is that you *must* possess this kind of seed, somewhere inside. Given that tiny seeds invariably produce huge results, it's not at all impossible that you took a morbid interest in someone's problems for only an hour or two at some point in the last few years, and the result is returning to you on a much bigger level.

A very common seed of this type is the one planted with the person in our last relationship. We had some strong feelings for them when we were together, and whatever broke us up probably created some even stronger ones.

Almost all of us have trouble keeping some feeling of kindness for our ex. More often, deep down we are holding those car-crash feelings for them: a subtle (or not so subtle) wish that they would fail somewhere, somehow, in their new life. And so, strange as it may sound, you're going to bring the fire back into your relationship by very carefully watching your own mind for any wishes that anybody else not get the things they want.

Spend some quiet time at home or out in a coffee shop, and go one by one through all the people that you know—ex-partners, or people at work, or other people in your family. Check yourself to see how you would feel if you heard that they had just won the lottery, or had just been fired from their job. Examine the deep emotions that come up in you at that moment. Life is hard, and it would be a lot harder if we didn't have the support of other people. Never withhold that support; for then love—and loving—will never be withheld from you.

Question 18

When we are being intimate, my partner and I seem to have trouble communicating to each other what would please each of us most. What's the karma to be able to talk comfortably about these things, and have the other person listen?

The reason that most of us have trouble talking about sex and our sexual needs—even with our partner—is that, deep inside, we have some kind of perception of sex as being dirty, or unclean. The sexual urge is, undeniably, one of the most powerful forces of the human psyche, and the desire for sex can make the most reasonable person the most irrational one, deceiving themselves and hurting others.

Like all powerful forces though—like fire, for example, which can cook your food or burn your house down—the human libido can be channeled for great good. This fact is recognized in advanced teachings of the Buddha known as the Diamond Way. These teachings describe an inner body which exists parallel to the gross physical body.

This inner body consists of a network of tiny inner channels made of light itself, and within these channels rides a subtle energy which provides the basis not only for life, but for our very thoughts. Here is the place where the mind meets the body, like a breeze on a blacksmith's anvil.

The deepest of these channels are normally inactive, blocked by the constant clutter of those 84,000 negative emotions. Because the energies which flow within the channels are the foundation of thought, there are certain thoughts that we will never be able to have, unless we open these channels up. And these are the highest kinds of thoughts: feelings of love for the whole world, insights into the very workings of reality.

In a normal person, these deepest channels open only on two occasions during the length of their whole life. One is at the moment of death, when the entire body loosens involuntarily and all the channels open—which is why urine and feces are released on the deathbed. But the deep channels also open during the act of sex, in the heights of an orgasm.

The ancient Tibetan scriptures say that—for a few seconds during each of these two experiences—we come close to those two highest thoughts: compassion and ultimate understanding. If we knew what to look for, and if we had the high intention to do so, then during the deepest moments of physical love we might even gain a glimpse of God.

Perhaps this helps explain the power of the sexual urge itself. Perhaps we sense, once we have tasted the sexual experience, that there is something deeper here, a potential for the highest flights of the human soul.

And so we can see sex, like fire, from both sides: as a very destructive and debasing force, when it is performed without love or kindness, or as a crucible for the elevation of the human spirit. Sex, and every other experience in the world, is like the pen that we talked about—it can be seen in two vastly different ways, depending on the seeds we have within our mind.

We have to plant seeds, then, to experience the uplifting side of the physical relationship that the two of us share; naturally then we would have no hesitation in discussing the most intimate of matters with one another. An easy way to do this is to think of ways in which the two of you, if your hearts were bonded closer through the bonding of your bodies, could serve others more than either of you could ever do alone.

Intimacy will inevitably bring you even closer together, and together you can do more. Consciously plan things that you can do together to help someone else; a good example would be going together to see the older woman whom we talked about earlier, to plant more seeds to keep the two of you tight. And remember to top it off with Coffee Meditation. The same seeds will ripen into a growing ease with talking to each other about your needs in bed.

Together you can do more

Question 19

About ten seconds after we have sex, my husband falls asleep, just when I would like a few last caresses and hugs. How to keep the man up?

To understand how we keep your husband from petering out, you'll need to understand more about how karmic seeds are planted, and the different ways in which they ripen.

Remember that we start each exercise with identifying the essence of what we want. And what we want this time is energy; or rather, to see more energy, in our husband. You might think that this involves giving him more energy, but that's not the way it works.

Generally speaking, there is no way that we can plant a karmic seed in another person; they can only do it themselves, and this is the nature of seeds. As much as we might want to plant for them, there is no way that we can give another person any of our own seeds. The ancient Tibetans have an interesting way of proving that this is true.

Only we can plant our own seeds

They say, first of all, that there are countless beings in the universe who have already succeeded in planting the highest of all seeds, and have already become angelic creatures of immense power. As you're already sensing, the better you get at planting seeds the more compassionate you become—it's just the nature of a person who spends a lot of their time looking for other people to help. Angels then are the most skilled planters of seeds, and the kindest of living beings.

It follows that—if there were any way for one person to give another person their seeds, to pluck a seed out of their own mind and insert it some how into the mind of another—then these angels would have already done so, a long time ago. And then people like you and I wouldn't be having any problem with our spouse in the first place, because beings of compassion would already gladly have placed in our minds the seeds for our spouse to possess inexhaustible energy.

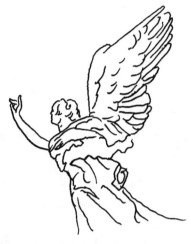

And so keeping your husband going would seem an impossible task—unless we understand the four ways that karmic seeds ripen. These are called the Four Flowers.

The first way is the one that we've seen most often so far, to make things happen the way we want to. If we give companionship, we will receive companionship; if we are friendly, affection will come to us; if we help others reach financial independence, we too reach our independence.

And so if we want energy—if we hope to be able to maintain or increase our own energy—then we need to help others do the same. The one thing that most drains energy is any kind of negative emotion: anger, jealousy, a hope that others might fail, a willingness to hurt someone else to get what we want. If we hope to have more energy, then we need to work at stopping our own negative emotions, and help those around us to stop theirs.

The way is easy. Simply remember that the pen is coming from us: anything that someone says to upset us must be coming from us, because we said some small thing of the same kind to someone else—last week, yesterday, this morning. And if we stop, then they stop.

The second way in which seeds ripen is in our habitual patterns: we may hesitate to tell our first serious lie, but the second one comes much more easily—and lying soon becomes a habit.

The fourth way in which mental seeds ripen comes later, as we die. During the death process, the seeds that we have planted most consistently during our lifetime come up to the front and begin throwing a new reality out ahead of us. And then we move forward into that reality. These are just more of the same kinds of seeds that are going to create your next five minutes right now, and the next five lines you read of this book.

As we die though, the power of certain seeds within us is multiplied thousands of times—enough to create a new world ahead of us; thus they are considered a different class of seeds. If for example we have constantly lied to others around us, we enter a life where the people around us are constantly trying to deceive us.

But it's the third way that seeds ripen that we're most interested in with your husband; something we've already touched on back in Question 3. We can call it an environmental effect of karmic seeds. If for example we frequently lie to others, then we will start to see lying all around us. I often meet people in my travels who want to know why government corruption is such a problem in their country, and this is the answer.

Here's where we can change your husband's energy, even without giving him our seeds. The karma to have more energy ourselves comes from using what we understand about seeds to stop our own negative emotions, and to help others do the same. As we make more and more progress in this effort, the different ripenings we've described above will begin to manifest themselves.

Instead of seeing more lying going on around you, you'll see the people in your life enjoying more energy—including your husband. So now you know where you have to put your efforts.

One last note. If it were possible for us to put a seed in our husband's head, then he would see himself having more energy at the same time as we see him having more energy because our own seeds have changed the world we live in. And in fact if he does help others get more energy, by helping them overcome their own negative emotions, then he will from his own side see himself have more energy.

But it's also entirely possible that—because we are helping others—we see our husband having more energy because he is part of our own increasingly energetic world; while at the very same time he perceives himself as more tired. It's all the pen thing, and you need to get used to that.

The Four Flowers

1) You get back the same

thing that you gave

2) Doing it becomes a habit

3) What you do creates

the people & the world around you

4) It also creates the world

that you step into next

TRUST

Question 20

When we first got together my partner was very free and easy, but lately he's started to get insanely jealous—he pounces on me whenever I get a text on my phone, and recently I think he broke into my emails to check them. What's the karma to create a partner who trusts me all the time?

I don't know about you, but my lama informs me that I have a very bad habit of judging other people constantly as I pass through my day. For example, there was a person at work who I always felt disliked me, because she constantly said so many negative things to me. Later on I found out that she had a serious problem with her back, which kept her in pain just about all the time, and her moods had nothing to do with me.

So in my mind I had written a story about this person; about who they were, and what our relationship was. And the story was wrong. It wasn't that I was thinking very evil things about them, just sort of a constant background noise of small judgmental thoughts. Which gets us into the concept of low-level radiation.

Once during a business trip to Hong Kong I came across a beautiful new gemstone, a rare sky-blue color in a gem of exceptional crystal sparkle. I asked the dealer what the stone could be, and he answered that it was a blue topaz.

Now I had seen topaz before in many different shades—brown, yellow, orange—and sometimes a kind that was almost colorless, like water; but all these stones had a certain dullness or cloudiness to them. I was aware that blue topaz did exist—again, with a certain shadow hue—but that it was extremely rare, because it took this color only when a colorless stone had accidentally lain underground next to a source of radiation for thousands of years.

The dealer told me that someone had discovered a way to turn colorless stones into blue, by purposely exposing them to the radiation produced in a nuclear reactor. He said that the process was secret, and that the person who had discovered it was making a killing in the market. So naturally our company decided to figure out how to do it ourselves.

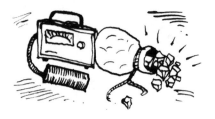

This led to some trial and error. We found a nuclear facility that would help us, for a charge, and after many experiments we learned to produce a beautiful blue. For safety, each stone had to be checked with a Geiger counter as it came out of the nuclear "oven," and we had to learn how to avoid over-radiating a stone—nuking it so heavily that it would be decades before its radioactivity would drop to what the reactor administration deemed a "reasonable level."

I began questioning them about this "reasonable level" of radiation. And I made some calls around to the various government regulatory agencies.

"Look," I said. "I need to understand this radioactivity thing. I mean, how can I be sure that a stone is safe?"

"Oh there's no problem," the technician assures me. "I mean, maybe just once we've seen a case where someone went a little overboard on a stone, and it burned the skin of the lady who wore it home in a ring."

"But how does it work?" I ask. "How does the radiation hurt somebody?"

"Oh," says the techie. "Particles in the stone get stirred up by the radiation treatment, and then they start flying out from the stone at odd moments. These particles are extremely powerful; they can pass through wood or plastic or human flesh as if they were thin air. Sometimes they fly through a person's body and hit a tiny DNA chain in one of their cells. They break the chain and then the cell starts to over-divide itself, which creates a tumor...a cancer."

"So how many of these particles is an 'reasonable level'?" I ask. "I mean, I've got pregnant women working in my office; is there any danger to people here?"

"No no," says the scientist. "We're talking really low levels of particles being emitted."

"But you just told me that a single particle coming out of a stone could cause a cancer in somebody; what's a 'reasonable' number of particles if even one can kill somebody?"

The techie backpedals furiously. "Of course our facility isn't making any guarantees, and we assume no liability; we're just following the government guidelines, you know." And then he goes on to tell me how a single bag of low-level stones becomes, you see, a high-level source of radiation—even though each stone by itself is legal.

Watch out for low-level radiation

This is how the idea of low-level radiation ties into your husband's paranoia. You didn't create this jealous habit of his by making up a little story about one or two people, or with one big story that destroyed a single individual. The point is that you've been making tiny judgments about people constantly, all day, day after day. The combined power of these tiny seeds, all thrown into the single bag of your subconscious, has created the cancer of a husband who refuses to trust you.

As usual, the karmic solution here—if it's done right—is a really fun thing. I want you to think about three or four of the people that you work with on a regular basis. Go into your mind and pull out the story that you've made up there about each of them—a whole set of tiny assumptions that together have become an entire novel.

To give an example, I used to work with a diamond dealer named Hasad. He was from Iran. I had him pegged as a hopeless materialist whose pursuit of money would end in the intensive care unit after the usual stroke from overworking, while members of his family descended on his office to dismantle his business and sell off all the hard-won assets.

One day though he asked me if I didn't want to come visit his mosque with him. I had a chance to talk to a lot of the people worshipping there, and learned that Hasad had pretty much built the mosque, and that he also led all the prayers. The reason he had gotten into the precious-stone business was so that he could build and maintain a place of worship for his entire community, as well as meet his traditional obligation to donate a specific percentage of his income to the needy on a regular basis.

He was an angel in disguise; which brings us to the art of writing stories which are divine.

The Tibetans, over many centuries of practice, have figured out a way to derail the constant flow of tiny judgmental thoughts which is creating your husband's jealousy. First learn to collect those stories of three or four of the people with whom you work: the stories you've made up to fit how they appear to you.

Now I want you to rewrite each one of these tales, turning them into an epic, or a romance—into a story of chivalry and nobility, like the story of Hasad the capitalist shifting into Hasad the imam, the inspired Muslim philanthropist.

Who knows if the stories will turn out to be true? That's the whole point of the exercise, to admit to ourselves that we never really know one way or the other what someone else is thinking. All you need to realize is that your new, beautiful made-up story fits the observable facts just as well as your old, negative made-up story did.

Someone at work seems to drink a lot of coffee, and you figure that they have given into a nervous habit. Now write a different story. At home is their samurai master, who trains them in swordplay to defeat various criminals in the bad part of your city. On some nights they duel with other secret samurais until dawn; on other nights they are out protecting people like your own family. Drinking coffee is the only way they can pull these 24-hour superhero shifts.

Don't be afraid that your stories, like the one we just mentioned, seem a little impossible. The Tibetans talk about a practice named *Takpay Nel-njor:* the Yoga of Make-Believe. The idea is that if we make up a beautiful fantasy and then fantasize about it long enough, this in itself plants seeds in our mind. In time these seeds ripen, and help the fantasy become reality.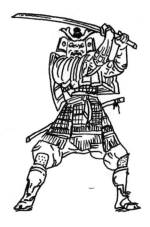

Notice the difference between this and the wishing thing we talked about back when we said that—even though the pen is coming from our mind—that doesn't mean we can just close our eyes and wish it into becoming a big diamond ring. When we fantasize that a person that we've been making judgments about is actually up to something epic, we keep our mind on how the seeds work: on how an habitual fantasy is planting seeds for the real thing to come later, when these seeds ripen within our consciousness.

Wishing is fine, but it only comes true if we plant the necessary seeds for it to do so. And for that we need to do something to help someone else, even if it's only wishing them well, wishing that they were more than they seem to us right now.

Question 21

I feel like there are a lot of things that my partner doesn't share with me: sometimes I come into the room and he's texting on his phone, and he gets really defensive if I ask him who he was texting. I'm not trying to pry or control his life, but I just want him to be more open with me. What's the karma I need to collect?

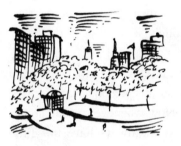 This question got popped on me by a friend named Michelle as we walked down the street to meet her significant other near Union Park, in New York.

"I mean," she continues, "we both text a lot for work and with friends, but it seems like something's going on with somebody."

"Like what?" I ask.

"Well like," she says, "he'll be staring down at his phone and punching keys furiously with this huge dumb grin on his face."

"Grins are okay," I note.

"Yeah, but…we're talking *intense.* Like my boss called me the other day and said he was thinking about firing me. I get off the phone and my guts are twisting with the anxiety, and I look across the breakfast table at John. He's texting and he's got that dumb grin again.

"I tell him like you know, I'm about to get fired, and we won't be able to pay the rent, and *he doesn't even hear me.* Yes I guess it really irritates me when he looks so happy and it can't be about us, because as a couple we're not doing so well. But to have a partner sitting across from me who's not even there, when I really need him to be…that kills me. I feel like I really need some answers."

"Okay," I start off where we always start off: with the first of the Four Starbucks Steps. "So tell me, in a single sentence, what you want." (And you'd be surprised how many people answer with about ten sentences.)

"I just want him to tell me the truth. The truth I can do something about, I can get used to, I can find somebody else. But not knowing the truth is killing me."

"Okay then. That's easy."

"How so?"

"You want a watermelon, you plant a watermelon. You want people telling you the truth, you gotta *tell* the truth."

Michelle looks relieved. "Okay then, I'll just start telling the truth to everybody."

I shake my head. Ah, if only it were that easy.

"Wait a minute," I say. "Just what do you think it means to *tell the truth?*"

"Well you know," she says, "like…don't lie."

"Not enough," I say. "Here's how the old books of Tibet describe what it is to tell the truth. Suppose somebody—like that mean boss of yours—says something to you at work. Something a little rough."

"Ok, that's not so hard to imagine," she grimaces.

"And then later on you want to tell someone else in your office about the little fight that you and the boss had. So you corner this person near the coffee machine and start to tell them what happened. Now whenever we tell somebody about something that has happened to us, we always have this little picture or video going in our mind about what it was like—our own memory of what happened."

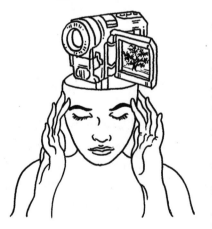

Michelle thinks for a minute. "Yeah," she says. "That's right."

"Good," I say. "And then when you tell somebody else what happened, you're really just describing this scene to them, as you see it in your own mind."

"Right," she says.

"Okay now," I say, "here's the part about what it means to speak the truth. As you tell your friend about what the boss did, a little scene—a little video— starts playing in their mind too, about what happened."

Michelle gives it some more thought. "Yeah, that's right. I never thought about it that way, but yeah—we've got two parallel videos going: one in my mind, one in hers."

"Right," I say. "Now here's the question. *How much does the new video in her mind match the original video in your mind?* While you talk to her, you're choosing words, and those words are helping her form the new video, her own impression of what happened. *Telling the truth* means that you choose your words so carefully that she gets exactly the same version of the video in her mind that you have in yours.

"And it's not like this doesn't really matter," I continue. "It *does* matter, because when you talk to somebody about something—especially about something that you feel strongly about, something that upsets you—then you are planting seeds for how people talk to you, in the next few weeks. You're planting seeds for how much they care that you know what they know: that you know the truth as they see it themselves.

"Including your partner," I conclude. Then I shut up for a while...people need time to process this sort of thing.

"Ah," she says, and I know she gets it. "Telling the truth that well—trying to guess how another person hears you, and trying to make sure they end up with exactly the same picture that you have about something—now *that's* going to be hard."

"But that's what truth is," I nod. "And if you plant truth-seeds carefully for a few weeks, say with everyone at work, then when you come home he's going to be honest with you. No negotiations, no arguments, no need to ask him."

Michelle nods. Then I get this feeling coming from her that maybe she doesn't really *want* to know the truth.

"By the way," I add, as we reach the The Grey Dog, and spot her partner at a table, with a couple of coffees waiting for us. "You can also plant seeds so that the truth he tells you is something happy to hear—like that he hasn't actually been texting at all, but was just downloading songs for you all along, to play on your birthday next week. But to make this happen, you're going to need to know about the seeds to make him loyal..." and I tell her what I told you, back at Question 6, about having your partner standing next to you all the time.

LOOKS

Question 22

I love my husband, but to tell you the truth—and I know it's kind of silly—I've always felt like his ears were too big. I don't suppose karma can do anything about that?

The best (or worst) version of this question I heard one day treading water with a friend named Jeff in the ocean off a beach, at a resort where I had been asked to give presentations to a big group of businesspeople.

"So Jeff," I ask, "when are you going to tie the knot with Rita? I mean, it's been like how many years, and I know she's up for it."

"Ah," he says, looking a little sheepish. "She's a really great girl, but… well, I just always thought it would be with someone a little more…" And then he just sort of sputters out.

"More what?" I ask. As far as I know, he's not shy about anything.

"Well, you know…" he says, looking in at the beach, where she's sunning herself. "I always thought it would be someone who…like, you know… filled out a bikini a little better."

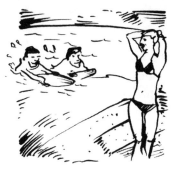

I gaze in at Rita with new eyes. "Jeff, let me get this straight…you're going to pass up this amazing and attractive woman *just because of the size of her boobs?"*

"Uh," is about all he can get out. I'm really disappointed in him, but then it dawns on me that this is probably going on between couples all the time, and they just never speak to me about it. I mean, after talking to hundreds of couples I've realized that either the man, or the woman, often wishes that their partner looked a little different in some way or another, even where the relationship is going well and they really love each other.

Now again I know what you're expecting me to say. After all, I'm a Buddhist monk, and the last thing we're supposed to do is to judge someone on their appearance.

Unless…you could just *change* that appearance, any time you wanted to.

Everything can be changed

I can hear what you're thinking: Now he's gone too far. You expect me to believe that I can make my husband's ears a little smaller, or my wife's breasts a little bigger?

Come on! Didn't we go through that with the pen? You've got to understand one thing. The way everything around you looks is coming from *your* side, not from *its* side. And that includes the way your partner looks. If your man's ears were coming from your man's ears, then no…you could never change how they look. But if your man's ears are coming from the seeds in *your* mind, then of course you can change them. And you can.

"Look, Jeff," I start out. I gotta say this carefully, for him and for you. "If I have a pen in my hand, and a dog comes in the room, do they see it as a pen? Or something else?"

Jeff nods. He's heard The Pen Thing like 500 times at my talks. "To the human it's a pen, and to the dog it's a chew-toy. And they're both right."

"Because…" I say.

"Because how they see it is coming from them. In fact, the fact that they see different things *proves* that it's coming from them. Otherwise the dog would write a novel, or the human would eat his pen."

"Which also proves…" I say.

"That you can change how you see a thing—*you can change what a thing is*—just by planting different seeds in your mind."

I wait a bit for this to sink in. Jeff gets this big grin on his face, and glances in at Rita on the beach. "Nah…" he says. "Really?"

"Just like anything else," I nod.

"Okay so…how do I put this…what's the Boob Seed?" he asks.

If you think this is a dumb or impossible question, then I beg to differ. Everything around you really *is* coming from the seeds in your mind. *Everything.*

And that means that *everything, everything, can be changed.* Miracles are not at all impossible, if you know what you're doing. If you know about the seeds.

I saw a cool video online not too long ago, recommended by a friend who's a sometimes stand-up comic. I don't remember who the comedian in the video was, and I hope he's not going to sue me for repeating his routine here. But it was just too good.

Two guys get on a plane, and as fate would have it they end up sitting next to each other.

The plane takes off, and once they're in the air the flight attendant makes an announcement. "We're pleased to inform our valued customers that our airline is the very first to offer free wireless internet during the flight! Enjoy!"

Oohs and *ahs* throughout the plane. In about ten seconds, 30 laptops pop out of nowhere. Everyone is online, including one of the two guys. The other one is trying to read the newspaper.

"Damn!" says the guy with the laptop. "I can't believe it! This thing is so frigging slow! They call this wireless?"

Guy #2 slowly looks up from his newspaper.

"Let me get this straight. No other airline in the world has wireless internet on the plane, and you're complaining that it's *too slow?"*

"Dang right I am," says Guy #1.

"So...millions of people have been flying on commercial airplanes for like a hundred years, and you're on one of the first flights in history where you have the power to communicate instantaneously, for free, with almost anyone in the world, and you're worried that it's *too slow?"*

"Dang right," insists Guy #1.

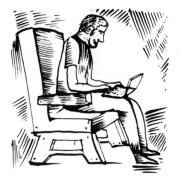

Guy #2 starts to get a little hot. "I mean, I can't believe it! Look!" He grabs #1 by the collar, and points to the sky. "Do you have *any idea* how far that little signal has to travel to get to where it's going? We're talking a satellite, and it's *a hundred and fifty miles up in the air above us,* and your little email has to get up there, and bounce back, *and you're upset that it takes like two seconds to do it?*

What's *wrong* with you, man?"

Guy #1 by this time is just staring into #2's eyes, like scared, like he just sat down next to a psychopath. He can't say anything.

"And *furthermore,"* says Guy #2. "Couldn't you have just a little bit of *wonder* about the freaking *miracle* that's going on right now? Do you realize that *you are sitting in a chair,* and that chair *is made out of solid iron,* but you are flying *through thin air on this iron chair,* just like a bird, like zillions of times faster than a bird?

"Doing something that human beings have dreamed of doing for *the entire length of history*—for two and a half million years? *Flying through thin air?* HAVE A LITTLE RESPECT FOR MIRACLES MAN!" and he drops the other guy's collar in disgust, and goes back to his newspaper.

We're like Guy #1. We have practically no awareness *that almost everything around us is already a miracle.* The sky is a miracle. Water is a miracle. Life is a miracle.

Miracles are going on all the time, all around us. And it's the seeds—the seeds in our minds—that keep them going.

Which means that one more miracle is no big deal. Just plant the right seed.

Miracles are possible, if you use the seeds

Okay, so in this case the seed is a little unexpected. In the end, it makes sense, but it's not something you would have guessed immediately.

What you want is to create a seed for beauty where you don't see beauty right now...whether it's the ears or the breasts. To have beauty come back to you, you're going to need to give some beauty. One way to do this lies in how you talk to people.

As you go through the day, take every little chance you can to say something nice to someone else. Encourage everyone around you: look carefully for something they're doing which is good, which is wonderful, and let them know about it, rather than looking for the bad. You don't have to make things up. There are lots of miracles out there, once you start to notice them.

Make this positive reinforcement of others a strong habit in your life. Let it become second nature. Constantly think of the seeds you are planting, and consciously send them to the person you want to see more beautiful.

They will change.

But here's the frustrating thing. I tell all this stuff to Jeff, and then like six months later he's on the phone asking me if I can come to the wedding.

"What wedding?" I exclaim.

"Me and Rita," he says, with surprise. "I mean…it was always meant to be, anyone can see that."

"But what about…" I don't know quite how to bring this up. "I mean, do you remember our little swim earlier this year?"

"Sure I do."

"And…do you remember…telling me about Rita in a bikini?"

"Sure I do! I've never seen anyone prettier in one! That's just one of the million things I love about her."

"Yeah Jeff, okay" I sigh, but I know what's happening. When you change a seed, when you do it right, it's not just that you change what you see in your partner right now. You also change the way you remember how they've always been. For Jeff, he thinks—and in a way now he's right—that he *always* thought Rita's figure was perfect. Fixing a seed is so powerful that you even fix the way it *used to be.*

The only problem I have with that is that I never get any credit. People don't even remember the problem they used to have before we talked together about the seeds to fix it!

Oh well, just an occupational hazard, in an otherwise very pleasant job— of seeing people get all the things they ever wanted.

COMMUNICATING,
PART ONE

Question 23

Whenever my husband and I try to have a conversation, he ends up doing about 90% of the talking; and he even interrupts me during my 10%! I've pointed this out to him many times, but he just seems to forget once he opens his mouth again. How can I work on this karmically?

I got this question from a lady named Mary one day in San Diego, while I was visiting my stepmom and also catching some classes on anatomy, to help my yoga teaching. So first of course I'm trying to get her to narrow down what she wants to a single thought.

"Basically, Mary, your husband is just completely self-absorbed, and isn't even aware that he's doing all the talking, or thinking that you might have something to say too. And that's also why he interrupts you while you're talking. If we work on the interrupting, it's going to backwash and make him aware that he's so self-absorbed.

"So can we say, in a single sentence, that what you want to change is your husband's habit of interrupting you?"

"Yes," she says quietly. "I mean, I want you to know that I really really love him, and I'm really interested in the things he has to say. I just want him to be more sensitive to the fact that I might have something I'd like to say too."

"Okay then," I say. "Let's start with the Four Kinds of Food."

"Food?" she asks.

"Yes! The ancient books of Tibet, you see, talk about four different kinds of food—four different kinds of sustenance that we all need to be healthy and happy."

"Which are…" she replies, obviously wondering where all this is leading to.

"Okay, well here's one version of the four. The first of the Four Foods is called 'bitable' food, which just means physical food—anything you can bite off and chew, like a piece of an apple. We obviously need physical food as fuel to keep our bodies going.

"And then a second kind of sustenance is sleep: deprive somebody of sleep for more than a day or two, and they start to go cuckoo. The body and mind definitely need regular sleep.

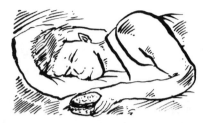

"The third of the foods is hope, and the ancient books describe it like this. A horse is stuck out in the middle of the Sahara Desert, and wanders for a few days in search of water. Just as he is about to die of thirst, he smells water; he crawls on his knees over a hill, and down below he sees an oasis with a sweet small lake.

"The point is that—no matter how far gone he is—the horse will make it down to the water. He won't die in sight of the water that will save him. His body may be finished, but hope is enough to sustain him for the last hundred yards. Hope keeps him going, it keeps all of us going.

Mary thinks about it for a moment and nods. "Perhaps we've never thought of it that way, but hope *is* a kind of food," she muses.

"And now the fourth food," I say, "is simply uninterrupted moments of concentration. We thrive on those moments when we are lost inside of something, when we have deep peace and quiet; whether it's listening intently to a song, or reading a book which we really enjoy, or sitting in the arms of that special someone.

"And whenever we are torn away from these moments, whenever the feeding tube of deep focus is ripped away from us because the boss shows up with one more job to do, or one of the kids starts crying, then it really hurts us, inside our body and our mind. A person who is constantly interrupted becomes as cranky as a person who hasn't slept for a few days.

"So what I'm saying," I conclude, "is that you really do need to be able to finish what you're saying before your husband interrupts you—it's not just a point of good manners, it's actually important for your physical and mental health."

Mary nods again; it sounds right, and she looks up at me again with a question in her eyes.

"We all do it," I continue. "We are all guilty of interrupting others—it might be talking over somebody at work, or just turning away during dinner to send a text on our phone, or writing too many texts or emails in the first place. Even just how much noise our shoes make as we step across the floor, or how quietly we close a door behind us, or the tone and volume of our voice as we utter a single sentence to another person."

"So I have to be super-careful about not interrupting anybody else then," says Mary, "because it's coming back to me through my husband." I nod.

"Even in very small ways," she continues, "because the big interruptions I get are caused by the very small interruptions I give…seeds grow bigger!"

"True, true," I agree. "And one more thing."

"What's that?"

"You should go at it from the positive side too. It's one thing to stop planting bad seeds, by not interrupting other people; it's another thing to set up moments of deep peace and quiet focus which other people can stop and enjoy.

"Think of one thing you can do every day, for example, to create a situation where your children have a chance to enjoy something deeply, in silence. Perhaps get into the habit of going out together somewhere where there's grass and trees, or open water, or free sky and wind—see if slowly you can get your kids to appreciate a few quiet moments of rest, away from the videos and music downloads, just to enjoy a few moments of quiet. This is actually very close to meditating."

"To do that," she says ruefully, "I'm going to have to learn to enjoy a quiet moment myself once in a while."

"That's the idea," I agree.

Question 24

For some reason, my husband sometimes just goes into "ignore" mode, refusing to reply to anything I say. What's the seed for getting the communication to flow between us?

Just about all of us who've been in any kind of close relationship have found ourselves in this place. Maybe one of us doesn't sleep so well the night before, and then in the morning at the breakfast table you can already feel some sort of disconnect—not a lot of cheery conversation going back and forth.

And then by noon there are already a few hard words passed back and forth; and throughout the afternoon several longer, heated exchanges. One of us then gets so angry or frustrated that they decide they'll refuse to talk at all. "I don't want to say anything else that might hurt you," when actually we know that not talking is often just another way to hurt.

We can open up these blocks to communication between ourselves and our partner if we really start to understand the cause and effect that's going 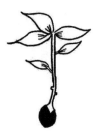 on here. On the surface of it, the lack of sleep created the first disconnect at the breakfast table, and then that escalated into the argument of the afternoon, and the silence by evening.

And so to stop it, well, I just have to get more sleep. Right?

Not really.

Look at how cause and effect works in a tree. A tree works itself up out of the ground in stages: first the seed splits open under the soil; then the sprout pops up into the open sky; next a little trunk, and the first lower branches. Then come the higher branches, and finally the leaves and the fruits.

Think of how the lower branches of a tree relate to the higher ones. It's true that the higher limbs come after the lower ones, connected by the same

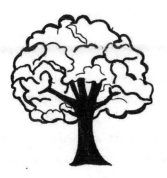

trunk of the tree—in the same way that the argument in the afternoon precedes the spiteful silence in the evening of the same day.

But we can't really say that the lower branches have *caused* the higher ones, in the sense of growing into them. There is a stream of events where one followed the other, but the lower branch went its way and the higher branch went the other. They are connected to each other, but it's through the trunk, which itself has come from the original seed.

What I'm saying is that we have to get past what we think is happening when our partner refuses to talk to us in the evening. Maybe it didn't come from the fight in the afternoon, or the crossed wires in the morning, or even from the trouble getting enough sleep the night before.

Maybe it's all coming from one deeper seed

Maybe all of these events—maybe all of these branches—are all just really coming from one big main seed, down below them all. Maybe what happens in the morning doesn't cause what happens in the evening. Maybe they are both coming from a single older thing.

And that's the point here in the Karma of Love. There are bigger and older seeds which are causing everything that happens to us throughout the day. Don't blame your husband, and don't blame your mattress. They are both coming from something further down, something that you yourself planted before.

Now you can work on the seeds for not getting enough sleep, or you can work on the seeds for seeing someone refuse to talk to you. Learn to separate out all the different seeds contributing to a situation, and go at them one by one. Don't try to tackle them all; there are too many of them going on. Get in the habit of picking one and working on it until it's finished, then go on to the next one.

Ultimately, all these seeds are connected, back in our original failure to understand where all the events were coming from. And that means that finishing off just one of our problem seeds already weakens all the others.

You know the exercise by now. Let's work on the silence thing, because in a way that's worse than the not sleeping. (And now we know that one didn't necessarily cause the other; have you never spent all night out with companionable friends and enjoyed perfectly wonderful conversations over croissants and coffee the following morning?)

The ancient books of Tibet make a big deal about answering people promptly and considerately, whether it's a question about what's for dinner, or where the universe came from.

Make it a point then, for the next few weeks, to listen very carefully whenever someone asks you about anything, and be sure to respond with a thoughtful answer. We avoid some questions (and we're including emails and texts here) because to answer is difficult or demanding; we avoid other questions because they seem foolish, or uninteresting, to us. You can be sure though that—to the person asking a question—it is important, and deserves a good answer.

And remember to do Coffee Meditation on these new seeds when you get home at night.

If you take the time to listen, you will find a grain of intelligence behind almost every question anyone ever asks you. Answer with grace, and your husband will stop the resentful silence thing—without being asked to, without any tension.

Question 25

My girlfriend ignores every suggestion I ever make, even if it's a really good one, or just a tiny one. What seed do I need to plant to have my ideas considered?

If you don't know my friend Tony, you know someone like him. You don't have to be a genius to see where the seeds are coming from—you can talk all day but he just doesn't seem to *listen*. And of course that means that I'm not listening either.

"Well maybe you're not listening so well to other people's suggestions," I start.

"Like what?" he blurts accusingly.

I sigh. Well, let's give it a try. I make a mental note to be more open to suggestions today; maybe that will be enough of a seed to get him to open up a bit.

"Look, Tony—you know all about the seed thing, right?" I know he does; he's been coming to my talks for over a decade.

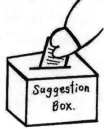

"Yeah…" he admits.

"So what kind of seed do you have to plant to get somebody to start listening to your suggestions?"

"I guess I have to stop ignoring suggestions myself," he replies.

Now, I've learned enough to know that you can't just leave it at that. There has to be a plan, some specific detail. And it's a lot more fun to start with *doing* something, rather than *not* doing something.

"You're a supervisor in your department at work, right?" I begin.

"I am," he says.

"Okay, so we're going to go through three steps," I say. "Is there any big project that you're working on right now?"

"There is," he answers. "We're doing some marketing videos, and there's a big debate going on about what software to use for the editing."

"Okay then, here's step one. I don't want you to just stop ignoring other people's suggestions. I want you to go through your team, one by one, and ask them if they have any ideas about the software that they think might help."

"Okay, no problem," says Tony; but his answer comes too fast. Sounds like his own supervisors at work have asked him a hundred times to get suggestions from his crew, and I can guess where those suggestions ended up.

"And next week," I continue, "we're going to meet up at Starbucks, and you're going to tell me about three of the suggestions that you thought were pretty good. That's step two."

"Okay," he says. There's a hint of a frown on his forehead—I can see he's not used to actually *considering* the suggestions he asks his staff for.

"And then the third step," I add. "A week after that, you're going to start *implementing* one of those suggestions."

I can see that now I've gone too far. Time for a reality check.

"I mean, you *do* want your girlfriend to start listening to the suggestions you have, right?"

That seems to do the trick. "Okay," he says. "Okay," he says with some resolution, hunching his shoulders. He thinks we're done, but we're not.

"And about the credit," I add.

"What credit?"

"I mean, you want to plant a really strong seed here—you really *want* your girlfriend to start listening to you seriously—so there's one last thing you've got to do. Don't just *ask* for suggestions from other people; don't just *consider* them carefully; and don't just *implement* the best suggestions you get.

"When you do try someone's suggestion, and it works, then I want you to make sure that they get the credit for their suggestion—*all* the credit."

Because, you see, all of us have this natural resistance to the whole process. First of all, we each have our own logic for how we're behaving in our life—for the things we've decided to do, and the things we've decided not to do. Chances are, we've already considered a lot of the suggestions that other people might think to give us, and we've already decided that they won't work out, for one reason or another.

But there are also a lot of ideas we avoid just because we don't feel like putting in the work involved, or the mental effort to think through them. If we really want people to be more open to our own ideas, then we've got to admit to ourselves that some of the suggestions we've gotten from others in the past have worked out pretty well, when we actually tried them out.

At the very least, we can be considerate enough to try out the first step of someone's suggestion, or see how we can incorporate it into a plan that we already have. Start looking for ways that you can collaborate with other people, especially those who work for you—people that you're supposed to be managing in some way.

And don't be afraid to give them full credit for ideas that work out. This is a great seed for getting credit from your own bosses—including your girl-friend.

TENSION

Question 26

I seem to go through this pattern with almost everybody I ever get involved with—sort of a natural decay, or aging of our relationship. At first we both feel excited, like we've finally met the perfect person. And then slowly we begin to see a few problems in the other person, which get more and more serious. After a while we start fighting with them, and finally we end up really disliking each other. Is there any karmic way to stop this kind of repeated downward cycle?

This isn't a question that first came from somebody else. It's a question that I asked myself, over and over, watching my parents' marriage crumble and going through my own first attempts at a relationship, in high school and college. It just seems that there is a natural and unavoidable aging to relationships, in the same way that everything else around us ages: a tree, a new car, the human body.

Except that with relationships it seems as though the process is often much more painful. It's not just that the relationship grows older—it's not just that things get stale, or that we lose interest in each other. You know it as well as I do: we oftentimes end up hating the person we once loved, more than anything else.

This repeated downward cycle has always disturbed me deeply. In fact, it's one of the reasons that I decided to take the vows of a monk: I had become one of those people who sincerely believes that it's the fate of every relationship to go bad, that a relationship which stays sweet only happens in the movies. And a part of me thought—as I think a part of you may also feel—that there was just something wrong with me, that deep down I might be incapable of keeping a relationship going.

Once you really understand the Diamond Cutter Principles, you can throw out all that baggage. It's *not* inevitable that relationships go bad, and you are *not* a bad person. It's not you who made the relationship go bad. *It's the seeds.* Left untended, the seeds for any relationship grow old, and then the relationship itself *must* get old, in the same way that trees or people do.

The birth of a thing kills it

The ancient books of Tibet put it very bluntly: **The birth of a thing is what kills it.** You can take a child fresh out of the womb, and you can lock her in a huge underground bank vault, and you can feed her organic vegetables and vitamins for her whole life. She will still age; she will still get old, day by day; and she will still die. What kills her is *simply the fact that she was born.*

But there's a way out of all this. It's called *reinvesting the seeds.* Here's a real-life example.

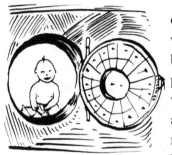

We know now a very successful method of planting a seed for a relationship. Since what we want is companionship—no more being lonely—then we need to provide companionship to someone else first. We saw this work back in Question 2: Ann paid visits to an elderly woman to plant the seeds for a new relationship, and created her future husband. We left her in Manhattan, at the wedding.

But there was more.

I walk up to Ann at the reception; we're in her parents' living room, everyone having refreshments after the ceremony.

"So Ann," I say, looking down into my vegetable-juice cocktail. "Visiting the old lady—Mrs. Taylor—it really worked, didn't it?"

"Oh it *did,* Geshe La," she gushes. "And I'm so grateful to you."

"Well," I give the standard reply, "let us thank the teachers of the lineage, for passing this wisdom down through the last few thousand years."

Ann nods contentedly, looking around at the wedding guests. It's time for me, right here at the beginning, to try to make sure this marriage doesn't begin to wear out a year or two down the line.

"So," I say nonchalantly, "how *is* Mrs. Taylor?"

Ann pauses a moment, looking a little guilty. "Well, Geshe La, you know—with the wedding and all—I haven't had a chance to visit her for a while. And…"

"And what?" I ask.

"And well," she says a little sheepishly, "you know…I mean, it *did* work, after all; and now I have John."

I hear what she's saying, and I knew it was coming. *I have John now; I have someone to spend my time with, someone to give me companionship. And so I don't have the time, and I no longer have the* need, *to visit the old lady much any more.*

"Big mistake," I say simply. "Your time with Mrs. Taylor planted the seeds for John, true. But every hour that you spend with John uses up some of those seeds. It's like the time with Mrs. T. charged up the debit card of your relationship, and now you're using that card up, as the seeds ripen and cause you to see John standing next to you.

"If you just let things go on like that, then those seeds are going to wear out, one by one. And there will come a day that John forgets to kiss you good morning, and a day when he doesn't make it home for dinner—a day for the first fight, and a day for the last fight. We don't want that to happen, Ann."

Now I've got her attention. She looks at me with true concern. "You're saying that it's going to wear out? That it's *got* to wear out?"

"Wear out, yes," I reply. "But not that it's *got* to. It won't happen, if you reinvest the seeds."

"Reinvest?" Ann asks.

"Right," I say, and I start to talk a little faster, more excited. Because you see, it took me so long to figure this part out, and it's so very important for all of us. "Let's take a different example. You're looking for some financial security in your life, so you have to plant the seeds. You invest some time helping *someone else* reach their own security. And then prosperity just comes to you; you couldn't stop it, even if you wanted to.

"But the seeds, you understand, they wear out; and sooner or later every job, every new company, every soaring career falls back to the earth. Unless…"

"…unless you reinvest the seeds," says Ann, and I can see from her face that she gets it. "Take some of the money that comes back to you, set it aside, use it to help new people reach their own security. Create an upward cycle—new seeds replace the old seeds, as the old ones wear out."

"Exactly," I say. "And that's how we're going to keep your and John's relationship from getting old, from wearing out. You need to *use* your seeds to make new seeds…" I wait to let her pick up the thought.

Ann considers for a minute. "Okay," she says, "I've got it. By keep-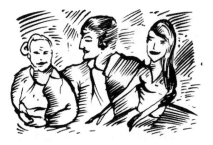ing Mrs. Taylor company, I created the seeds for John. Now John and I need to work—together this time—to keep those seeds going. We need to plant some new ones, and we have to keep planting, if we don't want to see this love wear out."

I wait for the light to come on in her head. And it doesn't take more than a second to come.

"I have to keep visiting Mrs. Taylor…for the rest of my life," she whispers. I nod.

"And John has to come with me."

She's right.

Reinvest your seeds

Question 27

Here's a scenario: We're standing in line at the grocery store, and my wife makes a rude remark to the check-out lady, who then glares at both of us. I can't say anything to apologize, or my wife will get mad at me. But if I don't say anything, then I get lumped together with my wife as the bad guy, even though I don't want to be. This happens over and over, every day, and every day I feel more and more like I'm in a little prison— like I don't have any say in my life any more. How do I plant the seeds to feel like I'm my own person again?

I look across the coffee-shop table at my friend Anthony. I feel for him; I've been there. In fact, I guess I've been just about everywhere, but I guess that's why I'm writing the book.

"Anthony," I start, "tell me what the word *counter-intuitive* means."

"Well," he says, "there's a problem, and someone gives you a suggestion for fixing the problem, and maybe it's the exact opposite of what you might have expected."

"Exactly," I say. "So basically, what you're feeling—and I know what it feels like—is that your wife has taken away all your independence, all your existence as a separate person. Everywhere you go, you get lumped in with her, with what she's doing, good or bad. It almost feels like there's no more you."

"Exactly," he says softly, with that grateful look of someone who's met someone else who actually understands their problem.

"And it's not like you need to be the boss," I continue. "You're fine with being part of a couple, you're fine with working together. But you want to work together in a way where you're also acknowledged as an individual, as who you are, with your own hopes and needs."

"You've got it," he says gratefully. He leans close to see how we're going to work this out.

"Okay," I breathe. "So here's the counter-intuitive part. To get back some of yourself, to be more empowered, you're going to have to *give up* some of the power you already have. I think…" And then something comes back to me—a moment at a talk in southern China.

"Look Anthony, I was in Guangzhou last year."

"Okay," he says, obviously not sure if Guangzhou isn't a new fusion restaurant on the west side of Chicago.

"It's a city, in China…just on the other side of Hong Kong. People with money in Hong Kong start businesses that make most of the stuff in the whole world, and the factories where they make this stuff, you see, they're all over in Guangzhou, because everything's cheaper there. You can hop on a subway in downtown Hong Kong and cross straight over to Guangzhou to check on your factory in like an hour."

"Okay," he repeats, a little less quizzically.

"And we're giving a big business seminar in Guangzhou to this big group of big business owners, and I'm explaining how—if they want to make more money themselves—then they're going to have to help some other people make some money of their own. This is going on for like two days, and everyone's starting to get it, and everyone's excited, and then this one lady raises her hand to ask a question."

Anthony: "Okay."

"'Geshe Michael,' she says. 'I didn't come here to learn how to *give* money. I came here to learn how to *make* money.'" Anthony and I share a chuckle.

Your old instincts are wrong

"And that's the counter-intuitive part," I continue. "If you want something to come to you, then you have to give the same thing to someone else, first—even if you don't have a lot of it to start with…*especially* if you don't have a lot of it to start with.

"So in your case, you need to empower people: give them a chance to show what they can do, give them a chance to be themselves. And then your wife will let you be yourself.

"Look, life at your job is stressful—I know, you talk about it all the time. Just too much to do, like 300 emails to answer every single day, and a pile of financials that need checking. I also know that you have some amazing people working for you, and that some of them are actually a little bored doing the same menial jobs every day.

"So turn it around: give them a challenge, and take some of the load off yourself. Create little areas of responsibility that your people can become owners of: one of them answers all the email inquiries you get about product; two others go through the financials for you independently of each other, and you see if they catch the same mistakes in the numbers."

Anthony hrrumphs. "Two problems with that. I mean, first of all, the *reason* that those emails and financial reports come to me is that I'm the only one who can really deal with them properly."

I smile. "Anthony, old man, this is a number I call the Baby Manager Syndrome: no one else is as good as me at what I do; they'll just mess it up, and I'll have fix it later.

"Look, no one is irreplaceable. Everything you do can be done by someone else; if you were to quit your company today, there would be someone else sitting in the same chair within a week, reading those emails and checking those reports. And they'd probably do a pretty good job."

Anthony grimaces. "Uh, well actually…that's the second problem."

"What's that?"

"Well, if I let other people at work have real responsibility for some of what I do, then it won't take long for the management to figure out that they don't really need me."

I smile. Another version of the Baby Manager Syndrome.

"Look, Anthony. Suppose you owned the company. Suppose you had a senior person who was obviously always doing the best for the company… like training other people to do what they do, so the company has more depth and talent, so the company makes more money. And then suddenly a VP position opens up. Who do you think you're going to give it to? Who already has enough strong people around them that they can take a step up to something bigger?"

Anthony looks off to that golden horizon. "Me," he smiles.

"Right," I say. "So empower the people around you—at work, and in your family too. Give them a chance to be their own person. And then…"

"And then," he says, standing up from the table, "maybe I won't be stuck in my wife's shadow, in the checkout line at the store."

Question 28

My wife demands that I always be around the house and close to her, and that I don't talk much with other people, which seems to make her feel insecure. How can I change this karma of feeling trapped in a box inside my own house?

So many of our wounds are self-inflicted. I'm in a pizza parlor, trying to talk to my friend Charles about this problem he's having with the box thing, and I can barely get his attention. His head is pretty constantly buried in his cell phone, searching the web voraciously but strangely never quite finding anything that satisfies him for more than a few moments. I grab his arm.

"Charlie, listen to me. You can get out of this thing—you don't have to be unhappy day after day." With the other hand I push his phone under the table. "You know about the seed thing, right?" He nods. He's been around.

"Now almost 100% of the time, we need to plant our mental seeds with other people," I begin. We saw this back in Question 16, where we compared karma to an echo, or a basketball: you need a wall, you need a floor, to bounce it off of. "Think of the people around you as the soil, fertile soil, in which you plant your seeds. The Tibetans say you can't plant a seed in thin air; it has to be in the earth."

Charlie nods, although I dare say that in his entire life he's never planted a seed in the soil once.

"But there are exceptions," I continue.

"Like what?"

"The ancient books insist that your body and mind are like a temple—a precious temple, a vehicle which allows you to travel to the greatest heights of the human soul. Without a strong healthy body, without a bright clear mind, we can't get around in the world, we can't do the things we need to do to get enlightened, to become a truly good person."

"And?"

"And if we hurt that body and mind—especially if we hurt it purposely—

then we are actually hurting others: the people that a good person could be helping."

"And?"

"And so you see, you can plant a seed in your own mind, by hurting your own mind. I think that's the key to what's going on with your wife, this feeling that you're trapped in a box."

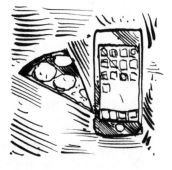

"So how am I hurting my own mind?"

I glance at his cell phone, which has mysteriously made its way back on top of the table, next to a few surviving pizza crusts. It's almost as if the phone has a mind of its own. But it's always better to go at things gently.

"Look," I say. "You've gone through some of the meditation training, right?"

Charlie nods. We have a component in our business seminars where we teach executives how to develop deeper powers of concentration, using an ancient meditation chart covered with monkeys and elephants.

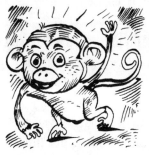

"So what's the monkey represent?"

"The monkey is your mind, when it gets too distracted. When there are too many things pulling at your attention while you're trying to concentrate."

"Like what?"

Charlie looks down at the table, where the cell phone has nestled up to a gooey piece of pizza. He picks it up lovingly and wipes off the tomato sauce.

"Like when you're trying to concentrate on texting your boss, and your friend pushes a piece of pizza under your nose," he smiles at me. "And so you learn to tune everything else out, and fight your way back into the text you're writing." He demonstrates, crunching over the table, hunkering down over his phone.

I nod. "That's right. Now there's a good place of concentration that you can reach, and there's a not-so-good place. The good place feels bright, and happy—like when you're watching a really good movie, or listening to your favorite song.

"But if you push too hard," I stop and dig my finger into the furrows between his eyebrows, "then you go into a not-so-good place of concentration. It's not like you've popped out of your concentration—you're still there looking at your phone, and not at the pizza—but you've struggled so hard to be there that your mind is tired.

"And because your mind is tired it goes into sort of a little box, and stays there, sort of half dead. You might just stare at the screen for a while, you might wander around to twenty different websites without really getting anything accomplished.

"And this shallow, fuzzy focus hurts your mind, because you get used to *not* focusing deeply, and *not* really enjoying where you are in the moment, even though you're still there on the screen."

"So what's this got to do with my wife?" says Charlie.

"Okay," I say. "So you've been squeezing your mind into this little box, over-concentrating, and making the mind tired and uninspired in the process. It's not that you're planting seeds by hurting someone else; instead, you're hurting yourself, and the point is that you plant bad seeds all the same.

"And then your wife…" I pause to let him pick it up.

"And then my wife puts me in a box, and forces me to stay there," says Charlie. He nods, and I can see that he's looking at the cell phone in a little different way, as if it's not the friend he used to think it was.

"So what to do?" he says, looking up.

"You need to plant the opposite kinds of seeds," I reply. "You need to let your mind have some space; let it be more spacious, more expansive.

"I once translated for the Dalai Lama's doctor for a while," I remark. "And one day he gave someone the most amazing prescription. They had a problem like yours, too much time spent in too tight a place. And they were waiting for the doctor to give them some kind of pill, but he just flipped through this ancient book of medicine, carved in wood and printed on Tibetan paper, until he came to a certain page.

"And he said, 'The medicine I want you to take is to walk outside every night, after dark, and just look up at the sky. See how big it is, see how many stars there are. Stand still for five minutes and don't think about anything else except how many stars there are, how many other worlds there might be out there in the universe.' Charlie, I think you could try the same."

The way it actually ended up was that Charlie needed a little more stimulation than just looking up at the sky. We got him a pretty nice little telescope, not too expensive, and a glow-in-the-dark map of the constellations. He did get into the habit of going out most evenings, and just drinking in the *big-*

ness of the night sky. And his wife has changed completely; there is that lovely balance between them now of enjoying each other's company intensely, while at the same time being able to be out on their own, spending close time with their individual friends and family.

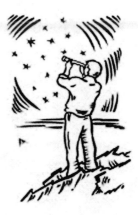

DEPRESSION

Question 29

Sometimes I just get sad or depressed for no special reason; and when I do, my partner gets really irritated, almost as if I *meant* to be depressed! How can I get some support at these times—and what is the karma behind this sadness, anyway?

Back in Question 23, we talked about the four kinds of food, or sustenance, that we need in order to live—and one of them was hope. We need hope as much as we need to eat. Depressed people have lost their hope, and they are starving.

Linda is one of the wealthiest people in the world. I've been her friend for a couple of years, working together on some projects to help the poor. I've been to her house a million times—but there are still whole wings of the place that I haven't even seen yet. Her husband Frank is a good friend too; they seem to be doing really well as a couple, and then one day she pops this question on me.

"I mean," she says quietly, "there are whole days when I don't even get out of bed. I'm so depressed that I can't see any point to it. And then on top of that he walks in and rants at me for not doing anything, which just makes me more depressed."

In my position—sort of a parish priest whose parish is the world—you get used to unexpected revelations; you've heard so many heart-rending stories that they begin to repeat themselves. So luckily I have the answer ready right there, in my spiritual toolbox.

"You know about the seeds…" I begin. Linda smiles tightly and nods her head sharply; you can't be in our circle of friends for more than a few days without hearing deep and sometimes heated discussions about the seeds, perhaps several times a day.

"That's what makes depression one of the most difficult problems of all," I continue. "What's the first thing you need to plant a seed?"

"Well," she says quickly, "first you need a clear idea of *what* you want, because to plant a seed you're going to have to provide the same thing to someone else, first."

This isn't where I was planning to take her, but I go with the flow. "Right," I say. "Starting with the one-sentence thing: the first of the Four Starbucks Steps. You've got to be able to express what it is you're looking for, in a single sentence."

Linda pauses, and then she gets it. "I guess there are two different problems here," she says. "And it would take two sentences."

I nod in agreement, and wait for the two.

"First of all," she says, "I need to plant some seeds that will work against the depression. And then secondly I need some seeds to see my husband show a little more concern about how bad I'm feeling when I'm in the middle of it."

"Right," I say. "So let's go at them one at a time. What's the opposite of depression?"

"Hope," says Linda immediately, without even pausing to think about it.

"So we need to supply hope…"

"…to someone else," she finishes.

"Aye, but there's the rub," I say. "The reason why it's so hard to plant seeds to stop depression is that a depressed person is completely and entirely focused on their own needs, on how bad *they* feel. Unless they really understand what's going on—unless they're well trained in the Diamond Cutter Principles—then the last thing they're going to do is take an active interest in someone else's needs.

"So first you have to struggle against this one thing: this resistance to even *thinking* about someone else. There's a very simple way of doing this, which is just to remember the second Starbucks step: planning who to plant your seeds with, and where."

Linda looks a little unsure. "Uh, remind me how that goes."

I nod. "You know that to plant a seed, you need somebody else. Other people are the soil in which we plant our seeds. The idea that you could plant a seed without doing something towards another person is as crazy as the idea that you could plant a watermelon seed in mid-air in front of you."

"Got it."

"So when somebody asks me for some kind of help in their life, I like to tell them that they should plant a seed for what they want. Then I tell them to take somebody else out to a Starbucks, because this is just an easy way to make sure that they have a place to plant their seed—that they are working with another person."

"Okay."

"Alright, so we're going to have you take somebody else to a Starbucks. And what are you going to do with them?"

"I don't know, help them in some way—help them with their depression, I guess."

I look away for a second and then come back. "You could think of it that way," I say, "but it feels better to me if we make it something positive."

Linda pauses. She's also one of the most intelligent people that I know. "Help them with something positive—help them find hope."

"Good. And I would say more than just hope. I would say help them with their dreams. Let's look for someone in need of a dream."

She pauses again. "I have a nephew, and…you know, the kind of problem we tend to get in our family is that we all have enough money to do or get just about anything we want, even at a very young age. Even if we do decide to work, we don't have to work, so we usually don't have much intensity about the work—no big goal in mind."

"No dream," I agree. "So yes, when you're depressed, those are the steps that I would work on. First, fight your way to a place where you can think about what somebody else needs—try to think of a person that you can help. Pick somebody who doesn't seem to know what to do with their life. Talk to them, help them figure out what their dream is, even if it's a dream they don't know they have—*especially* if they don't know.

"You don't have to solve all their problems. Just talk to them, give them some support, once a week, or once every couple of weeks. Small seeds make big trees." I can already see it. Linda plants such powerful seeds that later on she doesn't even remember that she used to be depressed. She brings me back by clearing her throat.

"And about Frank?" she asks.

"Say it in one sentence."

"I want him to notice how I'm feeling; I want him to sympathize a bit, rather than criticizing me when I feel so bad."

"Basically then you want him to make some effort to make you feel better."

"Right."

"Okay, so the seed here is to make it a habit to make *other* people feel more comfortable, day to day, hour by hour." I think about it for a second.

"Look," I say. "I was out getting my car fixed the other day. The mechanic was amazing. He sat down with me and took me through the problem

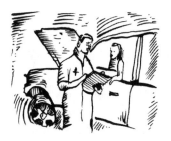

step by step, made sure that I knew what was wrong with the car. And then he told me, without getting too complicated, each thing he was going to do to fix it.

"He was really concerned that I should feel comfortable, that I would feel at ease. One of the best ways to put other people at ease is just to tell them what we're going to do, at any given time, ahead of time.

"This plants comfort seeds—seeds to have somebody care about how we feel, rather than berating us for not feeling well enough to fit into their own plans for the day."

"Got it," she says, and it looks to me like the clouds of her depression have already parted a bit, just thinking about

ALCOHOL & DRUGS

Question 30

Sometimes my husband and I have a glass of wine in the evening, and it really seems to help us both loosen up, especially before being intimate with each other. But I've seen alcohol destroy so many relationships and families that sometimes it scares me. What's your take on this?

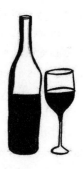

This question means a lot to me personally. I grew up with alcohol—it destroyed both my parents' lives and health, and it destroyed our family. The Buddha himself once sat with his disciples in a meadow, granting them a teaching, and was asked about alcohol. He plucked a piece of grass and pointed to the tip of it. "No one who drinks the amount of alcohol that you could hold on the tip of this blade of grass, or who serves that amount to another person, should ever say that they are my follower."

That's because even a small amount of alcohol is extremely addictive—more than we ever imagine over a glass of wine at a restaurant. And for good reason. Alcohol *does* make us feel better: it seems to take away the aches and pains of the day, it seems to loosen up the inhibitions that prevent us from connecting with others. There's a reason why people enjoy a glass of wine over dinner.

Now I could harp on the downside of alcohol here. It's not just addictive, it's also really unhealthy. You can make jokes about what it's doing to your liver, but when the damage is done and you're walking around with a constant pain in your guts, shelling out half your paycheck to the doctors every week, the jokes don't seem so cute.

Alcohol is not just a strain on your body, it's a strain on your finances. Much as with designer clothes, a mystique has been artificially created around liquor by those who make money from it—and in this case, from the misery of others. Truckloads of rotten grain are packaged in expensive bottles and advertised by expensive movie stars, to be served in expensive restaurants.

And so it would be really nice if we could get the same relaxing effect somehow without having to use the glass of wine. Perhaps we can get some ideas from a discussion which I once had with His Holiness the Dalai Lama.

I was still in college, and had just heard that my mother was dying of breast cancer brought on by alcohol and cigarettes, which seems to be a really virulent combination. I requested a sabbatical and took off on a journey to India, seeking some wisdom about the human condition. I ended up studying with Tibetan monks in the foothills of the Himalayas. One day I got a letter from my mother, who was a devoted schoolteacher, saying that the cancer had advanced to a point where she had gone into an epileptic seizure at work. She had been asked by the school not to return to the classroom, which we both knew was already like a death for her.

One of my teachers urged me to bring my mother to India; she could be treated by the Dalai Lama's doctor (which was how I first got to know him), and if the disease were too advanced for a cure, then the lamas could instruct her in how to pass through the realm of death to a better place. I wrote to my mother, and she quickly agreed, although she had never travelled outside the country at all.

I made the journey down to Delhi to meet her at the airport. The security guards wouldn't let me into the baggage area to assist her, but I found a place where I could watch for my mom through a window. I saw her struggling across the floor with her suitcase, barely able to stand, pushed and shoved in the typical Indian mob of screaming passengers. She came out and fell into my arms; we got her into a cab and laid her down in the back, then I used a lot of my remaining money to pay the taxi to drive day and night straight to Dharamsala, the small Himalayan village where His Holiness was living.

She spent several weeks recovering from the journey; we did visit the doctor, who came out and told me that she was gone beyond what he could treat—we should rather consult one of the senior monks, who could train her to make her journey gently. And so my mom began an extraordinarily brave course of daily study, propped up against the wall in a small room. In the afternoons we would move her bed out into the sun, and before long she had gathered a group of children who would come each day for drawing lessons, since of course she had brought a large bag of crayons and paper, knowing that the refugee camp would be teeming with children, and that she could have her classroom back.

Towards the end, my closest teacher encouraged us to go and meet His Holiness, for his advice. In those early days he was not the celebrity he is now—you could pretty much just walk up to his house, and he would come out on the porch to talk to you. It was a miracle then to sit down with two of the people I most loved in the world, but whom I had never thought would meet each other. My mother surprised me right off by pulling a crucifix out of her bag and offering it to His Holiness; I was mortified, but he graciously accepted the cross as if it were something he would use every day. And then it was time for me to surprise my mother.

His Holiness turned to me immediately, and his first question was: "So, have you ever used drugs?"

I glance over to my mom. I was not a regular user, but of course in college I had tried marijuana with friends, and had once done a spirit quest on a Native American drug called mescaline. So basically I'm in a situation where I either have to lie to the Dalai Lama, or embarrass my mother in front of him. I decide that it's better to tell the truth.

"Yes," I admit. A sharp glance from my mom.

"Oh!" he says with his usual affection. "What was it like? What did you see?"

I share a few experiences that had come to me, ranging from slight euphoria to some really wondrous moments in a hidden canyon in the Arizona desert, where I grew up.

"Good, good!" he booms. "Now you should keep here to this path, and learn to meditate! You can get to the same places, without the drugs!" My mother nods her approval, and His Holiness recommends a particularly qualified lama—with whom I am to spend the next 25 years.

The point of the story is that we can have the uplifting feelings and special experiences of alcohol, or drugs, without the downside of addiction, damage to our body, expense, and the destruction of our relationship with our partner and our family. Now I know you're expecting me to tell you that you can just learn to meditate, and that will be as good as the glass of wine—but this is not where we're headed. We're going deeper.

We start with a single crucial idea: The good feeling that you get from a glass of wine *isn't coming from the wine.* There's nothing *in the wine* that can make you feel happy. And this needs some explaining.

The good feeling isn't coming from the wine

It's probably clearer if we go at it through a different kind of drug—an aspirin. I like to talk about it in terms of Planet A and Planet B.

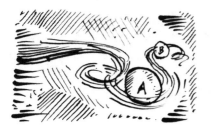

Now look, I'm actually from a place called Planet A. We perfected star travel long ago; we have extremely good tele-scopes, and we are very curious about other inhabitants of the galaxy. We've given your Earth the name "Planet B," and we've been watching you.

Our anthropologists are particularly intrigued by certain behavior exhibited by the mothers of your race. They haven't quite been able to figure it out, and they have sent me in person to ask about it. I hope you don't mind.

All right. So with our telescopes (which can see through the roofs of your houses, but don't worry—we never look when someone is dressing),

we have observed a particular scene played out. A mother is in a room with two of her younglings. Suddenly the young ones begin to howl and fight with each other, much like the creatures that you call "coyotes."

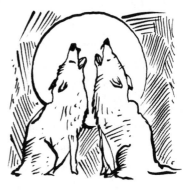

The older female speaks to them, and seems to be trying to reason with them. They are quiet for a while (especially if placed in front of a large box filled with moving pic-tures), but then usually the children start the coyote howling again. And then oftentimes the mother will begin to clutch her forehead and make strange whimpering sounds.

Here is where it gets strange.

The mother will then sneak into the small room which we know is nor-mally used for eliminating waste and washing the body. She opens a cabinet behind the mirror there and takes out a bottle. The bottle is filled with white pills.

She takes out one of the white pills and swallows it down, with a sip of water. And then she sits on the low chair where people eliminate their waste, but she leaves the top down and just sits there for a while. We're not sure why.

Sometimes after a while the wrinkles on her forehead start to soften, and she stops whimpering and clasping her head. Then she stands and composes herself and goes out to meet the little coyotes again, but with much more calmness.

But at other times she continues to rub her forehead, and then she gets up and opens the mirror cabinet again; pulls out the same bottle of tablets; and takes one or two more of them. Then she sits down on the top of the low chair again and waits, and sometimes she seems to get some relief, and sometimes not. Our scientists are dying to know what's going on; can we talk it over?

"What are those pills?"

"They are medicine."

"What does the word 'medicine' mean on your planet?"

"Medicine is something that you take to remove illness or pain."

"So what kind of medicine are those pills?"

"They are headache medicine; we use them to take away headaches."

"Do they require sitting down on top of the toilet seat to work?"

"No, no, she's just sitting down until they start to work—until the headache goes away, and she can face the children again without getting upset."

"So...why does she sometimes sit down once, and sometimes twice?"

"Sometimes the first aspirin you take works on the headache; and sometimes it doesn't. If it doesn't, then you take more."

"So why is she sometimes still clutching her head when she goes back to the little howling ones?"

"Well sometimes the aspirin doesn't work at all."

Long pause from the Planet A person.

"I don't understand. Are you saying that *sometimes the medicine doesn't work at all?*"

"That's right."

"So...some of the pills must be defective, right? I mean, in the factory they weren't made the right way, they are missing some ingredient? But in our telescopes we have never observed anyone taking the bottle back to the drug store and demanding a refund for the pills that didn't work."

"No, no," you laugh. "We have government agencies to check on that sort of thing. All the pills are made exactly the same; they all have exactly the same amount of the active ingredient."

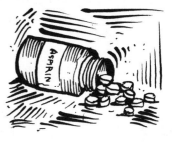

"*Active* ingredient? What do you mean by *active* ingredient?"

You chuckle and pull out a bottle of aspirin and stick it in my face. "Look, right here on the side…it says, *aspirin, 325mg.* That's the active ingredient."

"And this active ingredient is contained in every one of the pills, in that same amount?"

"Yes."

Another pause from Planet A. "So…what makes the ingredient *active?"*

You seem to be getting a little impatient with me now. "The *active* ingredient is the one that works—the one that takes away the headache. *Active* means 'works,' or 'acts.' You don't need a whole pill of the active ingredient, just a tiny drop, so they make a pill out of some neutral stuff that won't hurt you in any way—that's just filler—and then they put the exact same amount of that active ingredient in each one of the pills. They're very careful about it."

"So…sometimes the active ingredient is *active,* and sometimes it's *not?* I mean, sometimes the pill *works,* and sometimes it *doesn't?"*

That condescending smile on your face seems to waver a bit. "Well, you know, there could be a lot of other things going on…"

"But basically, can we say that sometimes the aspirin works, and sometimes it doesn't?"

"That's right," you admit.

"And you're telling me that when the aspirin doesn't work this poor woman has to go out and spend the rest of the day with a couple of howling children in the middle of a smashing headache?"

"Right."

"Then what you're saying is that people on your planet don't really *know* how to stop a headache; I mean, stop it for sure, stop it every time."

"Right," you say, and then you condemn the level of evolution upon your entire world because you add: "I mean, nothing works *all* the time. Not aspirin, not cars, not planes or strategies in a business or a relationship."

This stuns the Planet A person. "You mean…you people haven't figured out *what makes the active ingredient active?"*

Now it's getting confusing. "No, the active ingredient is just…active, by itself."

There is nothing inside an aspirin that works

Now it's time for the Planet A person to laugh. "Oh, I get it. *You think that what takes away the woman's headache is* **inside** *the aspirin.*"

"Well of course it is, it's that drop of active ingredient."

Planet A shakes their head sadly. So many people, so much pain. Unnecessary pain—a planet, and a planetary history, of unnecessary pain, all the way back to the beginning.

This is where we circle back to the glass of wine. Get this. If the ability to take away a headache were *inside* an aspirin, then the aspirin would work every time: every time you took an aspirin, your headache would go away. And if the ability to loosen us up were *inside* the wine, then every time we drank a glass of wine it would loosen us up.

But it doesn't. In fact, sometimes the wine gives us that same headache.

Something else must be going on here.

It all goes back to the seeds. It all goes back to the discussion we had about the pen in Question 1. We see a pen because we have a seed in our mind to see a pen; looking at the very same object, a dog sees a chew-toy because they have a seed in their mind for that. Some people see the aspirin work on their headache because they have a seed for this to happen; others don't because they don't. Same with the wine.

Now it's just a question of figuring out how to plant the seeds that make the wine work. And then maybe we wouldn't necessarily need the wine, and all the damage to our health and our pocketbook that comes from wine. What kind of seed do I need to plant to feel more relaxed, to feel less inhibited with my partner, especially when we're being intimate?

Look for somebody who's under stress in their life, who's under pressure for some reason. Why we could just take the example of the mother with the two children. Almost every parent feels a lot of pressure, juggling work and children and spouse. Purposely (and the more purposely it is, the more powerful the seed) look for opportunities where you can help take pressure off of someone with children.

Offer to pick up some groceries for them when you go out for your own; bring a bag of fruit along when you drop by, which in the end will save them a bit of money—and also bring along a comic book (a healthy one) that provides you an excuse to sit with one of the children quietly, and give the mom half an hour off.

What will happen? Since you have planted the seed for the pressure to come off—since you have planted a seed for being more loose and relaxed—then you'll begin to find peace and openness in more places than just the wine. A good cup of coffee will start to give you the same "buzz" and, as you plant more seeds, a cup of herbal tea will "work" exactly the same. And later, a few quiet moments under a particularly beautiful tree.

COMMUNITY

Question 31

My wife and I have a very close and good relationship, but sometimes I feel that our home has become like a little fortress, and that we are shut off from our community, and the rest of the world. How can we learn to reach out a bit? We feel a little nervous to try.

This question came out of the early years of a relationship between one of my best friends and his wife. After my parents' divorce, my brothers and I were shared between them; my dad lived in San Diego, and we all began surfing at a young age. My friend Jim and I really used to enjoy hitting the waves together after work.

That is, until he got married. And then suddenly everything changed, and yes their house did become like a fortress. She didn't really approve of him splitting for a few hours every day, and sitting on the beach waiting for us as it got dark quickly got old. Jim and I gradually drifted apart.

It seems like when we bond tightly with another individual, a kind of wall can go up between the two of us and the rest of the world. I've noticed that when I travel in a foreign country alone, people are very likely to approach me to help with getting on a train, or struggling to learn the local language. But when I'm travelling together with someone else from my own country, a kind of invisible wall goes up between us and others, and people tend to keep some distance from us. The same thing happens when we become a couple, and it feels as though we've lost something, some kind of contact with others in our life.

One basic fact of life, when we're dealing with things by using the seeds, is that nothing has to be the way it "usually" is. We all know people who get into a relationship and then seem to open up even more to the whole world around them. We just need to figure out the seeds that are going to drop the walls between the two of us and others, once we become "an" item. Perhaps the most beautiful thing about the Diamond Cutter system is that it automatically means we are dropping walls. Here's how Jim and I worked it out one day, sitting in his back yard—rather than on the sand at the beach, where we used to hang out together.

"So," says Jim, "how do you think I can work on this fortress thing? It's really starting to bug me; it's not just that I can't get out of the house to see old friends—they also seem to drop by less and less."

I consider for a moment. "Okay," I begin, "let me ask you a question."

"What's that?"

"I mean, we worked on the seed thing a lot at the very beginning; when you were looking for someone, before you met Amy."

"Yeah, I mean...Don't think I'm not grateful about that. It was a lot worse sitting around the house alone. I feel like now I couldn't live without her. It's just that, well, the whole point of working with seeds is that we not only use them to create a partner, but after we get the partner we can keep using the seeds to perfect them, to make the relationship everything we could ever want. Am I right?"

"Right," I say, "exactly right. Once we know how to use the seeds to make things happen the way we want them to happen, then we never have to settle for less than exactly what we want, ever again."

"So what's the seed for dropping the walls?"

"Well that's why I went back to the first few months, when we first got you to visit Mrs. Miller, to plant the seeds for Amy to show up. Let me ask you something about that—about the first day in the coffee shop, when we were going over the seed thing."

"Okay."

"I mean, I want you to think back. When I first brought up the idea of planting seeds for companionship by giving companionship to an elderly person, was there anything at all about the idea that bothered you?"

Jim doesn't need to think very long. "Well yes," he says, "there was... and to be honest I still think about it sometimes."

"And it was..."

"It was, frankly, that the whole system seemed to have a pretty serious flaw to it. I mean, ever since I was a kid, my parents and teachers talked about doing good things for others—but they always added that I should do so for unselfish reasons, that the purest kind of giving was when you didn't expect something back for yourself. But the whole Diamond Cutter thing seems *aimed* at getting something back. In some ways it seems really selfish."

"Exactly," I nod. "It *does* seem selfish. It seems like helping other people is reduced to some kind of business deal: I'll visit you so you won't be lonely, but only because I want to find a wife."

Jim nods enthusiastically; he almost seems relieved that I've brought it up myself, and that he's not alone. People all over the world approach me with the same question, which in a way is comforting. People all over the world are concerned that their giving should be pure, and not just one more exercise in selfishness.

"Alright," I say. "Let me ask you some questions—follow this line of thinking." He nods again.

"You go to the nursing home: you visit Mrs. Miller, keep her from feeling lonely.

"And this plants seeds in your mind. If you plant them the right way—understand *how* to plant them the right way—then on a visit to the bookstore..."

"...Amy comes right up next to me and starts going through the very same books, on the very same shelf—like, I've made myself a partner who's as wild about American history as I am...is that amazing, or what?"

"Right," I smile, happy that he appreciates how miraculous it is when any seed breaks open and begins to grow. "And then three months later..."

"...we're getting married, and you're my best man!"

"Right," I smile again. "But then there's the thing with Steve..." Steve is a mutual friend on two counts—the three of us surf, or *used* to surf, together pretty often; and we also like jamming together on our guitars.

"Yeah, well Steve comes up to me at the wedding and wants to know my secret; like, how did I get this amazing woman—where do I buy my clothes, what kind of workout do I do, whether I've found some new cologne that works better than the others when you're trying to approach a girl in a bar."

"And?"

"And, well—you know. I teach him about the seed thing, and..." Jim actually grimaces, like he's about to describe how some guy started hitting on his wife in the line for popcorn at the local movie theater. "...And then he actually starts visiting *Mrs. Miller,* rather than finding his own old lady to keep company!"

"And..."

"...And he plants the seeds, and that's how he met Francis," he concludes.

"Right," I say. "And what you don't know"—here I get this weird little hesitation, like I'm about to tell my best friend that his wife's been cheating on him—"is that he's got James Johnson taking care of her garden, and Eric

Sitman buying her groceries."

Jim looks a little shocked, but he rolls with it okay. "Well!" he hrrumphs. I can see that Mrs. Miller is going to get a lot more attention from him this week than last.

"But do you see what's happening?" I ask. "You have the courage to try something completely new, to find the woman you want. You score big, and then the rest of us are like, Wow! What's this guy doing? I mean..." I falter a bit.

"Yeah, I know," says Jim. "Like, you were all probably wondering why a loser who couldn't get a single decent girl to go out with him for three years suddenly has this beautiful, sensitive, intelligent wife."

Time to shift subjects. "Well yes, but...Jim, do you realize that because you had an open mind, because you were willing to try the seeds, we've got like six friends who are enjoying great relationships? You were the pioneer, the example, and everybody else is following you!"

Jim starts to perk up, to look proud—obviously he hasn't thought of it this way before.

I jump on the opportunity. "And look, *anyone* who uses the seeds to make something good happen in their life is being the same kind of example, sort of a role model for everybody else around them. You use the seeds and then something amazingly beautiful comes to you, and everyone else sees what's happening and starts to try the seeds too.

"Before you know it, you're at the epicenter of this big explosion of happiness. Your friends copy you, their friends copy them, and pretty soon..."

"Pretty soon," growls Jim, "visiting Mrs. Miller is gonna be like taking a trip to 31 Flavors. They're gonna be handing out numbers for half-hour slots to plant your seeds. One guy to take care of her garden, another who buys her groceries, someone else handling all her doctor's appointments, somebody else hogging all the trips to see a movie." He looks genuinely put out; nobody would guess that the center of his jealousy is 85 years old.

I grab his shoulder. "Yeah, you can look at it that way," I say, "but that's just planting jealousy seeds. And then Amy is on your case every time you say 'Good Morning' to anyone who's not a guy. You've got to realize something, Jim. You say you're tired of feeling like you're locked up in a fortress, but you've already got a way that you could plant seeds for the opposite.

"Just take a few minutes once a day—I would suggest while you're wrapping up your day, and getting ready for bed—to think about the revolution you've started; we call this Coffee Meditation. I mean, this thing could get big. You have no idea how fast being a really good example—a *success-ful* example—spreads a new idea.

"You don't need to go around preaching about the seeds, trying to convince people to pay more attention to elderly people who are lonely. Amy is a living testament to your new worldview, the view that the world is coming from seeds in your own mind—seeds that you put there purposely.

"Just *using* the seeds to achieve your dreams—just trying a method which finally works, every single time—is going to change the lives of hundreds of people around you. They'll give it a try too, and it will work, and it will bring them happiness.

"Look at it this way, try to look at it this way, and the one action of trying to help one old lady becomes at the same time an act of service towards hundreds of people around you.

"And that's not selfish. It's the *opposite* of selfish. It's the most *unselfish* thing you will ever do. And doesn't that feel right, isn't that the way you always thought it would be? That the action you take to serve the world also turns out to be the same action you take to find your own happiness?"

Jim nods, in a sort of wonder. It feels good to save the world. The seeds to drop the walls were right there, all along.

It's not selfish, if it helps everyone there is

SECURITY

Question 32

**I'm in a great relationship; which rather than making me happy makes
me feel totally insecure at times—like the whole thing is going *too* well,
and is bound to break down any minute. What's the karma I need to
plant if I want to reach a feeling of security, lasting security?**

My friends Andy and Nina, from Vancouver, had been together for six
years; Nina asked me this question while they were picking me up at a dock,
which needs some explaining.

Some other friends of mine were about six months into a 3-year silent
retreat, and they had asked me to come and counsel them on how to go deeper
(which we covered by sitting and writing notes to each other in their retreat
cabin). They were doing their retreat on an island in the Pacific Ocean off
the coast of Vancouver; they said I could get there by plane, and so I agreed.

What they didn't tell me was what kind of plane. They wrote that Andy
and Nina would be driving me over to Vancouver International Airport, but
instead of taking a right turn into the airport parking lot, they turned left, and
stopped near a busted-up old dock on the river.

"Okay," says Nina cheerfully, "they'll be here in a minute. We can wait
in the car."

"Uh," I say, confused, looking around.
"What do you mean? Who are 'they'?"

Andy points up to the sky, and I can see
a tiny plane circling over the other side of the
river. Suddenly it swoops down and lands *on*
the water—and now I see that it's one of those

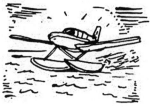

seaplanes with pontoons on the bottom, instead of wheels. Soon we are yelling over the roar of the propellers as the plane glides to the dock.

"Can I ask you a question when you get back?" shouts Nina.

"Sure!" I reply, trying to sound unconcerned. I stagger out and squeeze
myself into the cockpit.

The pilot is an old, crazed German hippie who likes to show off flying with no hands. He demands that I sing along with him on Louis Armstrong's "It's a Wonderful World" as we coast into a cove on the other side. I make the return flight just before dark; Nina is waiting for me, and we sit in their car to talk. My hands are still shaking from the plane ride—I tuck them into my coat pockets.

"Yeah," she says, "like…it's great. We have a wonderful relationship going, but because it's wonderful this other problem has popped up. I worry so much about what would happen if we ever split up that I can't really enjoy being together."

I look out the window to the west, and despite myself I feel an intense awe in the beauty of the golden sunlight spilling over the sea and the emerald peaks of the offshore islands, covered in dark green forest. But I'm still more than a little irritated that my friends put me through the plane thing, which now counts as my nearest-death experience.

I begin, as always, with the first of the Four Starbucks Steps. "So say it in one sentence."

"I want security—I want to *know* that Andy will still be with me next year, and every year. I don't want to ruin the happiness we already have by obsessing on how unhappy I would be if he ever left me." A bit more than a single sentence, but it will do.

Because that's the problem, you see. Even if by some miracle we get ourselves into a great relationship, we still don't know if our partner will be around in a year. We never know. And deep down that makes for an entire lifetime of anxiety, because we never know what's going to happen with anything else either. Try to appreciate that there are 7 billion other people in the world who are trying to get by in the same state of uncertainty as you.

In that sense, we are all cavemen.

Okay, so the cultivation of crops has been going on for well over 10,000 years. But try to appreciate what a breakthrough it was when the first crop ever was planted. The invention of the airplane or the electric light was pretty amazing, but the invention of agriculture was a much bigger deal. And here's how it happened.

The greatest invention ever invented

Woklok the Caveman kisses his wife Bookduk goodbye at the mouth of their cave one morning, and then heads off to work. For Woklok, of course, "work" means scrounging around in the forest for whatever food he can find—he's what the historians who come along a hundred centuries later will call a "hunter-gatherer."

If you think your work life is stressful, try to imagine Woklok's. In addition to the pressure he gets from his wife (which hasn't changed any), he just basically has a lot of pressure on him not to starve to death. Every day he wanders through the forest looking for an occasional stalk of wild rice popping up in between all the other plants. If he finds enough wild rice here and there, he and his family survive for another day. If he doesn't, they all die.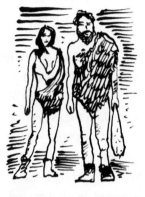

On this particular day—which turns out to be one of the most important days in the history of human kind—Woklok is pretty lucky. He's headed home with a whole handful of rice, but then disaster strikes. Around the bend on the path not far from the cave, he runs straight into a dinosaur. The dinosaur is also a hunter-gatherer, and right now he's hunting Woklok.

Woklok drops the rice and fights for dear life against the dinosaur, who eventually decides that this feisty little morsel is not worth all the trouble. Problem is, after Dino leaves, the caveman can't find much of the rice that he

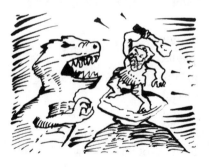

dropped, 'cause he and the critter kicked up so much dirt that all the rice got covered up.

He's got hell to pay with the wife, of course, who doesn't want to hear about the dinosaur. For all she knows, he stopped by the bar on the way home and spent all the rice buying beer for the boys.

Five months later Woklok is headed off to work, down the very same path. Right in front of him he runs into the biggest bunch of rice plants he's ever seen in one place. He leans over to pick the grain, and then he recalls that this is the exact place where he had the battle with the dinosaur. He squats next to the rice plants and contemplates for a bit—and then a light bulb goes off in his head. As he returns from his hunting/gathering that day, he bumps into his wife just outside the cave.

"Check this out!" he babbles excitedly. "I just found a big patch of rice plants, right where I dropped the handful of rice when I punched out the Tyrannosaurus Rex!"

Bookduk rolls her eyes. "Quit with the dinosaur story already. I didn't believe it then, I don't believe it now."

Woklok lets it go. "Yeah, but look!" he yells, holding out his take for the day: another whole handful of rice.

Bookduk nods. "Okay, so what's the big deal?"

"Watch this!" announces Woklok proudly. He throws the rice on the ground and kicks dirt all over it.

His wife thrashes him to within an inch of his life. "Are you crazy?" She sends him to bed with nothing but a piece of cold banana.

Now people who try new things need to be persistent. They have to have guts, and they have to be a little bull-headed. Woklok waits out the five months, then takes his wife outside to see the nice rice plants that have sprouted up all over the front yard.

"See!" he crows. "It works! Now we can have rice, as much rice as we want, *any time we want!* We just *plant* it!"

"I told you so!" says his wife—and thus begins the history of men laboring over plows to grow rice, women cooking the rice, and both of them fighting over who's going to do the dishes afterwards.

You get the moral of the story. Farming really was invented at some point, and it changed life on our planet completely. Try to appreciate the *anxiety* of wandering around the forest, hoping that you might come across some wild rice plants, knowing that if you don't then you and your family will starve to death. Then along comes Woklok the Great, the first farmer, and suddenly we pretty much *know* how much food we will have next year. *We just plant it.*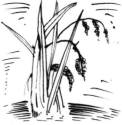

And on top of not starving, *the worry is gone.* Not knowing what's going to happen next year is gone.

With the wisdom of the Diamond Cutter, we can stop worrying about every other part of our life. Our income is coming from seeds; our health is coming from seeds; and our relationship is coming from seeds—all right on time, like rice after five months and babies after nine. Right now we walk out into our cities every morning like Woklok leaving his cave to go look for wild rice. Maybe we find some, and maybe we don't: maybe the boss gives us a raise, maybe the company goes under. Maybe Andy stays, maybe Andy finds someone else and leaves.

As children we learn to live with this uncertainty, and as we get older the people who cope with it the best are considered the most well-adjusted among us. But maybe that's a mistake. Maybe we've been programmed to accept random failure, maybe we've been brainwashed into believing that it's not even possible to predict what's going to happen in our lives.

Which means that we will never have any security at all, about anything. No wonder Nina can't enjoy the good times with Andy, knowing deep down that it could fall apart at any moment.

"So we need to plant some security," I tell her.

"How so?"

"You know the exercise. Decide what you want—get it down to a single sentence—and then go to Starbucks Step 2: put up your antennas and start looking for someone you know who needs the same thing. You want money, help other people to get it; you want health, help other people be healthy. You want security…"

"I need to find someone who needs security: someone else who feels insecure."

"Right. And then Starbucks Step 3—help them find security. Look, it starts with just listening, just having somebody to listen to. By the time your friend feels somewhat sure about you, somewhat secure in your friendship, then you can tell *them* about planting the seeds for security, with someone else they know."

We pause; Nina looks off towards the sun—a tiny bit is still visible, just above the horizon—and she starts the car for the ride home. As we get on the road, I add a little more.

"It will also help if you're generally just very dependable; if people can count on you. Make it a point to be on time everywhere you're supposed to be in the next three weeks. If you tell someone that the two of you should do lunch, then follow through on it. If you're sending birthday cards or holiday gifts to others, make sure they get them on time. Answer the emails you've promised to, when you've promised to. Help make others' lives a little more predictable."

"Got it," says Nina, and I get this strange feeling—which comes to me from time to time, almost everywhere—that she's made up the whole conversation so I can face my own feelings of fear on the seaplane, and figure out where they came from.

Through the traffic home we each settle into our own silence.

A HOME

Question 33

I think it's time that my husband and I tried to buy a house, but he's afraid to make such a big commitment. What's the karma to get him more interested in building a nest together?

I get a lot of variations on this question from people all over the world, especially since so many of them are interested in a spiritual path. It's not just a question about buying a house or not, it's a question about the role of possessions in our life, and the meaning of desire.

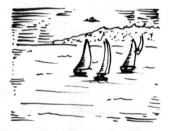

Kaye is asking me this question as we enjoy a rare quiet moment on one of my teaching trips to Vietnam; she and her husband Alex are on staff this time, and we are all sitting in a little coffee shop on the edge of a beautiful lake amidst a thick forest of trees, watching the locals herd their kids towards little sailboats that the families rent for the day.

I turn to Alex to get his take on it.

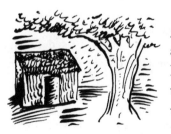

"It's not that I'm not committed," he begins. "It's just that I have serious questions about owning such a big thing. I mean, Geshe Michael, you're the one who taught us what the Buddha said about a place to sleep, and all that..."

I nod. In the early days of Buddhism, back in India, the Teacher was pretty insistent that people—monks especially—go light on possessions. The reason you see Tibetan monks wearing that maroon cape is because it doubled as a sleeping bag at night; scripture stipulates that a monk shall "make his home at the foot of whatever tree he is passing when it comes time to sleep."

Alex continues: "And that thing about the hard disk, and throwing out anything you haven't used for six months."

This is a teaching on simplicity that I try to get people interested in. If I ask you how many pairs of shoes you own, your mind goes back home to your closet, especially to the *back* of the closet. You see each pair of shoes—the color, the style, and the degree of wear—in your mind's eye, even if it's been ages since you wore them. And you are able to see this because you have an inventory of all your shoes and other possessions right there in your mind, as if it were all stored on a hard disk inside a computer.

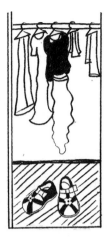

Your hard drive is not unlimited

And the hard disk of the mind, like the one in the computer, has limits to it. Only so much storage space is available. That's why I like to share with my friends the idea of throwing out anything they own that they haven't used for six months. Otherwise there's no *room* in your mind for the spiritual realizations which many of us are seeking.

At least, at Level One.

"That all comes from the Vinaya," I reply to Alex. "The rules that the Buddha set down for monks and nuns." I pause. "A lot of the people who try out the six-month thing come back to me with the same question."

"Which is?"

"I mean they come across something that they haven't used for six months, but which they think might come in handy later on, and so they're keeping it in their house."

"Like?"

"Like I don't know, we could say a wool scarf that you only wear on the three coldest days of the year. But when those days come, you're really glad that you didn't throw it out.

"Look, let's go back to the Vinaya. So monks were only allowed to have two sets of robes, no more. But then there was An Incident. Monks have over 250 vows, and for every one of those vows there was An Incident. Which means that at first there was no rule against doing a certain thing, and then something happened, and they had to make the rule.

"Which is to say, what do you do if you are only allowed two sets of robes, but one of them is starting to fall apart, and someone gives you enough cloth to make a new set? You're supposed to get all the use out of a set of robes that you can, which means wearing it until it actually *does* fall apart. I mean—knowing that the robes will probably fall apart in a month or two—are you allowed to store the cloth until you need to make the new robes?"

"Well, what did the Buddha decide?"

"The Buddha decided that it was probably too dangerous to allow monks and nuns to start storing stuff that they might need later. And so normally you had to *need* a new set of robes and you had to sew the cloth into robes within 10 days, or you had to give the cloth away to somebody else who needed it. Otherwise you start getting into storing things, keeping things that you think you want or you think you might need, and then *things* take up your mind, and your house."

"Right," says Alex, raising an eyebrow in Kay's direction. "And just having the *house* itself is like the biggest drain on your mind of all."

During our training in the monastery, we spend up to four hours a day outdoors, in a park called the Debate Ground. Here we learn to question each other in shouts and screams, while we execute moves that look a lot like martial arts; in fact, one day while I was in the Debate Ground a passing farmer called the police to report that the monks were having a riot. So anyway, we learn to love a challenging question.

"Ah," I say quietly, "but there's always Level Two." I give Kaye a conspiratorial glance that sets her at ease.

"Level Two is the path of the bodhisattva: someone who is pledged to work for the happiness of the whole world. Which often happens out in the world, and not just in a cave meditating—although the cave thing is important because it helps and supports the work in the world.

"There is a separate set of vows for those on the bodhisattva path—vows which build upon those of the ordained. One of these vows stipulates that a bodhisattva is not allowed to refuse a material gift that he or she could utilize in the service of others. A monk or nun cannot keep a small piece of cloth for more than ten days without using it to make robes for themselves; but a monk or nun, or anyone else, who has committed themselves to the bodhisattva path is required to accept an entire warehouse filled with cloth, and if necessary to store the cloth for years, until they can use it to clothe the poor."

"So we *should* buy a house," crows Kaye.

"Yes and no," I return. "Alex is absolutely right that a house can be a tremendous drain on your mental and spiritual resources, unless it is dedicated to a higher purpose. But if as you purchase the house you both commit to using the house to help others, then the whole thing turns around. Every day that passes while a bodhisattva is in possession of a warehouse full of cloth which they intend to use for others, massive amounts of good seeds are planted in the bodhisattva's mind, even if they haven't done anything yet with the cloth."

"Committed to help others?" Kaye looks a little dubious—I figure she thinks that I want them to start a soup kitchen or a homeless shelter in the new house.

"Level Three," I say simply. "It's more a matter of vision."

"Vision?"

"It's called the Diamond Way—the highest path of all. You start in the Vinaya with learning to live a simple life, and this gives you the foundation for the bodhisattva code, training to serve all living beings. Those who are well along in this training then enter the Diamond Way."

"And how does this relate to the house?" asks Alex.

"In the Diamond Way, the house becomes a headquarters."

"Headquarters for what?" asks Kaye.

"Superheroes," I reply. "Superman/Wonder Woman/Iron Man/Spiderman…and the Goddess.

"That would be you," I smile, nodding at Kaye.

"Goddess?" they chorus back.

"A woman practicing the Diamond Way might take a piece of the same cloth, get it sewn into a beautiful gown, and walk around the house all day pretending to be an angel."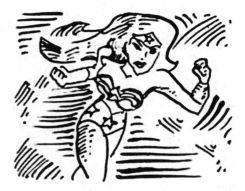

"Which helps others…how?" asks Alex.

"Sort of using the goal as the path; the first time she steps into the new house…"

(Kaye smiles.)

"…she walks around the place slow, with a vision that she and her husband are already using the house as a warm and happy home base from which they serve other people."

"Which I suppose could mean," Kaye says softly, already looking more regal, "a dinner say once a week for homeless people in the neighborhood. That's what an angel would do with their house."

Alex nods, and it looks like the deal is done.

DOING THINGS
TOGETHER

Question 34

I've gotten interested in yoga, and I feel that it would really help both me and my husband to lead longer, more active lives—but he's just not interested, and he won't even try a class with me. What seed do I need to plant to get him interested?

Elizabeth asked me this question in the living room of her home; I was visiting her and her husband Jeremy, who are both over 60 years old. Actually a visit to Elizabeth and Jeremy is mostly just a visit to Elizabeth, because after waving "Hi!" when you first walk in, Jeremy goes back to the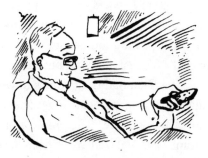

TV room—where he has sadly spent most of his life in recent years. Getting Jeremy to do even ten minutes of yoga is going to be a real challenge.

Thinking for a moment about how I'm going to approach this challenge, I reflect on all the huge mistakes I've made in the past, judging which partner is at fault when people I know are having a relationship problem. Nick and Tammy come to mind—Nick has a real temper, we all know it, and he just gets completely out of hand at times. Tammy left him, and for about a year he was non-stop furious, making wild claims about how she had cheated on him. We didn't see any other man suddenly show up, so we assumed he was just being spiteful. But something like two years later, Tammy confessed to me that she *had* been cheating on her partner—and I learned a lesson about judging other people's relationships.

Moral of the story: Jeremy in front of the TV might *not* be the one at fault for this stuck relationship. Maybe it's *never* the person it seems to be.

I start heading Elizabeth towards Starbucks. "So say it in one sentence," I ask her. "In one sentence, tell me what you want."

"I want him to be more open to trying new things, especially things we can do together. How can I get him to listen? Should I get tough with him, like stand him up on the scale in the bathroom and yell at him for eating so poorly; or should I bribe him, offer to take him out to ice cream afterwards if he goes to yoga with me?"

I smile to myself. A classic Diamond Deal. Which needs some explaining—about Bottom Feeders in the diamond business.

The center of the diamond business for the whole United States is 47th Street in New York City, mostly between 5th and 6th Avenues, down the street from icons of fashion like Saks Fifth Avenue, Tiffany's, and Bergdorf Goodman. Most of the movement of diamonds into the country goes through the upper floors of 580 Fifth Avenue, on the northwest corner of Fifth. Down below in the first-floor storefronts are the Bottom Feeders.

Bottom Feeders are playing on the fact that The Street is known for the big diamond deals going on upstairs. They stand out on the sidewalk and collar unsuspecting tourists into jumping for big savings at the epicenter of the world's biggest diamond business.

The Diamond Deal comes in when a young couple enters the store looking for an engagement ring. The salesman shows them one stone which is noticeably yellow. The groom-to-be is suffering from Male Shopping Syndrome, eyes glazed over from inspecting 200 engagement rings already, down the whole length of The Street. Without really looking he immediately declares the stone a Good Deal.

The bride is invariably a little tougher customer. She picks up on the yellow hue right away.

"Oh," smiles the salesman. "You want a *white* diamond."

"Right," she says righteously.

The salesman hands her a stone with a white body color, but peppered with huge black spots on the inside. She sees the spots but she doesn't have a chance to open her mouth before the salesman yells, "So which one do you want, the *whiter* stone or the *cleaner* stone?"

Don't fall for diamond deals

This time she does manage to open her mouth, but the salesman is all over her with another choice: "And will you pay cash or credit card?" He follows up immediately with "And do you want that in a red box, or a blue one?"

Faced with a pile of decisions to make, most people will just go ahead and struggle to try to make them, without asking themselves if they really *need* to make a decision. Remember one thing: *In the Diamond Cutter system, almost every decision we ever make involves two bad choices.*

And so "Elizabeth," I ask her, "does it always work with Jeremy when you criticize him? Do you always get what you want?"

"Well, no, but it works sometimes."

"And if you bribe him with a sweet to get him to do what you want, does *that* always work?"

"No, but again—it does work sometimes."

I leave that debate for later.

"So look; neither one of those choices seems so good to me. Why don't we just get to the root of the problem?"

"Jeremy's addiction to television?"

"In a way," I say. "Where do you think it's coming from? Why do you have to spend your life around somebody who would rather watch the news than ask you how your day went?"

"I don't know," she says honestly. "When I first met him, we had a lot of fun together: we went on a lot of trips, he was laughing most of the day."

"So what kind of seed do you think you might have inside your mind, that you see a person around you who has practically zero interest in anyone else in the room? I mean, what things are *you* doing that might make you see him this way?"

Elizabeth considers this for a moment. "Well one thing's for sure. I have never in my life sat and watched television all day."

I smile. "A watermelon is a lot bigger than a watermelon seed. Is there any *tiny* thing in your life that you're doing which might involve ignoring other people around you?"

Elizabeth pauses again, this time quite a bit longer.

"To be honest," she says, "I ignore people all day long, in little ways.

"I mean, somebody at work starts telling me a long story about her own husband, and I just start to zone out. I mean, I'm careful to be polite—I don't just walk off the minute they go on for the hundredth time about how their husband never washes the dishes. I sit down and look at them and try to concentrate on what they're saying."

"But?"

"But I mean, after a few minutes I just don't want to hear about somebody else's problems—I have more than enough problems myself, already. So I do stay and I do listen but sometimes I just zone out...or maybe I start thinking about what groceries I need to pick up on the way home after work."

Inside, I laugh at this. We talked about it a bit back in Question 14. It's *hard* to really focus on what somebody else is saying, simply because they're usually talking about what they want, and *we're simply more interested in what* we *want*. And Elizabeth has just mentioned the two great obstacles to meditation, without even knowing it. The first is distraction—thinking of something else (groceries) while we're trying to focus on one thing (our friend's problems). The second is zoning out: getting dull or sleepy, and losing the object of our focus altogether. A good way to fight both of them is a Tibetan practice called *dakshen jewa;* let's see if we can get Elizabeth to try it.

"Look Elizabeth," I say. "The key to planting seeds is to provide someone else with the same thing that we want, first. To do that, we need to *find out* what it is they want. To do that, we need to *listen* to them, and listen carefully.

"When you first try this seed thing—when you first take someone else out to the coffee shop to listen to their needs—it's very natural to discover that you have a noticeable resistance to listening to other people's problems. And there's a very clever trick that the Tibetans use to get around this resistance."

"What's that?" she asks.

"Make it into sort of a game. What's the name of the lady at work who wants to talk about her husband?"

"Mary."

"Okay, Mary it is. Now look, we're all a lot more interested in ourselves than in anybody else. It's an almost impossible habit to break. So don't even try.

"Continue to focus on what Elizabeth wants, but just switch names with Mary first."

"Switch names?"

"Yeah, switch names. Now Elizabeth is Mary, and Mary is Elizabeth. Then after that you just keep focusing on what Elizabeth wants, which will make it completely easy to sit and listen carefully to your friend at work."

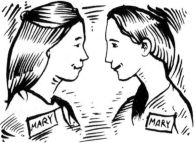

"Hmm," says Elizabeth, arching her eyebrows. "That's pretty weird."

"Weird, but it works," say I. "Try it."

"And…if I just keep paying careful attention to…to Elizabeth, who's sitting next to me in the cafeteria at work and telling me about all her problems with her husband, this is going to plant the seeds for Jeremy to suddenly ask if he can go to yoga with me?"

"Exactly. That is, he will finally *listen* to you. Because you've planted the seeds for it, by listening to others."

Elizabeth nods, as if all of this makes perfect sense. Which in fact it does. Then a little cloud passes over her features.

"But if I can change how Jeremy responds to me, by changing something in my own behavior…" she pauses.

She gulps and finishes: "…then the way he's been acting, all that sitting in front of the TV, was coming from me the whole time."

"Right. Which is to say, everything and everyone around us—all the time—is coming from us: it's *all our own fault*. Which also means that everything good is because of us too. Which means in turn that we each have the power to change the entire world."

SLEEP PROBLEMS

Question 35

My husband and I like to sleep in the
same bed, but we often have problems
getting a full night's sleep: he has to get

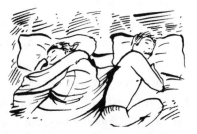

up and go to the bathroom, or else (so he claims) I pull the sheets off
him—or maybe one of us starts to snore. Can karma change this?

Karma can change everything, and nothing else can change anything

There's one thing you really need to grasp at this point, and it's not easy.
Karma can change everything, and nothing else can change anything. That
is, nothing that does anything ever does it unless we have the seeds for it to
work. And if we don't have the seeds for it to work, nothing can do anything.
This is always the case, with everything there is.

Which means that we can definitely get a good night's sleep for both of
you—in the same bed. No problem; just plant the necessary seeds. Which
begins with getting down to the essence of the problem, and saying it in a
single sentence.

This is what I challenged Phyllis to do, when she and her husband Jessie
met me in a small café in Brive, in central France. They were just getting
back from a vacation in the French countryside that ended early when a pair
of grumpy partners started getting on each other's nerves, because neither one
had had a good night's sleep in almost three weeks.

If you've ever been in this situation, you know that at the time you can't
see how bad it is, because you haven't even had enough sleep to know how
foggy your own mind has become. Lack of sleep in a relationship is not just

an inconvenience; it can sabotage the whole partnership, without either one of us really being aware of it.

Phyllis pauses over a *pain au chocolat* pastry and Jessie stares down at his own croissant politely; but his ears have obviously perked up—he definitely wants this problem resolved, starting tonight if possible.

"I guess," she begins, "you could say that I want to be able to get a whole night's sleep, without it being interrupted. Really it's all just about not being interrupted."

Now we covered the idea of how we all need some uninterrupted time back in Question 23. We said that moments of uninterrupted focus are as important as healthy food for maintaining a happy and well-balanced state of mind. But let's take it specifically to how we conduct a conversation.

"It's pretty serious," I say, "when your sleep keeps getting interrupted— I mean, if it goes on long enough, it can make almost anyone unhappy and irrational." Jessie's head comes up suddenly, but he has the wisdom to hold his tongue.

"Right," Phyllis replies.

"So we look for what caused it: something smaller…" I prompt her.

"Something *much* smaller," agrees Phyllis, "than getting shaken out of your sleep night after night."

"Right."

You know that people are starting to get the seed thing when they pause and stare off into space looking for the real cause of something, then get a sheepish look on their face when it occurs to them that they themselves might *be* that cause. Phyllis glances over at Jessie.

"I interrupt people a lot," she says.

"In fact, we *both* do." And I see another light go off in her head.

"Can two people make a seed together?" she asks.

"Yes and no. I mean, no one can make a seed for another person. If that was possible, then I wouldn't have gotten my teeth drilled at the dentist last week."

"How so?" asks Jessie, and I can see he's getting drawn into the conversation.

"I mean, there have been lots of good people in the world up to now, right?"

"Well, sure."

"I mean, and there must have been really good people in the world who figured out the seed thing, like a long time ago: the Golden Rule—do unto others what you would have them do unto you; reap what you sow; all that sort of thing.

"And if it were possible to give someone else a seed—like, pull a seed out of your head and hand it to someone else—then these people would have done it already, right?"

"Seems like."

"And if these really good people who lived before and who live around us now could just pull a getting-drilled-by-the-dentist seed out of our head, or just stick a healthy-teeth-that-don't-need-to-get-drilled seed into our head, then I wouldn't have had to go the dentist last week. Am I right?"

"Right."

"But I *did* have to go," I conclude. "Which proves that they can't. Nobody can. We can't share a seed."

"But what about the fact that we both get interrupted out of our sleep?" asks Phyllis. "Doesn't that mean that we're sharing the same seed?"

"You can both have the *same* seed, but that doesn't mean you're sharing it. What I mean is, suppose one of your friends comes over to the house for dinner and wants to tell you guys all about her last vacation, but you both keep interrupting her; and so she finally gives up trying to talk, and is forced to listen to you two talk about whatever you want to talk about.

"I mean, suppose you don't even *notice* that she's trying to say something—and you don't notice together.

"Each one of you then plants their own similar seed, in their own mind, to have some pretty serious interrupting ripen in your perceptions later on. And then…"

"And then he gets up to go to the toilet, or I pull the sheets off of him. Each of us experiences our own interruption, from separate seeds that we planted at the same time."

"Right." I pause. "So maybe you could just start with watching other people's faces really carefully when you're having a conversation with them. Try to pick up on any indication that they would like to say something, and don't speak yourself until they've obviously said all they have to say. If you're very conscious about planting it, this new not-interrupting seed will get down there into your subconscious and short-circuit the old seeds for having your sleep interrupted."

A companionable silence ensues, and I can see that both Phyllis and Jesse are tired enough of being tired that they're willing to make a conscious effort not to interrupt other people while they speak. They also look like they're ready for a Thanksgiving Meditation—an old Tibetan practice which is like a miracle cure for insomnia.

So "There's another trick for getting a really *good* night's sleep," I say.

"What's that?" they chorus back.

I point down to their two empty plates, where only the crumbs of two heavenly French pastries remain.

"I mean, just think about the work that went into those two pastries. You know, a few months ago I heard someone claim that this patisserie in Paris called 'Le Moulin de la Vierge' had the best croissant recipe in existence, and that they had just published the recipe in a book on French baking. It seems like croissants are so difficult that Julia Child doesn't even try to teach them out of a book.

"So I get in a cab and give the address to the driver and we drive for almost an hour to get to this place. I ask him if he'll wait for me, he says okay. Inside the bakery they sell me the book. I stuff it into my shoulder-bag and take two croissants to go.

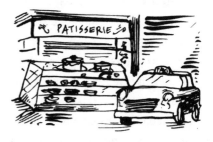

"Back in the taxi I try to give one of them to the driver and he shoots me this really grumpy look. He refuses the croissant and starts the long drive back. 'There are *other* patisseries in Paris, you know,' he sniffs. 'You took me all the way out here *for two croissants?*'"

Jessie chuckles. "Like there's a bakery on every single corner in Paris," he says.

"Yeah, so well I get home and really want to try out the croissant recipe. But first I have to type every sentence of the French into Google Translator, so I can get the English. Then I sit down to make myself a croissant for breakfast.

"Except that it turns out to be for dinner." I turn to Jesse. "I mean, do you have *any* idea how long it took to make the croissant that you just polished off in five minutes? We're talking like an hour to go to the grocery store and buy all the ingredients. You come back home and roll out the dough and then sit around for two hours while it rises. Then move the dough to the fridge and wait for another half hour.

"You roll *the butter* out into a huge flat square (and hey, we're talking about more than a quarter pound of butter here, in a single batch of croissants); flatten out the dough; wrap it around the square of butter; and fold it all up a special way—then back to the fridge and wait for another half hour.

"Roll the dough out again, cut it into triangles and roll out the croissants, brush with a coating, sit around for another hour while they rise some more.

"Sit around while they bake, because you gotta watch if they change color the wrong way, and if they do then you need to fool around with the temperature. Pull them out and sit around while they cool. I mean, I was wrestling with those croissants for like six hours!"

"Wow!" says Jessie. He looks a little guilty at eating the thing so fast.

"And so somebody around here," I wave my arm vaguely, "was up before dawn to bake you this croissant. Somebody else had to go to the store and pick up all the ingredients, fresh. Somebody else unpacked all that stuff from the delivery truck; somebody else drove the delivery truck from the warehouse; someone else loaded it up there.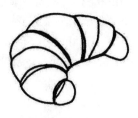

"Somebody else drove a truck to the warehouse to bring the wheat from the mill, and before that from the farm; somebody else was out in the hot sun or pouring rain to harvest the wheat; someone else planted it, someone tilled the soil, somebody watered the field and spread the fertilizer.

"And that's just the flour; it's the same for all the other ingredients. I mean, you just gobbled down like a year of work by other people, without giving them a single thought."

Jessie hangs his head.

"So where does the meditation come in?" asks Phyllis.

I nod. "So like before you go to bed, you plop down in an easy chair, or just on top of the bed. Bring to mind a single thing that you ate or used today: it could be a croissant, or a car, or your house.

"Then take your mind back one by one through all the people who had to work to bring you that thing. In your mind, thank the salesman who stood out in the sun at the car dealership and showed you the car. Thank the person who drove one of those big dangerous car-carrying trucks to bring the car to the lot. Thank the people who stood in the assembly line at the factory all day to screw each of the car's parts on; thank the people who stood in the factory to make that one part; thank the worker who stood over the molten steel that the part was cut from; thank the miner who risked his life to bring up the ore."

"But they all get paid..." begins Jesse. I cut him off impatiently.

"They are all spending the hours of their life, to make you the things you need," I whisper. "And no one, and no amount of money, can give those hours back to them. They are sacrificing their lives for us, so that we can live—so we can sit here and enjoy a single piece of bread.

"So this is meditation, and a real meditation. In this case, you don't need to sit there staring at a wall with your legs crossed. Just relax on your bed and take your mind back slowly, almost luxuriously, through the chain of people who offered their lives so that you could live today. Thank each one of them.

"As you get better at it, the chains get longer and longer. Not a dozen, but hundreds of people involved in creating this single croissant: laboring to build the roads that the delivery truck used; to maintain the truck's engine; to pay for the truck in the first place.

"And the act of gratitude, aside from being one of the most noble of all human emotions, itself brings us a great deal of peace. Each time you pause to thank someone, your mind becomes more gentle, more full of peace.

"Then lay your head down on the pillow. You can even continue the Thanksgiving Meditation there, but it won't go on for very long. You'll be into a deep, peaceful sleep that lasts till morning, and you'll wake up very quiet and clear."

"Two seeds then," observes Phyllis. "One for an uninterrupted sleep, and another for a peaceful sleep." She glances at Jesse, who is already smiling. We order some more pastries, so we'll have more people to thank for them.

Showing our gratitude makes us very, very happy

Question 36

My husband and I share the same bed, but we have different sleep cycles, so we often get into problems. I like to stay up late and sleep in, but he prefers to get to bed early and rise with the sun. He doesn't like to disturb me, but it's hard for me when I can hear him on his computer or up and around the house, before I'm ready to get up. Karmically speaking, how can we get our sleep times better synchronized?

If this were a regular book of advice for your relationship, I would either tell you that you should wear earplugs and he should get up when he wants to; or that he should lie awake in bed until you're ready to get up—that he could even use the time to do a little contemplation, like the Thanksgiving Meditation that we just talked about.

But that's just a diamond deal: two bad choices. I want you to get used to approaching problems from a whole new angle. Don't assume that the problem is there, and that the two of you have to make some hard decisions

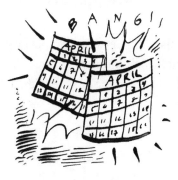

about who's going to get their way, and who's going to be nice and let the other have what they want.

That's not at all the Karma of Love way.

So I get this question from people all over the globe, just about weekly. I guess a lot of people really enjoy spending the night with another warm and loving human body next to them, even if they're on different schedules. We muddle through the problem, because a hug close at hand all night is worth an hour or two less sleep than we would really like to get.

"But why not have both?" I say to Chris, who I can see is having a real problem. The bags under her eyes are deep and dark.

"What do you mean?"

"I mean, have Tom next to you all night long, and also get a full night's sleep."

"But, I mean, the schedule thing…he likes getting up early, I like working late."

"So we have to bring you closer," I say. "We want him to get up a bit later, we want you to go to bed a bit earlier."

"But I don't *want* to," they both answer at the same time. We share a laugh. I'm glad they *can* laugh, because it means the problem hasn't gotten to the point where they resent each other about it. They just want to work it out.

"But if somehow your schedules *did* match," I persist, "wouldn't that solve the problem?"

Chris and Tom look at each other and nod.

"Okay. So if we had to say it in a single sentence…"

"We want our schedules to match," finishes Tom. "It's that easy."

"Okay, so it's a question of timing, isn't it?" I reply.

"Right," says Chris.

"So you're both going to have to plant seeds for better *timing*. And since the only place we can normally plant a seed is with another person, you're both going to have to watch your timing with other people."

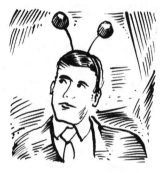

"Okay," says Tom, "but give me some examples."

"I like to call it 'putting up your antennas.' You're both going to be on the lookout for opportunities where you can help out somebody else, timing-wise. Somebody at work needs to get home on time today because their kid is playing in the big baseball game, and you offer to cover for them when the boss tells them they need to work late.

Keep your antennas up

"Let people know what time you'll be someplace where you're supposed to meet them; be on time, and when you first sit down try to find out what time would be best for them to leave, so that they can get on to the next thing they need to do today. Pay your bills on time, or early. Build a little extra time into everything you do and every trip you make in the car, so you can let others go ahead of you if they need to, or stop and help somebody who's having a problem getting where they need to go.

"Be very aware of timing even when you're just talking with someone. If there's something they need to know now, say it now. If there's something that might hurt less if you tell them later, then wait."

I pause and think a bit. "Ultimately, all this ties into a very cool meditation from ancient Tibet called *Je Michu, Dun Misu:* Staying in The Present Moment."

"What's that all about?" asks Chris.

"Okay, it starts like any other meditation: to get your mind calmed down, first you watch your breath for a while. Sort of like you've just put your car in reverse to back it out of your driveway, and then you need to stop and pause it for at least a second before you jam it into forward—otherwise..."

"Otherwise you strip the gears," laughs Tom. "My brother did that one day with our mom's car, banged into the gearshift knob and jammed the car into reverse while we were running down the highway. Not a pretty sight."

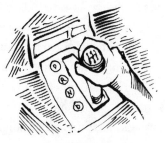

"Right," I say. "You need to put the car into neutral first if you want to change directions, and you need to put your mind into neutral first if you want to head it inward, into meditation. So first you count your breath: this is just a warmup, and not a goal in itself."

"Why not?" asks Chris.

"We're talking *content* here. The point of meditation is that whatever thing or person you bring to mind is going to be reflected in the mirror of the mind when it's very still. It gets burned there, the way that an object gets burned into a camera when the lens opens and you hold the camera still.

"Keeping your mind on your breath helps slow it down, take it to neutral—but it's not like the goal is to have a picture of your breath burned into your mind for the rest of your life. You slow the mind down, and then you move it on to something else, something more powerful."

"Like what?" Tom wants to know.

"Once you've followed your breath to get your mind calmed down, then you switch to an even more helpful meditation. To do that, you first split a little piece of your mind off of your bigger mind—personally, it helps me a lot if I imagine that this little part of my mind has stepped back a few inches, just a bit outside the back of my skull, so it can start to watch the main part of the mind."

"Watch for what?"

"In this case, just learn to step back and watch what thoughts your mind is thinking. It's like watching two other people have a conversation: one of them is listening to the other. At first, you just practice watching your mind listen to its thoughts. At this point, you're not doing anything *to* the thoughts. Not judging them, not trying to change them in any way. Just watch your own mind as it listens to its own thoughts.

"Once you get good at that, start to take a poll—it's like stopping people on the street, and asking them who they're going to vote for: the Republican, or the Democrat. Except that in this case we're checking the thoughts that come up, to see if our mind is listening to a thought about something that happened earlier, or something that's coming later.

"What you'll find—what I found, at least—is that a huge amount of our thoughts at any given moment have wandered off to something in the past, or something in the future. If we've just watched a movie the night before, then a lot of the thoughts that we see our mind listening to are going to be related somehow to that movie: to the past. If we're going into a tough meeting with our boss later this afternoon at work, then a lot of the thoughts that we watch our mind listening to are going to be future thoughts.

"It's like we're constantly living in expectations about the future or worries about the past—we're very rarely *here, now.*"

"So what's that got to do," asks Chris, "with getting Tom to come to bed a little bit later?"

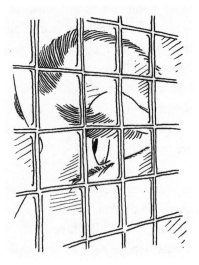

"Stay with me. We watch our mind for a few minutes to see which thoughts win the election: more thoughts of what did happen in the past, or more thoughts about what might happen in the future. We try to figure out if we have more of a problem with being stuck in the past, or worrying about the future.

"Then we know which one to go after first. If today—and it changes from day to day—we are worrying more about this afternoon, or next week, or next year, then we need to practice cutting our future thoughts off. A good way to do this is with a little trick of visualization.

"We focus on our forehead, and then imagine that we've built a wall of tiny bricks just in front of it. The bricks are transparent, like those walls of glass bricks that you sometimes see in office buildings. If you make the bricks out of something like clay or cement, then it's going to be dark in your mind behind the bricks, and you'll start to feel a little dark too. Keep the wall of bricks light, keep some light pouring in from the front of it.

"This wall blocks all thoughts of anything that's going to happen beyond this present moment in time. Any time the meeting with your boss this afternoon tries to come into your head, set in on the other side of the wall and keep it there, blocked. Now when the little piece of your mind watches your main mind, it only sees it listening to thoughts about the present, or the past.

"Now block thoughts of the past—which for a lot of us are stuck on something somebody did maybe a long time ago to hurt us. We do this by setting up the same kind of transparent wall just behind the back of our skull.

"This leaves you with thoughts only of the present moment. You are here, in this room, aware only of what's happening right now. And then something really strange happens…"

"Like what?" asks Tom.

"Like, you realize suddenly that the Present Moment—which is where we always are anyway, physically at least—is a place that we almost never stay in. We're constantly worrying about something somebody did to us before, or worrying about whether something we want in the future is going to come or not.

"Once we block the front and the back though, suddenly we have permission to just be here, right now. And it's a very *relaxing* place to be. Suddenly we are freed from expectations and worries—suddenly we can just surrender to whatever beauty or love is right in front of us, right now.

"This meditation as well is only a warmup, and we need to take it on to something else, to connect it to some real content. In this case we connect it to timing, because a person who's 100% present is infinitely more aware of what the person sitting in front of them needs—and when they need it. When they need us to talk, when they need us to be quiet, when they want to meet with us to talk, when they're ready to go home after we've talked.

"That is, strangely, a person who is truly here in the present moment is more present in what's coming and what's been—more sensitive to other people's timing, more able to match that timing and make other people feel comfortable. And those are seeds to see your own timing with each other, timing about your bedtime, straighten itself out."

Chris asks, "Just what will that look like—what will it look like when these seeds ripen for us?"

I smile. "That's the cool part. You can just about forget about trying to guess how those seeds are going to ripen, and how your timing with each other will suddenly become perfect. I mean, I know we talked about each of you changing your schedule—Chris earlier, Tom later—but it doesn't have to work out that way.

"One of the most exciting things about all these seeds is that, when they ripen, they will have to ripen within the context of millions of other seeds you already have waiting in line to ripen. It's a miracle of nature, the very nature of the seeds, that all these seeds as they ripen will mesh with each other perfectly. Millions of threads from millions of moments in your past will create the tapestry of a new and different Tom and Chris, as the new seeds for timing ripen.

"So just relax and don't try to guess or predict how the new seeds are going to solve your problem; just know that they will, that nothing can stop them. They usually ripen into some completely beautiful and unexpected chapter in your relationship. Enjoy not knowing how the miracle will come: just watch, and enjoy it as it unfolds—as surely it will."

Learn to listen to what your mind is thinking

CONTROL

Question 37

My wife is a real control freak, like even down to grabbing the menu out of my hands when we go out to eat, and insisting on being the one to order, and deciding what I'm going to eat too. What's the karma to see her loosen up a bit?

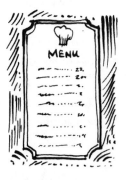

This is a really classic Stare Into Space question. People ask it quite often, but the case that I remember the best was with Sam and Dawn. I mean, it was so bad that Sam and I had no little trouble getting some private time together at a café to discuss it: Dawn wanted to "sit in" on our conversation and "give a few suggestions," which we both knew would end up with Sam retreating into a resentful silence while Dawn explained why there wasn't really any problem. As usual, I head him first to Starbucks 1.

"Say it in a single sentence, Sam."

"Well she just wants to control…*everything*. Every little thing. And it's not that I want to control her back. I just want us to be like, you know, a little two-person democracy where each of us gets a chance, and we each have a say in things. I mean, with the menu thing, I can't even remember what it's like to order what I really want—a long time ago I just sort of gave up, and nowadays I just automatically let her order my meal too, but the whole time I feel resentful. And then I spend a lot of my day just managing that resentment, trying not to explode at her."

"You want to be with someone who doesn't try to control everything."

"Right."

"Okay. So we have to look for seeds that you've been planting yourself, for having this happen to you. We have to be detectives, in a way, because the seeds for what you see her doing are going to be a lot smaller than what she's doing.

"So tell me: Is there anyone, anywhere, in your life that you tend to try to control?"

Sam stares off into space; a *long* pause ensues, which usually means that a person has found something.

"Yeah, yeah," he nods. "I mean, it's at work. I make people check in with me more often than they have to, when they're working on a project for me. To be honest, it's really just more that I feel a little threatened if they do a good job without my being involved somehow.

"So how does it work?" he asks then. "Like, do I have to go to Dawn and confess to her that I've been doing exactly the same thing?"

"You could," I nod, "but it's not really necessary. The nice thing about the Diamond Cutter system is that we can clean up our messes without having to confront the person that we have the mess with.

Use Third Party Loops

"Instead, you can use what we call a Third Party Loop. Dawn bugs me by being a *big* control freak, so I conduct a small investigation into my own life to see where I'm being a *little* control freak with somebody else—with a third party. I try really hard to change my behavior with this person, and that loops back to Dawn, and changes how she acts with me.

"The best thing here is that there's no confrontation with her: you don't need to talk to Dawn, because the way you see her treating you isn't coming from her, and talking to her isn't going to help. I mean, you might as well try discussing her control thing with the front of your refrigerator, for all the good it's going to do.

"Not only that, but you are freed from all the decisions you'd have to make otherwise. That is, for years probably you've been mulling over whether you should just grab the menu out of her hand, and scream that you're perfectly capable of ordering your own veggie burger; or whether sending her silent poisonous vibes over and over will suddenly sensitize her to how you feel.

"In the Diamond Cutter system, we ignore both these two choices: both are bad, because neither of them works all the time. We just plant the seed for what we want, by being careful not to be a control freak with other people in our life. Properly planted and tended, this seed *must* and *will* grow into a Dawn who treats us as an equal partner.

"And the cool thing is that we save all the wear and tear on our mind and emotions that results from agonizing over two possible responses to her overcontrol. That time and that mental space is now freed up for more productive thoughts."

"Like thinking about what *I* want for lunch," smiles Sam, reaching for the menu.

Question 38

I really enjoy having a girls' night out with my friends every week or so, but it really seems to bother my husband to be left at home by himself. Any karmic solution?

Kelly asked me this question at a prayer program we were having with some Muslim friends in Phoenix. Left unspoken between us was the fact that she was there only after quite a bit of negotiation with her husband Arthur, who was now standing over at the refreshment table.

Back at Question 17 we talked about the fact that there are something like 84,000 different possible negative emotions. And we said that the Buddha narrowed this down to a Top Ten list so that we could focus on the most serious and prevalent of these emotions. Kelly's problem is Number 8.

"What's that mean?" she asks. "What's Number 8?"

"It's a very strange habit that all of us have—the ancient Tibetans said that it was so bad that most of us have some form of Number 8 going on almost all day.

"I mean, you hear that one of your friends just got a promotion at work. They're going to have more money now for the things that they and their family really need; they'll be able to get caught up on the car payments, and enjoy an occasional evening out at a restaurant.

"And instead of being *happy* for them, you feel somehow irritated." I pause and lose myself in a thought that I whisper out loud: "I wonder why that is?"

"Why we feel unhappy when something good happens to somebody else?" asks Kelly.

"Right," I say. "I mean…why is that? Why don't we just feel happy that somebody else has managed to find a tiny bit of happiness in a world that can be so tough and disappointing?"

Kelly shrugs. "I guess we feel jealous," she begins, but then her voice trails off, and she gives it some more thought. "In a way," she continues, "it sort of calls back to a more basic problem. I mean, if we're unhappy that somebody else got something because *we* didn't get it, then it must be that we feel disconnected from them in some way."

"How so?" I ask.

"I mean," she says pensively, "I can only be unhappy that you got something if I see you as fundamentally separate from myself. If I felt very connected to you—if I even felt that somehow you and me were one—then I don't think it would be possible to have Number 8.

"That is, the closer I am to you, or to being you, then the happier I feel every time something good happens to you. If instead I feel *unhappy* that you've gotten something good, then it must mean that I see you as separate from myself."

I nod; I hadn't thought of that. And it brings my mind around to an old idea from about 12 centuries ago—the idea of a common enemy.

"There was this Buddhist saint from India," I say, "named Shantideva. He said that the closer we feel to others, the more we view unhappiness as a common enemy. That any time anybody in the entire world ekes a tiny bit of happiness out of life, it is a blow to the unhappiness which plagues us all.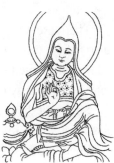

"It's nice to think of it that way—that we are all at war, all the time, with one big unhappiness that hurts us all."

"And calling something an enemy," muses Kelly, "implies that it can one day be defeated. For everybody."

"Exactly," I nod.

"So how is this going to get me a night out with the girls without coming home to a grumpy man afterwards?" she asks.

"You know the drill," I answer. "Whatever you want, plant a seed for it by providing the same thing to someone else, first. Whatever you don't want, stop that seed by stopping things of the same kind that you do to others on a much smaller level—since whatever you see being done to you has come from a much smaller seed than you yourself planted, in the past."

Kelly thinks for a minute. "So I must sometimes be unhappy—in a small way—that others around me get what they want; which makes Arthur unhappy that I would get what I want, which is a night out with my girlfriends."

"Right."

"So I have to look into my daily life, and figure out times and places where I'm doing this kind of thing myself?"

"You could do that," I agree, "but I think it's often a lot more fun and productive to go at it from the positive side. There's this thing they have in Tibet called a Celebration Meditation—I think that would be just the thing."

Kelly wrinkles her nose. "Meditation—sitting on a cushion on the cold floor, with your knees throbbing pins and needles. Something that's supposed to calm your mind but becomes just another guilt trip to disturb your mind: Oh! I'm a bad person! I didn't do my meditation this morning!"

I chuckle a bit; she's so right! "That kind of meditation, sort of a strict daily practice, has its own rewards, like exercising on a regular basis. Thing is, you're more likely to do your exercise if it's something you really enjoy anyway. Maybe you can force yourself to do 50 pushups and 50 situps a day, which can be really repetitive and boring. Or you can get just about the same amount of exercise if you go out riding bikes on a pretty country road with a good friend—and it's a lot more fun. That's what Celebration Meditation is all about.

"There are a lot of really sweet meditations that you can do just before you go to bed; this is one of them. So yes, oftentimes we feel bad when someone else gets something good that we didn't; but that's just a matter of habit, an old, habitual way of thinking. And we can turn it around.

"So forget the meditation cushion and the cold floor. Come home from work, have a nice dinner, take your bath and then if you want watch a little TV. When you're ready to go to bed, sit on the edge of the mattress or even lean back, and just stare at the ceiling and let your mind wander.

"Except let it wander towards the good things that you know have come to other people in the last few days. Be happy that Annie went out on a nice date; that Nick is doing well in school training for his new career; that a holiday is coming up, and people all over the country will have a day off.

Celebrate others' successes

"If you just do this Celebration Meditation a little bit for a few days a week, you'll find that being happy for others becomes a new habit. You'll catch yourself at the grocery store smiling at a child who's having a good time with her mom; you'll enjoy listening to a warm exchange between the cashier and a working man buying a pack of beer at the local convenience store. You become a happier person.

"You'll sleep well, because your mind is in a happy place as you're drifting off to sleep. And you wake up peaceful as well. The mind is particularly vulnerable and open as we fall asleep; now, as we put our head on the pillow, we're consciously rejoicing in other people's good fortune—instead of worrying about all the things that went wrong today.

"This plants a powerful seed to see others take joy in our own good fortune. Arthur..." and we see him detach himself from the refreshments and head back our way, "...will begin to enjoy how happy your girls' night out makes you. And that makes for more fun after you get home!"

Kelly smiles up at Arthur—it seems like the bedtime meditation might be even more of a celebration than we planned.

Question 39

I know it sounds strange, but my wife seems to get jealous if I'm deeply engrossed in anything—a book, or my computer work—and she finds ways to come and interrupt me, which really makes me irritated. How karmically can I get her to be happy when I'm deep into something I enjoy?

This is a lot like Kelly's question that we just covered, but it gives us a chance to go a little further into how to work on these kinds of seeds. The question, as you can guess, is pretty common—it could also apply to a shopping trip, when one partner or the other is ready to move on to the food court for lunch, but the other wants another half hour looking at books or curtains. In fact, I'm sitting on a bench in a department store with Tim on a DCI tour to Tokyo when he asks me this question; his partner Claire is engrossed in picking out a pair of gloves from a huge pile offered on a table nearby.

"Ever done any meditation?" I ask, as we lean back against some kitschy Hello Kitty displays draped across the whole back of the store.

"A long time ago," he says, "some TM—I still do a little of that from time to time, helps me calm my thoughts. Then a bit of Zen, which did teach me to sit still. And lately I've tried some Vipassana, which allows me slow down if I start to get upset, say at work."

"Okay," I say. "Those are all a good start—I've noticed that people who've had some experience in meditations like those definitely do better when they move on to the classical meditations which are more focused on content.

"So what I would suggest is planting some seeds to see Claire feel really happy when she knows that you're engrossed in something and enjoying it—even if what you're engrossed in right then is not her, or anything that she's into at the particular moment. You can plant these seeds with a very traditional Tibetan meditation called *Tong Len,* which means *Giving & Taking."*

"Okay," says Tim, but he says it in sort of a slow way that tells me he's another one of those people who aren't too excited about meditation. I think that's sad—I mean, first we people in the West didn't know about meditation at all, and then some meditation instruction reached our countries; but somehow meditation seems to have become just one more chore in our impossibly busy days. I feel like Tim needs some clarification at this point.

"But first understand one thing," I say. "This idea about meditation—don't let it get associated in your mind with lighting some incense and sitting on the floor and struggling to ignore the pain in your knees. We need to set up an atmosphere where you can just let your mind go—let it fly—in a way which is really enjoyable to you.

"When I say 'meditation,' I want you to think how you feel when you're propped up in bed with a pillow behind your back, reading the best part of the best book you've ever read. Or sitting on the edge of the seat in a movie theater, during your favorite scene in your favorite film. Hey, what *is* your favorite scene in your favorite movie, anyway?"

"Oh that's easy," says Tim. "There's this obscure film called *Date with an Angel*. At some point the hero falls down unconscious in a forest, and he gets saved by this Angel, and when he wakes up in the hospital…"

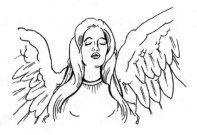

Tim stops suddenly, with this dumb smile on his face, staring up at the ceiling, remembering the best moment he ever saw on film.

"That's it!" I yell. Claire looks over for a second to see if we're okay, then dips her head back to the pile of gloves.

"That's what?" asks Tim.

"That's meditation," I enthuse. "You enjoy something so deeply, your mind is so deeply engrossed in something, that you forget what you were talking about the moment before."

Staring at the ceiling can be meditation

"What *were* we talking about?" asks Tim, sliding back to the pink world of Hello Kitty.

"How you're going to get Claire to enjoy it when you're really deep into something, rather than trying to derail it."

"Okay, yeah, a kind of meditation…"

"Yes, *Tong Len:* Giving & Taking. The part about giving is what will help you plant the seeds you need to change Claire.

"So again, let's just set up a pleasant spot in your house. You're home from work and you've changed into some more comfortable clothes, had a bite to eat. The layers of stress from the day are dropping off, you're sitting in your favorite easy chair.

"Lean back, scrunch your legs up any way you want, prop your head on your hand, stare at the ceiling—whatever. Just *relax,* and get your mind a little dreamy.

"Let the mind wander through a list of your friends, or people at work, until someone who really needs something comes to mind." I pause to let Tim do just that.

"Okay, got it," he says.

"Do you mind if I ask who it is?"

"No, that's okay. It's somebody I know who's between jobs, and between relationships. They really don't seem to know what to do with themselves. They get bored, and cranky, and because of that they begin to worry about things that they don't need to be worrying about."

"Okay, good. So what is it that you think they want in their life?"

"They want some sense of purpose, something to keep them happily busy, something that helps other people."

"Okay. So let's do a little *tong* meditation on them: give them what they want.

Tim starts to straighten up, and I grab his arm before he can cross his legs on the bench. "It's bedtime," I say, "and you're just going to let your mind relax, and lightly connect with this other person. No need to look like somebody sitting in a cave meditating in the Himalaya Mountains."

Tim smiles, and he gets it—he puts his elbow on the arm of the bench and sort of folds his body over towards it, gazing off somewhere towards the ceiling.

"Picture your friend," I say. "The one who needs a cause in their life. They are in their own bedroom, ready for bed. They are sitting on the edge of the bed, gazing lightly up towards the ceiling, thinking about their life.

"You are in the room too, sitting in a chair opposite them, but you're invisible—they can't see you.

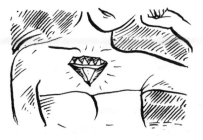

"Now imagine that there's a tiny little diamond in your chest, inside your heart. The diamond radiates a soft white light. Every time you breathe out, a little stream from this ball of light comes up your throat, and then out your nose with the breath. Concentrate on taking long out-breaths; this really calms the mind and puts it into a meditative space."

Tim nods, and closes his eyes. His breath slows noticeably.

"Focus on that soft diamond light in your chest," I say.

He's very quiet for a moment, then nods.

"Now imagine that, mixed with this light, there is an inspiration for your friend—a beautiful idea about where they want their life to go, and how to get there."

Tim is quiet for a bit longer, and then nods again.

"Now just breathe, long relaxed breaths. The diamond light, infused with life-inspiration, comes up your throat with your breath when you exhale. Watch as it leaves your nostrils."

Tim gets there, despite the noise of people in the department store.

"Okay, now make it longer," I say. "Usually when we breathe we have a mental picture of air coming in and out of nostrils, down into our lungs. But we don't much picture how the breath leaves our body, back into the air that we all breathe together.

"Now I want you to concentrate on that. Watch that stream of diamond light leave your nose, and head straight out in front of you. Try to exhale deeper and deeper, which is automatic if you try to imagine the stream of light slowly stretching farther and farther out across the room in front of you, each time you breathe out. Remember to hold on to the thought that this light is carrying upon it ideas which will help your friend out of their rut."

Tim gets even quieter; I'm happy for all the meditation he's ever tried in his life.

"Now here's the cool part. Imagine that your light-breath exits from your own nose and slowly stretches all the way across the room to your friend's nose. In the split second that it touches their nose, they happen to be taking an inhale, and so this medicine breath goes down into their own lungs.

"From there, the soft light reaches out to enfold their heart. And then suddenly they know exactly what they want to do with their life, and how it will be done. This is the Giving part of the meditation on Giving & Taking.

"Now keep your eyes closed, and try to connect with how they feel. For the first time in a long time, they feel that special joy that comes with knowing what you need to do with your life, what you can do to help others.

"And this is the part that will help you see Claire be happy when you are deep into something you enjoy. That is, spend a few moments to really enjoy how happy you've made your friend. Be very quiet for a few more moments and be happy in their happiness. That's all."

I try to sit as quietly as I can. I can feel Tim deeply quiet, I can almost see the seeds being planted in his mind. Claire looks over, curious, her eyes already somehow more supportive.

IN-LAWS

Question 40

My wife often drags me to family events, where I'm forced to sit with her parents and brothers and make small talk for hours. What's the karma to get her to understand how tiring this is for me, and to let me stay home sometimes?

I got this question at a little Mexican restaurant on Highway 17, in some deserted spot between Phoenix and Flagstaff. Samuel and his partner Viv were visiting the Grand Canyon from Finland; he had come to a talk in Europe a few years before. The owner of the restaurant, an old friend who comes from Guatemala and whose name is Jose, whispers in my ear, "These amigos—they're not from around here, are they?" I smile.

"There's a couple of ways we could go at this," I say to Samuel. "I mean, there are just plain seeds for consideration—for having someone consider your feelings, whenever you're doing anything together.

"But I think it would be more fun if we tried another angle. You know about the seed thing, right?"

Samuel nods; as is often the case, Viv is looking a little put out that the question was asked in the first place, but I know that once the conversation gets rolling she'll see how she can use the seeds too. The amazing thing is that—if two people both understand how to plant and care for seeds—then by some miracle of the world they both get what they want, even if what each one wants seems to be the opposite of what the other one wants.

"So let's take the case of beauty," I say. "What are the seeds for beauty: to see beauty around us, to have people see us as beautiful?"

"Hmm," says Samuel. "From what I understand, there are two different kinds of seeds, in general. When you want something to happen in your life, most of the time the kind of seed you need to plant is self-evident. You want to make money, you help others make money.

"And then some seeds are not so obvious. In the case of beauty, the seed is unexpected: to see beauty, and to be seen as beautiful, we need to watch our temper. The more we can be patient in situations where an untrained person might get angry, the more beauty we find ourselves in."

"Right," I nod. "And remember, the beauty is coming back to us through the seeds—we're not just saying that a person who avoids getting angry has fewer wrinkles on their face. The whole web of reality around them actually shifts, and what was not beautiful before becomes now, truly, beautiful."

Viv nods, and I can see from her face that she has grasped the difference. Not so sure about Samuel, but he'll catch up.

"So now tell me," I continue. "Can you guess what the seed would be to *hear* something as beautiful, and meaningful?"

"I don't know what you're talking about," grumps Samuel. He's visibly nervous that I'm trying to talk him into the joys of small talk with in-laws. "The things that people say are either important, or they're just small talk. It's pretty obvious which is which."

I don't say anything, I just pull a pen out of my pocket and wave it in his face.

"That's the cool part about the seed thing—that's the part I really like," Viv suddenly breaks in. "I mean, it means that every way we see every thing there is is coming from us.

Everything there is is coming from us

"Two of us can be listening to somebody talk, and the person next to me might be hearing what they say as meaningless small talk. At the same time, every single word can be striking me as something deeply profound. And the cool thing—the emptiness thing, I guess you could call it—is that 'by themselves' their words are just sounds, neither meaningful nor mundane." She stops suddenly, with a kind of awe on her face.

"Which is to say," she says slowly, "that nothing is even…itself, by itself. You could even go so far to say that a pen is not a pen." She looks at me to see what I think. I nod, but carefully—you could get a lot of misunderstanding, which could lead to a lot of thoughtless behavior, if you didn't get that last part just right.

"The point that always keeps us on the right track," I add, "is that a pen is not a pen until our seeds make it a pen, and those seeds always come from sharing with others, from being kind to others."

Back to Sam—I can see from his face that he's with us.

"I'll take a shot," he smiles. "I will hear the talk and other sounds in my life as beautiful, as meaningful, if I take care to speak kindly to others. Every time I feel like my in-laws are smothering me in small talk, it's my fault.

"If I want to fix it, I need to look into my own day-to-day life and see where I can speak more kindly, with more encouragement; more sweetly, to everyone around me."

I feel how the mood around the table has shifted entirely, into a very positive energy. This is what always happens when partners really get the seed thing—people start taking responsibility for their own lives, people are empowered to turn their lives to a new and beautiful course. Even in the moment, that wisdom is so powerful that the seeds around the table are shifting from moment to moment, sweeter and sweeter.

Jose walks over from behind the counter and plops down a big plate of sopapillas—Mexican pastries dripping with so much honey that no human being can eat one without spilling goo all over their lap.

"On the house!" he beams sweetly.

Question 41

I work a lot to make my husband's parents happy with me and our relationship, but he never reciprocates, and never shows respect or attention to my Mom especially. What karma do I need to do for him to see that we both have families we care about?

You may have noticed that a lot of these questions are asked in restaurants, but I don't want you to get the wrong idea—I'm not eating all the time, it's just that when couples need to talk about their relationship, I think it's often more relaxing over some cocoa or a nice salad, out where we can be around other people too, and appreciate having them in our lives.

Anyway, I got this question from Mina in a really nice outdoor balcony café in Kiev, in the Ukraine, where we were doing a DCI program. I shooed my two assistants off to another table so we could speak frankly. Mina's husband Rob was out with the ground staff looking for a weird power cord that we needed for the sound system at the talk that night. I look over at Mina, enjoying the open air.

"So look, Mina, what's like the best book ever written about the karmic seeds?"

She smiles. One thing about Mina, she knows her stuff—she has really taken the time to educate herself about these things, to do it right.

"Master Vasubandhu's *Treasure House of Higher Knowledge,*" she replies quickly. "And we're talking mainly the fourth chapter."

I nod. "So what then are the two most obvious ways to plant a seed in your mind—a seed to see Rob show a little more respect towards Mom?"

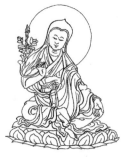

"Anything we say in our words, or anything we do in our actions; these are the most obvious ways of planting seeds," she rattles from rote.

"Right," I say. "And the kind of seed we want to plant here is…"

"A seed for him to show respect; which means, of course, that I have to show some respect myself."

"Towards...?"

"Well, it could be towards anyone; it doesn't necessarily have to be towards someone's parents, or specifically Rob's parents. If I just take care to show respect to my supervisor at work, for example, then I'll still be planting seeds to see Rob show more respect towards my Mom."

I nod. She's got the basic idea down pat. But we could go further.

"Yes, so, you think of respectful things you can say to people; or you think of actions which demonstrate respect for them. But what makes you do *that?*"

Mina does that staring-up-at the ceiling thing, towards the outdoor umbrella which covers us both at the table.

"Well I guess," she says, "it's just like Master Vasubandhu himself said, in his book. The things that we say, and the things that we do, do plant karmic seeds in our mind, to see the same thing around us later on.

"But there's always a state of mind that comes just before we do or say something: we *think* to say it, or we *think* to do it. Sort of an intention, or a motivation."

"And the kind of seed that this thinking plants..." I prompt.

"...is the most powerful," she finishes. She looks across to me, with a question in her eyes. "So what are you saying? What do you want me to... *think?*"

I look out across the street, to the buildings of downtown Kiev—sort of a mix of that atrocious Soviet non-architecture of the cold war, and some pretty cool places going up nowadays, which fit in nicely with the really old classical buildings.

"You get it," I say. "Doing something, saying something, these are just secondary seeds. But they're easy to track. We make a commitment to give an enthusiastic answer to our supervisor, at least once a day, when they ask us to do something. We promise to show up 15 minutes early to work, every day for the next two weeks, and ask if they have any special needs from us that day.

"These are things we can watch or hear ourselves do—easy things. And it's true that if you say and do them, you will gradually see Rob treat your Mom differently."

Mina cocks her head. "And is there...any way...a little faster than *gradually?*" she asks.

I nod. "You were right about what you said before. If you think about it, we are always planting two sets of seeds, any time we do or say anything at all. Because first we have to *decide* to act or speak, and that decision itself plants powerful seeds, *even if we never get a chance to actually do or say what we decided to do.*

"That is, of course it's much more powerful if we first intend to act, and then act—double seeds, in a way. But when we do fix our intention to act, that in itself is an action which takes place deep down within the human mind: *very close to the core of the mind,* which is where the seeds themselves are stored."

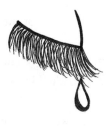

Mina points to her head, but I point to my heart. "The Tibetans say that the storehouse of the seeds, the core of the mind, is here, at the heart. Just in front of the backbone, within a channel that runs up and down the spine. Deep down inside there is a tiny sphere, a tiny drop no larger than the tip of a needle. It's called the 'indestructible drop,' and within it are all the seeds we've ever planted that haven't gone off yet.

"Every year, you create just about 2 billion new seeds inside this tiny space. And every seed you create doubles in its power every 24 hours while it's waiting for a chance to open. So there are billions upon billions of seeds there, stored at the core. And when you *decide* to say or do something, just before you do, then tons of new seeds are inserted directly into that tiny storehouse.

"And so the *reason* why you do something is actually more powerful than the doing."

Mina nods. "It makes sense. And it also explains a lot of other things. On the outside, people look like they're doing the right things, but we have no idea what they're thinking on the inside—why they're doing the things that they're doing, even when they're doing the right things."

I nod, and wait a second for her to work it out.

"So I…" she begins, "I have to figure out what it is that *triggers* respect in me, whenever I am respectful. That's the very essence of the seed to see respect around me."

"And faster than *gradually,*" I add. "Now come back to this specific seed: the seed to see Rob be more respectful to your Mom. Would your being respectful to *his* parents be a good seed?"

Mina nods, but she's already gone beyond that. Her eyes light up, and I know she's got it. "It would be good to act respectfully towards them—say, to be sure to buy them a nice present on their birthday. And it would be good to speak respectfully to them—to refer to them as 'Mom' or 'Dad' in a sweet way whenever I see them. But how I *think* about them..." she stops dead. Her mental jaw drops.

"But I *don't* respect them," she blurts. "I want to *show* that I respect them, I want to *look like* I respect them, but deep down I don't really respect them."

She gazes off towards a stand of trees, behind the balcony. "And that's the real reason why Rob doesn't respect my Mom," she concludes softly.

Now truth is a good thing, but if we don't use it for something it doesn't count for much. "Why *don't* you respect them?" I ask.

"Well...I guess...I guess that I just never thought about it much," Mina confesses. "I mean, if I think about it for a moment, there are lots of things to respect about them. But I guess the biggest thing is just how much they love people—I love how they love people, everybody."

There, we finally got to it. The root of respect, and it's love. "So Mina, what's the action plan here?"

She smiles. "Why, I guess, I just keep thinking of reasons why I respect Rob's parents—really respect them, a respect born in love for them. I have to *love* his parents—really love them, not just in words or actions, but in my most private thoughts, down close to that pindrop storehouse of the seeds.

"I have to love them as much as I love my own Mom...and then Rob will love her too, and I will see him respect her."

We finish off our lattes, I collect my assistants, and we walk down towards the town square of Kiev to buy a little something special for the elderly lady back home that I plant my own seeds with.

EQUALITY

Question 42

I don't feel like my relationship with my partner has any equality. As far as our finances, he can go out and buy a motorboat without asking me, but he gets mad if I bring home a new blouse without consulting him first. I'm not supposed to glance at a cute guy sitting at a nearby table in a restaurant, but he can draw my attention to a cute miniskirt walking down the sidewalk anytime. What is the karma for having equal rights in a relationship?

Juana is asking me this question on a DCI tour of Latin America; we're sitting in a waiting room off of a partly open-air auditorium in Guadalajara, Mexico, and workmen are putting up a thousand chairs outside… one of our largest talks ever. I think for a 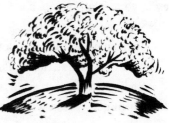 moment, looking outside at the jacaranda trees, in their full lavender bloom.

"So let me ask you something," I start.

"Okay." She looks a bit defensive already; I go slow.

"Have you guys taken any vacations lately?"

She looks up and counts. "Three, in the last two years or so."

"Where did you go?"

"Once to Mexico City; then Colombia, the coast. Last time we just hopped down to Vallarta."

"Why those particular places?"

"Mexico City to take in some of the walled gardens there, the old Colonial style, with the porches that have the arches and pillars; I love those places, and the mariachis that are usually hanging around. Colombia, we did a little yoga retreat up on the Caribbean side. And then in Vallarta we got out of town and went up north to one of the smaller beaches, just sat and swam and cooked a lot in one of those houses with the kitchen outside."

"So…how did you find out about these places?"

"Well, Mexico City because my sister is there; and Colombia because I met the yoga teacher on a trip to New York; and Vallarta I just found on the internet."

"And you did all the arrangements for all these places?"

"I did," she says with a bit of pride. "And sometimes it took a lot of work!"

I nod and slip in the question I really want to ask. "So…you picked all these places, right?"

"Sure," she answers, without thinking. "I always pick the places."

I stay quiet for a minute. It's almost always better to let people figure things out themselves.

Juana suddenly looks a little sheepish. "You mean me being the one who picks out the vacation spots and restaurants, and places like that, has planted some kind of seed for…"

"For you to see Gustavo deciding he gets to decide who spends the money in your relationship, and who gets to look at somebody cute walking down the other side of the street."

Juana pauses and considers for a moment. "But I've been deciding on the vacations for years…how many seeds is that? How long will they last?"

She's really smart, and she has a good heart, so I don't mince words with her. "Okay look, one time somebody asked the Buddha himself how many seeds we plant in a given amount of time. There weren't any clocks around 25 centuries ago, so fingersnaps were pretty much the shortest moment of time you could conveniently show somebody.

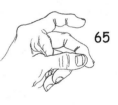

65

"Buddha snapped his fingers and said, 'There are 65 tiny moments inside the time it takes me to snap my fingers like that. And when you do or think or say anything, you're planting 65 seeds a second.'

"So figure—what—in the last few years you've spent maybe 3 or 4 full eight-hour days deciding the details of the vacations without Gustavo getting any say in the matter…I'd guess you've planted something like…" I pause to do the math in my head, "like over a hundred thousand seeds."

"Which will grow as?" she raises an eyebrow.

"Which will grow as him deciding, without asking you, how you guys spend your money."

I clear my throat. "But…it doesn't exactly end there," I add.

"What do you mean?"

"I mean, mental seeds are a lot like seeds in the ground. The minute they get planted—and assuming they get water and the other stuff they need—they start expanding, splitting and spreading out. The Tibetan scriptures say that a seed doubles in power every 24 hours between the time that it's planted and the time that it opens up into something you experience in the world around you—something like Gustavo!"

"So what's that got to do with me?" says Juana nervously.

A mental seed doubles in power every 24 hours

"Well, I mean," I say gently, "just from those last few vacations, you've now got something like a *hundred million* seeds floating around there in your head, for Gus to decide a lot of what happens in your life for the next few decades or so."

Juana looks a little stunned, and then asks the question that I've been waiting for.

"Uh, so is there any way to just…like…*cancel* those seeds, get them out of my brain, whatever?"

I shake my head. "Lord Buddha was pretty insistent that nobody could just cancel the seeds in your head. The Diamond Cutter system is fair—completely fair, complete justice…and you always get exactly what you deserve, good or bad."

I pause to let that sink in, and then add quietly, "Except…"

"Except what?" Juana jumps on it.

"Except there *is* a way to…sort of…mess with your seeds, kind of short-circuit them, in a way. I mean, they still go off, but not at all with the power they were supposed to have."

Juana waves her hand in a way that says "Ok then, let's hear it!"

I dive in. "It comes from an ancient book, something called *The Book of the Four Powers,* spoken by the Buddha himself, 25 centuries ago. This teaching gives four steps, four powerful steps, that you can use to work on your old bad seeds.

"The first power is called **Review.** You just review everything you know about how the seeds work—how they create the world and the people around you. This first power is even more powerful if you throw in some strong intention, which is really easy. Just think to yourself: 'If I figure out how to change Gustavo in a really positive way, then all my friends will get inspired to try fixing their own partners by using seeds, and I might end up living in a world where everyone treats their partner equally!'

"The second power is called **Intelligent Regret.** You've already got that!" I spout cheerfully.

"How so?"

"I mean, the moment you're aware that your old bad seeds are sitting there inside you, multiplying like a cancer, then it's no big jump to regretting them—to wishing you hadn't put them there in the first place.

"And this regret isn't some kind of guilt complex: 'Oh, I'm such a bad person!' Instead it's simply *intelligent regret:* 'I messed up putting those seeds inside of me, and now I must calmly do whatever I have to do to short-circuit them.'

"Which brings us to the third power: **Restraint.** This is the power that does the most to deflate the bad seed—so remember this one well. And it's just a little commitment to yourself that you'll stop planting this kind of seed in the future. That is, you promise yourself that you won't fail to seek Gustavo's input on the next vacation."

"Uh," wonders Juana, "does that apply to *all* the vacations we ever take again?"

"Better if it does," I nod. "But it's not the same with every bad seed you're ever trying to disable. If you've been getting mad at Gustavo every once in a while, that's not a great seed at all. But if you make too much of a commitment about it—if you swear you will never get mad at him again..."

"Then you'll just plant another bad seed," smiles Juana wryly. "Because you'll be sure to break this commitment, sooner or later."

"Right," say I. "So the great lamas of history—the ones who have passed this teaching about the Four Powers down through the lineage—always tell us to set a time limit, something realistic: 'I won't get mad at Gustavo for the next 24 hours, no matter what he does.'

"And this takes us to the fourth and final power: the power of **a Make-up Activity.**" I think for a moment and continue on, "Juana, I don't know what the custom is here in Mexico, but when I was growing up in America there was this thing in our elementary school called Detention."

Juana shakes her head. "What's that?"

"Okay, so...all through my early school days I had really incredible teachers, except for one: Mr. Riley.

"Mr. Riley was my 7th grade teacher, and he was the worst! He taught us U.S. History and we had to sit through these incredibly dull lectures every day, hearing about how Americans had invented everything ever invented, and how our country had always been perfectly right in every war in history, etc etc.

"So this is driving me crazy and I start making little paper airplanes under the desk while he talks." I take a piece of paper and begin folding it into the shape of a little plane.

"He's droning on and on, and I'm thinking what a cool little jet airplane I've just created. I forget I'm in his class and I'm just thinking to myself, 'I bet this thing can really fly!'

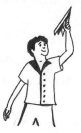

"I stand up suddenly, right there in the middle of the Civil War, and throw the paper plane towards the front of the room. It hits Mr. Riley right in the chest. His mouth drops open. All the other kids' mouths drop open too.

"Dead silence. And then Mr. Riley glares at me and says one word: 'Detention.'

"What that means," I explain, "is that I have to show up in Mr. Riley's room after school. I have to sit there—*detained,* like a criminal—for an hour or two and do some stupid thing that he tells me to do.

"In this case, he stands me up in front of a chalk board and makes me write 'I will not throw paper airplanes in class' like 200 times. Then he has to check that it looks nice and straight and then I have to erase it and do it over again, 200 times more—and then over and over again until my arms are about to drop off."

Juana nods. "Understood. We had something similar here in Guadalajara when I was growing up. But what's this got to do with getting Gus to treat me equally?"

"Ah yes." I struggle back to the point, which for me is sometimes a long round trip. "You need to do some kind of make-up activity: something to balance out the negative seeds that you've been planting.

"Notice that in the third power we are promising *not* to do something again: we are promising to restrain or control ourselves from doing this kind of thing in the future.

"With the fourth power, we're promising *to do* something, to balance out the negative. You've already made a commitment not to ignore Gustavo's wishes for your next vacation. Now you have to come up with something positive that will balance what you did before.

"And remember the 'Third Party' thing: the thing you do to balance out the negative doesn't have to be with Gustavo himself. It could be with anyone else, because the good seed will come around to your relationship with Gus just the same, if you send it that way with your intentions. So…do you have any ideas?"

Juana thinks for a bit, eyes gazing up in that nice unfocused natural way of meditation, of daydreaming.

"Okay, I've got something," she says with determination. "I visit my mom twice a week, and usually bring her something I've cooked. But come to think of it I usually decide what it will be. How about if, for the next three weeks, I call her up the day before and ask her what she'd like me to cook?"

"Great," I say. I glance through the windows and see that the space outside is filling up fast, and pretty soon I'll have to stand up in front of a thousand Spanish speakers and try to say something that will help them live their lives. The butterflies in my tummy start flapping. "And remember to send that seed to Gus, so you see him start to treat you more equally in your relationship.

"Anything else?" I ask.

Juana smiles. She can see my mind has slipped outside already. "Good luck," she says, and I know it's for both of us, equally.

The Four Powers for stopping old bad seeds

1) Think about the pen: Remember where everything is coming from

2) Strong decision to stop this seed before it multiplies inside of you

3) Make a promise not to make the same mistake again

4) Do something positive to balance the karma

SEX, PART TWO

Question 43

My boyfriend really enjoys oral sex, but sometimes it makes me feel dirty, and I'm not sure if it's a good thing to do. What's the karmic take on this?

Robyn is a nurse from Nevada who has shown up at one of our 10-day intensive retreats in the forest in northern Arizona. I don't usually have time to meet personally with everyone who comes, but I try to cover anybody who has what they consider a major challenge in their life, something they need to talk about *now*. I smile a bit about this particular Major Challenge.

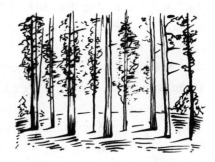

"Maybe it would help," I begin, "if we talk about the idea of right and wrong in the Tibetan tradition. And then we can try to apply it to this particular question."

"Seems reasonable," Robyn agrees.

"Okay. So you know about the seeds, right? How everything that we ever do, or say, or even just think is recorded inside of our own mind, in the form of a seed."

"I'm pretty clear on that." Robyn is no-nonsense level-headed clinical, the kind of person you'd want to be your nurse next time you need one.

"Alright. So the way that the Tibetans decide whether something is right or wrong is really interesting. If a thing you do plants a seed which opens up later as something that hurts you, then doing that thing is considered wrong. If a thing you do plants a seed that opens up later as something that brings you happiness, then doing that thing is right.

"So the decision of what is moral is connected to happiness itself. An action is *moral* if—in the end—it brings you happiness. And an action is *not moral* if it inevitably brings you suffering."

Robyn's forehead creases up a bit while she works out the implications. "That's really interesting," she begins. "Normally you'd think that an action is immoral, or unethical, when it hurts someone else. But here you're saying that it's immoral if it hurts *me*."

"Right," I nod, "but of course the two are connected. According to the Diamond Cutter Principles, anything you do that hurts someone else plants a seed that is going to hurt you. And the same with helping somebody else. I guess the point is that it's a lot easier to be moral if you know that being immoral—hurting someone else—is really just hurting yourself."

"Makes sense," she nods. And then a pause, and I can see the question in her mind: "So how does this apply to oral sex?"

"Okay," I say, "so deciding whether having oral sex with your boyfriend is okay or not really depends on deciding whether or not oral sex is going to plant a seed which comes back to hurt you later."

"And that depends," she makes the connection immediately, "on whether it causes harm to somebody else when the seed is planted."

Robyn sits with that for a while and comes right to one of the most important points in any discussion of this type. "I don't think my boyfriend thinks that oral sex would hurt him—that's clear. It makes him feel good; he really enjoys it. But there's lots of things that people do—drink liquor, or overeat at the dinner table—that feel good to them and hurt them at the same time.

"So I guess what I'm really asking is if there is any downside to the oral sex that my boyfriend enjoys. If there isn't, then I'm willing to do it, just to make him happy—even if I don't enjoy it so much myself."

I think this over for a minute. In the many years of my geshe training I had the opportunity to learn thousands of pages of ancient scripture from my dear teachers. People often assume that if there are over 100,000 wonderful ancient books in the Tibetan tradition, then every question you could ever think of must be covered. But an ancient opinion on oral sex is pushing it a bit—sometimes you just have to figure out a specific case by going to the general principles behind it, or by thinking carefully about what your own personal teacher might have said about it. I decide to combine the two.

"I think there's an upside," I begin, "and I think there could be a downside. That is, I think there could be a case where offering your partner oral sex—just because they like it—could plant a good seed, and bring you more happiness later. And I can also imagine a case where the same action could plant a bad seed, and bring you pain later.

"That is, the scriptures say that we have to be careful with activities which might be addicting—and sex is powerfully addicting. It's not that it's wrong, just that it's powerful; and we have to watch our motivation carefully around it. The test would be if we want some kind of sex so strongly that it would make us hurt someone else to get it.

"And so making your boyfriend happy would be a good thing; but doing something that increases his desire to the point where it might become an addiction is a bad thing. In the end you probably have to watch that he stays gentle and considerate about wanting it, and help him stay that way—help him not to hurt himself."

I think for a moment and decide that Robyn is ready for one more step here. "But let me ask you one last question on this. You know about seeds, and you know that they create both the people and the situations around you in your life." She nods.

"So what would be the seeds to see your boyfriend treat oral sex in a respectful and enjoyable way; and what would be the seeds to see him be addictive and unkind about demanding it of you?"

I see the understanding light up in her eyes. "If I see a person in my life who wants things in an addictive way, it's because I've been the same way myself. And if I see them simply enjoying something in a clean, kind way, then that's again for the very same reasons."

"Meaning," I say, "that if you needed to, you could change how he wants you, just by changing how you want things from other people in your life. That is, be careful how you interact with others to fulfill your own hopes and needs—make sure you're not using them, make sure there's a feeling of mutual consideration.

"Now give me an example," I check the time, "and then we're going to have to get to class!"

Robyn thinks for a moment. "There's a woman at work," she says. "I'm her supervisor, so it's true that she's supposed to do whatever jobs I choose to give her. But I think sometimes I push her a little too hard—beyond what's good for her, and beyond what she's required to do—just because I want to look good to my own boss.

"So in a way I'm sometimes putting her in an uncomfortable situation…"

"Which is not so different from the one that my boyfriend puts me in," she smiles knowingly. I nod, and we run. She knows where to take it from here.

Question 44

Karmically, what's the best form of birth control?

This is, not surprisingly, one of the most common questions that people ask me, all over the world. Tibetan lamas—at least the ones who trained me—approach the issue with a simple practicality which, to me, seems quite logical. This particular time the question is coming from a friend named Steve, on a twisting drive through the Swiss countryside to get to a talk for

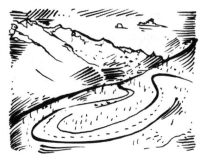

some bankers in Zurich. He and Susan are already married, and I know that children aren't part of their plans, at least for the next few years.

"I'm going to tell you," I begin, "how my own lama used to answer this question. I think this is a personal issue which each person has to decide on their own—and a lot of it depends on your

own cultural and religious upbringing; each person's answer will perhaps be different. But I can tell you how the Tibetans see it, and I do think it will give you some perspective."

"Fair enough," he nods.

"First of all, my own lama said that there was nothing wrong with birth control—that it was alright to prevent the conception of a child. Tibetans believe that we have lived countless lifetimes, and that each time we die we enter a spirit realm which they call the *bardo,* or the 'realm inbetween.'

"We can stay in this realm for up to 49 days after we die, and then—if we are to be born as a human—our spirit enters our mother's womb. It enters at the exact moment of conception: when the sperm of the father meets the egg of the mother."

Steve thinks for a moment. "According to that idea, then life would begin at the moment of conception."

"Right," I nod. "So if you're going to do some kind of birth control, then you need to prevent conception. Doing anything to stop life after conception would be taking a life." (We'll talk more about that one at Question 74.)

"So let's look at the options. Condom?"

Steve chuckles. "As far as preventing conception in the first place, I guess they're okay."

I nod, waiting for more.

"But not so reliable," he continues. "I mean, their failure rate in actual use is something like 20%, whether the man or the woman uses one. 'Failure rate' by the way means that, in one year of use, 20% of the women will get pregnant, often because the birth control method is used sloppily. If a condom breaks or slips—which typically happens about 5% of the times you have sex—then you're both also exposed to the chance of catching AIDS or other sexually transmitted disease. I mean, is a few minutes of pleasure worth dying?

"And if a condom does fail and something happens, then you're faced with deciding whether you're going to take away a new life, or start a family. "

"Which is a huge decision," I agree. "Having children—taking care of another human being for the first 20 years or so of their life—can be one of the most profound of all spiritual practices. But obviously it's something that you want to *choose* to do, and not have it happen by accident. Any other options?"

"What about birth control pills?" Steve asks.

"Also okay," I answer, "as far as preventing conception in the first place. The failure rate here, if Susan is perfect with taking her pills regularly (and it's both your business to make sure she does)—is way down around 3%.

"But the pills do have a profound effect on the woman, and I think it's a man's responsibility to acknowledge that and do the right thing. Pills first of all affect her hormones, which is going to give her mood swings, and make life less pleasant from her side.

"Many women are going to gain weight from the pills, which is going to affect her self-esteem in many cases. But most important of all, there has been a correlation drawn between birth control pills and certain kinds of cancer, as well as blood clots.

"Other women have reported chest pains and headaches; and of course there's no protection against stuff like AIDS.

"So again, in the case of pills, you've got to think if it's all worth the downside for Susan—you've got to think about both of you."

Steve nods. "How about an IUD? I've heard of them, but I'm not exactly sure what they are, or how they work."

Okay, so you're wondering how I know all this stuff. I consider myself lucky that I lived the life of a normal American boy all through high school and college, before I ever went to the monastery. So besides having Google to help (and the answers here have been researched carefully), I am not completely without personal experience.

So I answer, "Okay, an IUD is most often a little T-shaped strip of copper which is inserted by a health professional into a woman's uterus. It's not completely clear to scientists how they work, but it seems that they act as a spermicide and prevent fertilization altogether. The failure rate for an IUD is something around 1%.

"The way the Tibetans see conception then, it seems that the IUD stops pregnancy before, so you wouldn't be harming a living being by using one. But still the chance of AIDS, etc. Other choices?"

Steve looks a little unsure. "The rhythm method? Try to time your sex really carefully?"

"Failure rate of 10% or more even if you're pretty careful," I grimace. "Not good odds. But definitely prevents conception, because for several weeks she's not fertile."

"Pulling out?" Steve tries.

"Typical failure rate of abut 25%— in a single year, one out of four people trying it will get pregnant. And no protection against AIDS and the other sexually-transmitted diseases."

"Morning-after pill?" he asks.

"Well doctors recommend using them—they are usually a pair of pills—

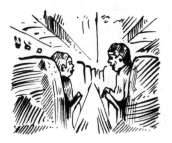

much sooner than the morning after. They sort of give a big dose of what's in the birth-control pills, to prevent an unwanted pregnancy after unprotected sex, or for example the break of a condom. If you use them right, 7 out of 8 women who would have gotten pregnant don't. Scientists aren't sure, but it looks like they work by disrupting ovulation, which would be okay as the fertilization hasn't happened yet. There's some chance that they work by refusing fertilized eggs a place to grow."

Steve's starting to look a little frustrated. "Outercourse?"

"What's that?" I ask. "Haven't heard of that one."

"You know," he says. "Just messing around. No actual intercourse—so no chance of conception."

"Any sperm that touches the outside of the vagina, even if it soaks through clothing, has some very small chance of entering the uterus and causing pregnancy...so just be careful that way.

"And there's always, you know, just plain abstinence." Then I'm recalling a conversation on a plane with my old boss at the diamond company— we're flying out to Japan to work with some customers, and suddenly he turns to me and says "Michael, can I ask you a personal question?"

"Sure," I say. We've been working together tight for something like 10 years, but he's always been pretty considerate of my personal life.

"Well, you know, there's that good-looking girl in the jewelry production department—Annie. I know she's been trying to get you out on a date..." he begins.

I roll my eyes.

"Yeah, well, you just don't seem to show any interest," he pushes on. "And I was just wondering—like...are you *gay* or anything like that?"

"Boss," I answer. "Just because you don't agree to go out with a cute girl doesn't mean you have to be gay...I mean, there are other options, you know."

He pauses for a pretty long moment and then his eyes light up. "Oh... like...you're *choosing* not to have sex?"

"Yeah," I smile. And that's an option too, if you can find the beauty in it. I'm not talking about some frustrated, bitter refusal of the opposite sex because you've had a hard time with one of them. I'm talking about a conscious decision to refrain for a certain period—maybe a week, maybe a month or two—when you *could* be having sex, but you choose not to.

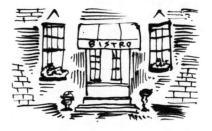

This can be an extraordinary wellspring of strength and vigor, a time to collect yourself inward and find some quiet there. Abstinence isn't the only choice, but it's certainly one that can be very inspiring and fruitful if it's done right. It's one of the reasons I personally have had so much energy to do the things I've always wanted to do.

And so I stop and do a little, gentle sales job on the subject of abstinence with Steve, just pointing it out as an option. Like most people, I think, he already appreciates how it might keep him from dissipating his inner strength for a while, and how much more focused his mind might be if he actually didn't have to *think* about sex for a month or two.

So those are my thoughts on birth control—no obvious, easy answer, but some pretty clear guidelines about what might or might not hurt another living being. We're just pulling up to the lovely bistro in downtown Zurich where I'm giving the talk to the bankers, and I throw him one last thought that my lama always used, in order to end this particular conversation.

"Rinpoche used to say," I add, "that there was nothing wrong with birth control, as long as you were preventing conception and not stopping a baby who was already conceived. But he did say something else too."

"What's that?" says Steve.

"He said that even though it wasn't wrong to prevent a birth, it was in a way denying a spirit a chance for a life—he said that life is incredibly precious, a priceless opportunity, and that if we're ready as a couple to have a child, it is one of the greatest kindnesses we can ever pay to welcome another into the world."

Steve nods. "Susan and I will keep that option open too," he smiles.

Question 45

Whenever I have sex with my husband, he just satisfies himself by ejaculating in a few minutes—he seems oblivious to the fact that it takes me a little longer to get there. What's the karma to see him be a little more attentive to my needs too?

Sandy's asking me this question during a break in one of my monthly talks in Phoenix. We've known each other for a long time, and I'm close to her husband Steve too. They're both comfortable with me answering the question, which I've heard a thousand times from others.

"I remember when I came back from my first-ever trip to India," I begin. "India was a hard place then; the poverty was extreme, hunger everywhere. And nothing was working. I was living with the Tibetan refugees in the foothills of the Himalayas. It was freezing cold and there was no fuel: no wood, no coal, no oil, and no transportation working anywhere to bring it.

"You couldn't find a single slice of bread, or anything like it. But you could buy a crude sort of flour, and the Tibetans taught me how to knead and steam a single piece of bread every morning, inside a tin can, with only a few twigs of wood.

"I spent about three months this way, learning to live on nothing, until the day before my air ticket back home to America was due to expire. Then I rushed back to New Delhi and took a bicycle rickshaw out to the airport. I remember getting on the plane, being served a hearty meal by an elegant airline attendant, the unreality of it all.

As soon as I got to my mother's house in Phoenix I went out to a grocery store; I recall walking down the aisles, slowly, completely stunned by dozens of brands of bread, hundreds of bars of deodorant.

"I walked home and went to my mother's room—she was watching TV. Strange things were happening; I was getting messages in the most unexpected ways. My mother was sick then, with cancer, and I sat down on the floor next to her bed just to keep her company.

"There was a Christian preacher on the TV—I guess normally I would have just tuned him out, but for some reason I caught some of what he was

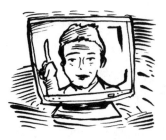

saying, and it struck me as almost a message from heaven: 'God doesn't care how you feel, God just wants you to do the right thing,' he said."

Sandy's looking at me patiently, but I can tell she's hoping that I'll get to the point. I try to head there a bit faster.

"I think the bottom line with your problem," I say, "is the bottom line for almost every problem there is. In a way, Steve is using you. Like every living creature there is, he wants to feel good—and making love with you makes him feel good.

"That's the way of almost everything we ever do with someone else: almost every human interaction is aimed at getting something for ourselves from someone else.

It is not wrong to like things, or to want the things you like

"Getting something for ourselves isn't wrong. It's not wrong to enjoy those intense moments of pleasure with our partner, any more than it would be wrong to enjoy moments standing by the sea, or looking at a sunflower. What *does* matter is *how* we enjoy these moments."

"How so?" she asks.

"Two people can feel the same pleasure, and have two completely different experiences of it. Those experiences of their pleasure decide how long the pleasure will last, and how full it is."

Sandy smiles ruefully. "Which in my case is usually not very long— never long enough to fill me up."

"Right," I agree. "So what's happening is that Steve is enjoying his time with you, and to be honest he probably has some kind of awareness that he has to try to bring you to the same climax that he reaches himself. But somewhere in there he forgets, and just ends up using you for his own pleasure. And that comes back to what the Christian preacher said on TV."

"How's that?"

"So what do you think is the karma for pleasure? What kind of seed do you have to plant to feel pleasure?"

Sandy frowns. "That's the whole problem. I mean, I've been coming to your talks for a long time—you know that. And I think I'm pretty clear on the Four Starbucks Steps: I know I need to plant seeds for the things I want, and I know the technique: the four steps that make them grow fast and strong.

"Looking at my life, I can honestly say that I enjoy taking care of other people's needs. I've always enjoyed it. I know that my own needs will be fulfilled if I take care of others' needs, and I do—I'm constantly taking care of my parents, my friends, and the people I work with. But it just doesn't seem to come back to me, and that makes me begin to doubt the whole idea of seeds."

I think a minute. "Or rather, can we say that it comes back, but it doesn't come back full? I mean, in Steve's case, you do enjoy the time with him, right? But it's never quite enough; it doesn't come to fulfillment for you."

"Exactly."

"So I think the answer here is somewhere in what the preacher was talking about. You say you *enjoy* taking care of others' needs. Do you *always* enjoy it?"

Sandy thinks for a moment. "Well no, I mean, I'm like anyone else. With my mother, for example, most of the time I do enjoy taking care of her. There are days though when I wake up a little tired and I just don't feel like going over to her house."

"And what happens then?"

"Well I call her, and make some gentle excuse; tell her I've got to run an errand for someone at work, something like that."

"And how does it make her feel?"

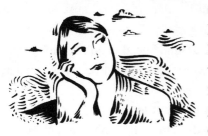

"Well she's disappointed, of course. I mean, in general we have a great relationship, and I know she's very happy with her daughter, with how much I care for her. But just sometimes she doesn't get everything she wants…" Sandy trails off, doing that gaze up at the ceiling.

"Really?" she asks then.

I nod. "Okay, here's the crux of it. You just thought of a small example where you give someone else pleasure—you fill their needs in a flow, but the flow is interrupted sometimes. It's not a big interruption, just a tiny one; but it's there.

"And then seeds you know, they grow. You serve someone else with small interruptions, and then you are served with bigger interruptions: with a never-quite-satisfied time in bed with Steve. And to change it, I think you're going to have to think about what the preacher said."

"'God doesn't care how you feel, God just wants you do the right thing,'" she quotes. "I don't quite get how that applies here, to me and Steve."

"The point is that serving others is a good thing—and it will always bring us what we hope for. But we have to look at *why* we're serving others, if we want that service to bring us *all* the pleasure we hope for; otherwise it might get..."

"...Interrupted," she fills in. "So how should I be serving others, if I want *full* pleasure coming back to me?"

"You said you enjoy serving. But then sometimes you don't enjoy it. And when you don't enjoy it, you don't do it.

"But how does your mother feel?"

"I don't know, I suppose she's disappointed."

"How do you *want* her to feel?"

"Well I want her to feel happy, of course."

"And do you want her to feel happy as much as *you* want to feel happy?"

A long silence...I can almost hear the gears turning inside of Sandy's head.

"To be honest, no" she admits. Another long silence.

"I come to her to make her happy," she says slowly, "when it makes *me* feel happy. When I'm in the mood. I mean, it's a good thing to do, it's a good seed, but I only do it when I *like* to do it—when I feel good, and when it makes me feel good." Now I see the light coming on strong, in her head.

I nod. "I've been thinking a lot about it," I confess, "because I have the same problem. I go around the world trying to teach people how to be happy, how to be successful. But then from time to time I need to do a reality check. I need to make sure that I'm doing it for *them,* and not just because it's what *I* want to do at the time.

"I mean, it's not wrong to do what you want to do. It's just that there might be times when somebody else needs something, and it might *not* be what you want to do. And then you should do it anyway, because we have a *responsibility* to make others happy.

"So it's this feeling of doing good for others, doing what they need or want (as long as it's a good thing to do, in general), because it's the *right* thing to do, whether you feel like doing it or not at the moment.

"When you're alone sometimes, when life is quiet, think about it. Think about the things that the people around you want, and think about the joy of giving them these things. Think of making others happy as your mission, and take responsibility for it, whether you *feel* like making them happy right now or not. Do the right thing, regardless of how you *feel*."

"And then Sal will shift out of himself, out of just paying attention to his own needs in bed," Sandy smiles.

"I'll give it a try."

Do the right thing, regardless of how you feel

SELF-ESTEEM

Question 46

Mostly my boyfriend and I get along really well, but every once in a while he'll say something really sarcastic to me—like "Oh, that was brilliant!" if I drop a plate on the floor. In a single moment he throws me into a big pit of self-doubt and low self-esteem. How can I stop this karma?

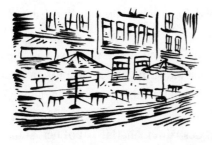

I'm writing this particular part of the book in an outside café in Sofia, Bulgaria. Our DCI teachers and I gave a talk here last night at one of the main theaters in town, and this afternoon we're headed out to the Ukraine. I got this specific question from a woman named Milena during a short break inbetween signing books and fielding questions on the Bulgarian economy.

"I had the same problem, at the beginning," I begin. "No self-confidence, scared to death of making a mistake in front of other people. A single critical sentence from somebody else would throw me off for the whole rest of the day.

"It all came to a head one day when I got a call from a radio station. We were doing a project of teaching children in the local elementary school about a fun custom in the Tibetan monasteries called *tsupa*.

"*Tsupa* is a kind of question-and-answer that Tibetan monks use for learning things quickly and thoroughly. It's more fun for kids because while you ask and answer the questions you jump back and forth and slap your hands, almost like Kung Fu, without the fighting.

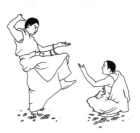

"I thought it might be really good to try it in a modern American school, and we got a government grant to do it for a few months. A radio station heard about it, and a talk-show host called me up out of the blue.

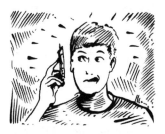

"Mr. Roach! You're *live* on KSBU! Tell us about your project to introduce ancient Tibetan educational methods into a public school in New Jersey!"

My jaw dropped, and my mouth moved up and down, but nothing came out.

"Mr. Roach! Are you there? Tell us a little bit about your project!'

Mouth still moving, but still nothing coming out.

"Ok then folks! Looks like we've lost our connection! We'll have to check in on this story later!" *Click.*

I was crushed. I sat on my bed for a while feeling like I couldn't do anything.

Milena nods. "That's exactly the feeling that I get. And in the same place: I go off to our bedroom and just sit. I might be there for an hour, just filled with some kind of despair, feeling that I can't do anything, and not even wanting to try anymore."

I can actually feel waves of that despair emanating off of her, at that very moment. "So yeah…I finally stood up, went upstairs, and told my lama what had happened. I thought he might be irritated with me, because we had been working pretty hard on the project together, and were still trying to fundraise some money to print a book written by the children. But instead of getting upset, he took me through the Four Starbucks Steps…"

I wiggle my eyebrows up and down, trying to cue Milena. She perks up and exclaims, "Oh! That's what you were just talking about, on stage. Step One would be…well, I guess you wanted more confidence, more self-esteem. So that would be your single sentence."

"Right. And the second step?"

"You have to go through all your friends and family and coworkers in your mind, and come up with somebody who's looking for the same thing: someone who wants to be more confident about themselves."

"Exactly. Step Three?"

"Take them to Starbucks!" and then she giggles, because the night before I got the usual question from someone else in the audience, asking me if I owned any stock in Starbucks. I told them no, but that the way our DCI programs were taking off in so many cities, I was thinking about buying some soon.

"Take them to Starbucks," Milena continues, "and help them out with their problem—make some suggestions."

She pauses then. "But it's not going to work," she says. "Remember that other question last night?"

I do, because it was a really good one. A woman in the audience first wanted to know why I was asking her to take someone to Starbucks and give them suggestions about finding a partner, so that she herself could plant a seed for a partner—Because if she knew how to get a partner, then she would already have one. And until she did get one, she could hardly claim to be an authority who could help anyone else get one.

"So…" I say slowly, "does a pen *work?*"

Milena nods yes.

"Does it work even if you don't understand why it works? If you've never even heard about planting seeds?"

Milena thinks for a moment. "Of course. There are people all over the world using pens who have no idea that a pen is coming from a seed in their own mind."

"So if you take a friend to Starbucks and you give them some suggestions about how to gain more confidence, will those suggestions work?"

Milena ponders for a moment or two. "I'm not sure about that. But I'm guessing the answer is that—if they have the right seeds—then my suggestions will work for them. And if they don't, they won't."

"Right," I agree. That's where the woman in the audience had gone last night: Okay, assuming I'm not an expert on this seed thing, I still do my best at Starbucks to give my friend some support. I make suggestions, but they are the kind of suggestions that don't necessarily work, because they're not altogether based on seeds. And suppose then that my friend fails to get, in this case, the partner they were hoping for. What happens to my own seeds?

"Either way," I say, "your seeds are good. 90% of the power of all seeds lies in the intention: If you do your very best to help another person get more confidence, then you inevitably begin to feel more confidence yourself.

"That's an important point to remember," I say. "Otherwise we can get disappointed, or lose our faith in the system. We try to help others, because it helps them and it helps us: it's win/win. But if they refuse the help; if even they get angry with us for trying to help; or because of their own bad seeds the help fails; then we have to relax and realize that we've done the best we could. We've planted our seeds. And there will always be others for us to help—there is no end to people who need our help." We pause for a moment and then look up at each other.

"Step Four…" we both blurt at the same moment. But I have a feeling she's not going to have a problem with that one: appreciating herself.

The Four Starbucks Steps, Again!

1) Say what it is you want in your life, in a single short sentence.

2) Plan who it is you're going to help get the same thing, and which Starbucks you're going to take them to, to talk about it.

3) Actually do something to help them.

4) Do your Coffee Meditation: as you go to sleep, think of the good things you're doing to help them.

FUN

Question 47

My partner and I used to have a lot of excitement in our relationship, but lately everything seems boring and repetitive. What's the karma for getting the thrill back?

During our DCI intensive weekends we spend a lot of time in small breakout groups, which are led by our senior staff teachers. There might be 10 or 15 of us stuffed into a little hotel room, planning these groups. And the rule of thumb for teachers is: If you're not sure how to answer a question from a participant, just say "Seeds!"

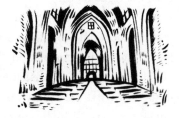

Any question can be answered with: "Seeds!"

So "Seeds!" I say, when I get this question from a friend named Claude, in a small French city called Montpelier; we've been invited to give a presentation there for over a thousand young business owners.

He frowns. "But what are the seeds for excitement in a relationship?"

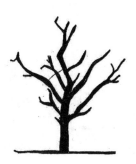

Back in Question 26, we talked about how seeds get old. "First of all, neither you nor Josephine should feel bad about the excitement fading. It's not that there's something wrong with you, or her, or the two of you together.

"The growing of a tree kills the seed that the tree comes from. The electricity in the first few years of your relationship kills the mental seeds that produced the electricity. This is, unfortunately, a natural progression in every relationship there ever was or will be. Left to itself, a relationship *must* get old; it *must* get boring.

Nothing is coming from its own side

"But remember, that's not coming from itself, any more than the pen is coming from itself. And that means that it doesn't have to be that way. If you know what you're doing, then a relationship can get *more* exciting each year, instead of less. It's possible that Josephine can turn you on, and you can turn her on, more in your tenth year together than in the first. But you're going to need the right seeds."

Claude looks at me with that patient expression that tells me, politely, that he knows all about the seeds and the Four Starbucks Steps. What he's looking for is the correlation. We talked about correlations back in Question 40, although we didn't use the word just then. Here it means that we need to figure out what the seed would be for something we want, when the seed is not so obvious. Which reminds me of Oslo.

Our DCI team was giving a presentation at the Museum for Folk Art in Hamburg, and our friends John and Liyang called us from Norway and asked if we could take a day off and fly up for an evening talk. That evening we went through the Four Starbucks Steps and then took some questions.

One young man asked, "I want kuss! What is seed?"

I cock my head and try to figure out what he means by *kuss*.

"You mean kids? You want to know the seeds for having a child?" I ask. I get this question a lot in China, but not so much in Europe. I start framing an answer where I can help him with the difference between a physical seed for a child (which is not so complicated) and a mental seed for one (which is what makes the physical seed *work*.)

"No! Not *kids*. I want *kuss!*"

"What's that like?" I ask.

"*Kuss!* You know, girl puts lips on my lips, and then…"

"Okay, okay, I got it," I say quickly. "You want to know how to get a girl to *kiss* you."

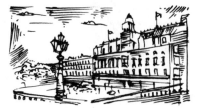

"Right!" he beams. He assumes that this is a common question covered in every Buddhist sutra over the last few millennia. I start scrambling mentally for an answer.

"Okay! Anyway, I know answer!" he breaks into this incredible smile. "I go up to Grand Hotel on Karl Johans Street! I walk in to the restaurant and kiss every girl I can find! That way I plant seeds for my girlfriend to kiss *me!*" The crowd roars its approval of this approach.

"Uh," I say, "it's not exactly like that."

And to Claude I say, "You have to think of the essence of the thing you're looking for. The essence of the spark that used to be there between you and

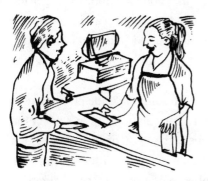

Josephine was *fun.* Plain old fun. To plant a seed for that, you'll need to bring some fun to others: to the people around you all day."

Claude looks dubious. "I mean, it makes sense, but..."

"How to do it?"

"How to do it."

"Look," I say. "Most of us are around other people all day. Friends, the people who work in the stores and other places that we visit, parents or children. And we interact with each of them.

"Just in the case of going to the store, we have a shallow interaction with the cashier. We start pulling our groceries out of the cart and putting them on the counter; the cashier is supposed to look up and say, 'Hi! How are you?' And then after we pay they're supposed to say, 'Have a good day!'

"But it's not like there's any *fun* going on between us. I mean, you tell me: How could you give the cashier some fun in this case—and plant a seed for some fun with Josephine?"

While Claude is thinking, let's say one thing. We've been talking a lot about the Four Starbucks Steps. When you try them out to achieve a certain goal in your life, it's best to stick to a single goal, working with a single person at a single Starbucks.

Sometimes though you'll want to try a different approach: many small seeds planted with many people throughout the day. A theme for the day that you return to, again and again.

"Okay, I got it," Claude pipes up.

"Let's hear it."

"I lean over the counter while the cashier's ringing up my stuff, and tell her I'm thinking to take my wife out to a movie tonight. And I want to know if she's seen any good movies that she might want to suggest. In the middle of whatever answer she gives me, I tell her no, no...we want a *dull* movie, 'cause we're gonna make out during the whole thing, and we don't want anything to distract us..."

"Uh, I guess that would work," I reply quickly. I don't know why I'm getting all this kissing karma this week. "I think that would be a lot more fun for the cashier, brighten up her day."

"And then I could ask her which aisle I'd have to go to if I want to find..."

I'm not putting you through the rest of this conversation. You get the point. It's not at all unnatural for the excitement to fade from a relationship... I mean, once you know all your partner's stories and jokes and once they know all of yours, conversation can get a little bit dry—not to mention intimacy.

As so often happens with spiritual things, the solution to the problem here is a joy in itself. If you want the thrill back in your relationship, it's never too late. Just plant the right seeds. Each and every time you have an interaction with anyone, all day long, work really hard on making it fun for both of you.

And then before you go to bed, remember to do your Coffee Meditation, reviewing every detail of all the fun you've spread today. Perhaps you can even get your partner into spreading the same kind of fun; and no matter what seeds you're trying to grow, you can both get a lot more mileage during Coffee Meditation time at night by reminding *each other* about the wonderful things you've seen the other person do in the last day or two.

That is, if you're not busy with something else.

Question 48

I love to get out of the house—to see new things and people, and especially travelling to exotic places—but my partner just considers it a disturbance and a hassle. How can I make my little couch potato more adventurous?

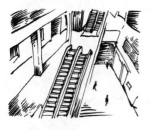 There's a cool thing in Buddhism called "skillful means." Basically it means tricking people into doing something good, and that's exactly what comes to mind when I get this question from Anna, in a waiting room before I give a talk at the MAMBA Museum of Modern Art in Buenos Aires. She and her TV crew have just finished shooting an interview with us, and she's lingering behind with a personal question, which often seems to happen.

"How can I plant a seed in him so he wants to get out?" she says.

"One thing about seeds," I begin. "You *can't* plant them in someone else. So in a way you can't 'make' anybody do anything. He has to plant his own seeds."

Anna frowns. "But I thought he was coming from me; and if he's coming from me, then I should be able to plant the seeds to see him be more active."

This time it's my turn to frown. "You can change how you see him; but when you talk about planting a seed *in* Luis, we're talking about how he's going to see himself."

"Won't those two always be the same? Won't they always match?"

"Not at all. We can perceive a movie star or a politician as being incredibly poised, and at the very same time they might perceive themselves as having panic attacks all the time."

"So I can't change how adventurous he feels?"

"I didn't say that; you can't plant a seed for him, but you can teach him how to plant a seed for himself."

Anna gives her head a good shake. "That's never going to happen. I've tried getting him interested in the seeds a few times, but he just doesn't buy it."

"So trick him."

"Trick him?"

"Yes—I had a similar sort of situation a while back. A woman with a son who is intellectually challenged. She wants to know how to help him, but when I tell her he has to plant his own seeds, she gets this look of despair.

"No problem, I say. He just has to help other children who have the same problem; maybe collect some toys and bring them to the hospital, to share with the others.

"She says that he could never make it to the hospital on his own, much less hand out the toys. I tell her just take him to the hospital, sit him down in front of another child, put her hands around his and pick up a gift together, then hand it to someone. After that, move on to the next child.

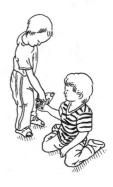

"He will plant a few seeds; no intention before, and no Coffee Meditation afterwards, appreciating his own goodness. But there will be the actual action, and this is a big part of planting a seed.

"Each seed planted this way makes a small change in his heart, his mind, his capacity for life. They build upon each other—each trip to the hospital is a little more conscious, and purposeful. In time his mind is healed."

Anna nods. "So with Luis, I do the same thing? Put my hands around his and trick him into doing something good? And what thing should he do?"

"He's pretty good with a computer, isn't he?"

"Yes—that's part of the problem, he's online almost all day."

"Alright then. Find a friend who is going on a vacation with her family. Tell Luis she's a klutz on the computer and that you promised to help her. Then get on your computer and after a while start making frustrated noises.

"Before long, Luis is sitting next to you and you're flipping through webpage after webpage of romantic Caribbean vacations and scuba-diving trips to Hawaii."

"You mean, something will catch his eye and he'll beg me to take him somewhere?" says Anna doubtfully.

"Not like that," I say. "It's really important to distinguish between what appears to be going on, and what's actually going on, at the level of the seeds. If he's not that interested in vacations, then tricking him into looking at vacations with you online probably isn't going to help much. It doesn't affect the seeds, and the seeds are running the show.

"No—what we want is that Luis himself starts planting some new seeds, by helping someone else plan their little adventure. Again, it's not as though there's a lot of intention before, or much rejoicing afterwards about what he did. But he *is* planting seeds, and that will start an upward cycle: one seed will build on another.

"Before long, you'll catch him on the internet planning his own vacation to Brazil."

Anna looks up, surprised. "But I was thinking of Paris!"

Question 49

Once a week or so, all of my husband's friends come over, and they hunker down in front of the TV for 3 or 4 hours watching football and drinking beer together. It really makes me feel left out, because I don't like beer or sports, and I have no idea what's going on in the game anyway. Is there any karmic fix for this? I don't want them not to have fun.

This question I got in the Ukraine, during a retreat outside of Kiev at a place called Irpin. And of course Natasha is talking about soccer when she says "football," but it applies just as well to the American brand.

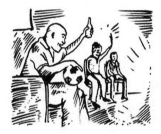

"It gets worse around the time of the finals for the European Cup," she adds. "At that point, Andrey pretty much expects me to be the out of the house by the time the game comes on."

"So you know about the seeds," I begin.

"Yes."

"And the Four Starbucks Steps," I add.

"Right," she replies. "Must help American economy!" This is a joke I sometimes make when encouraging people to take someone out to a specific coffee shop, and there's a Starbucks not far away in almost all the countries we visit.

"Okay, so Step One: first tell me what you want, in a single sentence. That will help us identify the essence of the problem, and that will help identify what we have to do."

"I guess to say it simply, I just don't want to be left out."

"Step Two."

"You mean, who do I know who wants the same thing?"

I nod.

Natasha thinks for a moment.

"Yes; at work. I often go out to lunch with the same two or three women in my office. There's a co-worker of ours named Olga who sometimes hovers nearby, sort of hopefully, but my friend Tanya—she sort of tends to decide everything between all of us—doesn't like her, so we never ask her along. But I know she would love to come."

"Okay then. So you know who you want to plant your seeds with. How about Step Three?"

"Well then, maybe it's time to tell Tanya that I'm bringing Olga along, and if she gives me any trouble about it I'll just take Olga out on my own."

"Good for you. Where will you take her?"

"There's a little Italian place on the first floor of our building."

"And *when* will this happen?"

"Well, today is Friday...how about Tuesday? That gives me Monday to ask her, and she'll have time to pick out what she wants to wear."

"Alright...so the details of the plan are there, and we really need them if we're going to plant a good seed. What about the vision?"

Natasha hesitates. "Uh, let's go over that again; I'm not sure I caught that part at the talk last night."

"Okay. When Olga comes out with you for lunch, it's important that you have a certain vision in mind. You're dealing with a problem that millions of other people in the world certainly share: Their partner is very much into football or a certain TV show, and when it comes on then they feel left out, excluded. And as you said, it's not that they want to deny their partner something they find very enjoyable.

"If the world were as it seems—if things *were not* coming from seeds—then it would be impossible to find a solution here. I mean, it could never happen that Andrey gets to continue enjoying his football shows with his friends and beer, and at the same time you don't feel left out.

"But the fact is that the world *is* coming from seeds: from how we have treated other people in the past. And if you fix the seeds, then a solution will come, all by itself.

"Take Olga out, and continue to *include* her. That will plant seeds in your mind to always be included, even during the football games."

Natasha grimaces. "Are you saying that suddenly I will develop a taste for beer, and for screaming my head off when our team makes a goal?"

I shake my head. "That's too simple. You're still stuck in thinking that the problem is coming from its own side—and so you think the solution will also be coming from its own side. You're seeing the situation as *this* or *that*:

either I drink the beer or not, either I sit in front of the TV with the boys or not.

"But your seeds are going to have to accommodate all the seeds of everybody else involved. Your and their seeds are locked together in this huge, inconceivably complicated network. The moment you step out of the building with Olga, billions of other seeds in the world shift.

"And so it's totally impossible to say *how* both you and Andrey will *both* get exactly what you want; but it is totally possible—totally true—to say *that you will*. What that is going to look like you cannot even imagine, but it will happen. Andrey will continue to get maximum enjoyment from his friends and football and beer; and in some magic, unpredictable way, you will find him including you completely. Don't worry yourself at all. Plant the seed, then sit back and relax, and let the magic happen."

"Sounds good," she says.

Question 50

I know spontaneous moments of fun when we're together are supposed to be spontaneous—but is there some kind of karma that we can plant to make these moments happen more often?

Most relationships aren't magical all the time, and we all know that. Problem is—as with so many other things—"what we all know" can be completely wrong.

If we sit back and think for a moment, all of us can remember one of these magical, unexpected moments of fun. The kind that sneak up on the two of us and leave us in each other's arms, overcome with big belly laughs, eyes full of happy tears.

Like maybe back when you first met each other, you were visiting a distant relative living in a southern California beach town. You're dressed in business casual because that's what Aunt Mabel likes when you have tea with her. You drive past a little surf shop and suddenly your sweetheart says to you, "Honey, can we just park right here and check out that little shop? It's calling me for some reason."

You take a sharp right and miraculously someone else is just pulling out of one of those impossible-to-find beachfront parking spaces. You swoop in and grab it and walk over to the shop. There are two goofy boys running the place; they talk you into renting a couple of surfboards *right now* and running down to the beach in some T-shirts and shorts that they happen to have laying around.

Pretty soon you're in the water and it's warmer than it's supposed to be this time of year, and the surf is just right not too big not too small; and just like the parking miracle there's another miracle in the water: there's not a single other surfer out at the moment; and the sun is going down in a crimson lightshow and you're both jumping on waves and standing up and falling down and here's the moment, you're dragging yourselves out of the water giggling uncontrollably and there's just a single minute of sunset left to hold each other soaking wet and kiss.

And then to top it all off, the boys back at the shop can't seem to work the math out as far as what to charge you and *they* giggle too and say "Hey man, how's about we just let it go this time," and then you're back in your button-down shirt and blouse, headed back down the highway to the hotel.

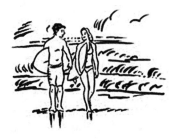

Question being, how come the two of us can't have these unplanned, magical moments all the time? Answer being, just figure out why the Sunset Surf Moment happened; as the Tibetans say, "If you figure out one, you figure out all the others."

I'm telling all this to Debbie and her partner David. They are old friends of mine who recently hooked up with each other—the kind of serendipitous collision of warmth that makes me and all their other friends wonder why we didn't suggest it to one of them years ago: sort of a romantic Titanic-hits-iceberg-in-the-middle-of-an-empty-ocean, if you'll excuse the metaphor. Anyway, they're both West Coast people and they appreciate the surf example, as we sit outside a little sandwich shop in Sedona.

"Right," says David. "We have that kind of thing happen to us too, but only like once in a month. Our question for you is how to make it happen more often."

"Personally," I reply, "I don't think the two of you should be satisfied with 'more often.' If we can figure out *why* any one magical moment happens, then we should be able to repeat it. And I think you should be able to repeat it as often as you darned well please. Like…maybe *your whole life* could be one long unexpectedly magical moment, if you really understood what makes one magical moment happen."

"Okay," smiles Debbie. "I'll settle for that."

"So we have to look," I begin, "for the seed that makes a moment magic. There's a specific practice for this in the ancient Tibetan scriptures—it's called 'Pretending the Path is the Goal.'

"The goal, in Tibet, is nothing less than to become an Angel of Light, one who can stand on many planets at once and help all the people there. While we're still on the path to this goal, we try to pretend that everyone around us is already an enlightened angel, and that everything they do or say to us is somehow meant to guide us further on our journey.

"So how would you get started on that?" I ask the two of them.

David looks up across the sidewalk—there's an older man in dark green overalls bending lovingly over a rose bush, trimming here and there.

"Okay," he says. "So that man over there is some kind of enlightened being in disguise. He knows we're having this conversation, and he's trying to think of some beautiful sign to send us that we're on the right track."

We all fix our eyes on the old gardener. Suddenly he reaches down and snips off a long-stem with a beautiful bloom on the top. He looks up and catches our eyes. And then he slowly walks over to our table.

With a flourish he offers the rose to Debbie. "I'm supposed to trim all these bushes down today," he says gruffly, waving off towards a whole row or roses. "It would just go to waste." He shuffles back to his charges.

Debbie smiles and looks at David. "So *pretending* that moments in the day are magical plants seeds for them to *become* magical later on," he says. "That one wasn't so hard to imagine."

To plant magic, see magic

I nod. "The challenge is when things *aren't* going so well. You're having a problem with someone at work; they say something bad about you in front of the boss.

"What's the message here? What are they trying to tell you? You may not be able to come up with anything right away, and there's no right answer really. But just *imagining* that something special could be going on plants the seeds you need…"

"…For surfing in the setting sun," Debbie smiles again, as she leans into David, hugging his arm.

A LOOK INTO
THE FUTURE

This whole book is going to work better for you if you learn about the Mandala: the Vision of a Perfect World. So let's pause for a few minutes, right here in the middle of the book, just after we left that perfect couple on the beach with their surfboards.

Anytime you do even the smallest thing with this Vision, the seeds that you create are, well, just about infinite. And that's because you are hoping that what you do will affect infinite numbers of people.

Anytime you use the Four Starbucks Steps to get anything you want, you can keep this Vision in mind, and things will work a lot, lot faster. In fact, anytime you use these Four Steps to make your own dreams come true, you are automatically helping everyone else make their dreams come true.

If you stay aware of how this works, every part of your life is the story of a Superhero, saving thousands of people. And if you think about it, this is nothing less than ultimate love.

So let's take a real example.

It's been like 5 years since you had a real boyfriend. Oh, some dates here and there, but nothing deep, nothing with real warmth and love. Then you pick up this book and read it

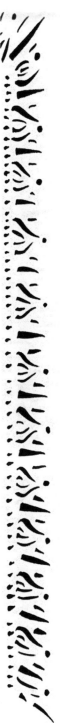

and decide to try planting a boyfriend, instead of looking for one.

You check around in your community and find a little nursing home that calls to you. You get over your shyness and walk in and talk to someone in the front office. You offer to come in once a week for an hour to visit an elderly woman who doesn't have any family to come see her—a woman who is especially lonely.

You keep this up for a few months, planting the seeds for your new beau, being sure to do Coffee Meditation every night when you go to bed. And of course it works, and you get a beautiful new man in your life.

Now it's time for the Superhero thing—for helping the whole world.

Call up three or four of your girlfriends and tell them you have a surprise for them. Ask them if they can meet you at a certain restaurant tomorrow night at 7pm.

Now call up your new partner and ask him if he can come over to your place tomorrow at 7pm too.

When he arrives, fill up three large glasses with water and ask him to drink all three, quickly. If he has any questions about that, tell him you'll explain later. Then go to the restaurant together.

Of course you're going to be about half an hour late, but that's all part of the plan. Your girlfriends are already seated at a table, wondering what's tying you up. They look over as you walk in the front door, arm in arm with the new boy.

"Who's the hunk?" one of them asks another.

"I don't know, but I doubt that it's a boy-friend. After all, she hasn't had a real relation-ship for what, 5 years now?"

"It's probably just her cousin," adds a third friend.

Walk him over to the table and pause, and then before you sit down take him in your arms and give him a big juicy kiss. We're talking a good French kiss, with lots of tongue and slob-ber.

"Definitely not her cousin," whispers one of your girlfriends, in awe.

You know what happens next. You sit down with introductions all round while menus are passed and everyone decides what they're go-ing to eat. Except there are a lot of sideways glances at the boy, over the menus.

Probably just about the time the food ar-rives, the boy is going to excuse himself and head for the bathroom—That's what the three glasses of water were for. And in the space before he gets back there's going to be a lot of heavy questioning and giggling.

"Where on earth did you find him?" squeals one friend.

"Yeah, where's the club? Was it a dance club?" asks another.

"No, it must have been a website!" yells the other. Napkins are tossed in front of you. "Write down the address for us, quick!"

You calmly write down the words *Nursing Home,* and pass them around the table.

"Huh? What's that supposed to mean?" they all ask. And then you go through the seed planting thing, in detail. You definitely have to cover the Four Starbucks Steps, okay?

Now not every girl at the table is going to believe you. And not everyone who does believe you is going to be willing to try it. But one or two of them will.

And of course each of them will each get their own beautiful new boy, because the seeds *always* work.

What happens next? Well, it doesn't require a genius to figure that out. They will take their new men to meet their own friends at other restaurants; and those men will excuse themselves to go to the bathroom; and this thing about nursing homes will start to spread to *their* friends, and to their friends' friends, and to *their* friends too.

Pretty soon, there are long lines of young women and young men waiting outside of nursing homes, trying to get in to spend some time visiting a lonely man or woman. Probably a good number of the boys and girls can get to know each other there, in the lines.

In time, everyone has the partner they dreamed of. And then partners visit the nursing homes together, to keep the seeds going. In time, no more lonely people. Anywhere.

Try to understand what happens, every time you use the seeds to get the things you want. You will *succeed,* and others will see it, and they will try the seeds too. And they will succeed, and others will follow them. You will change the world: just *deciding* to use the seeds changes the world already. There will be a perfect world, a Mandala, and you will be the one who started it.

So pause sometimes, and take a look at the future—a future which you are creating, for everyone.

ABUSE

Question 51

The husband of a friend of mine might have abused her physically. Do you think I should encourage her to leave him, or to stick it out instead?

I got this question from a friend named Lifen in Shenzhen—a city in southern China—but I've heard it from women in other countries, all over the world. And sadly they're always asking about "a friend" of theirs who "might" have been abused.

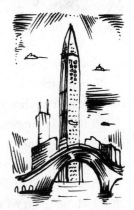

"First things first," I say. "If it's anything even remotely going on physically, she should leave the situation immediately—go stay with her mother, a sister, or a friend.

"As for solving the problem permanently," I continue, "you want to stop making decisions."

Stop making decisions

Now we've covered some of this back in Question 7, but it's time to go a little deeper.

"How so?"

"You've faced yourself...I mean, *she's* faced herself, with a decision. Should I leave him, or should I stay?"

"Well, what other choice is there?" asks Lifen.

I think for a moment. "Look, how do you guess that this whole situation feels to her—when she thinks about this decision, how does it make her feel?"

"It must make her feel terrible. She's been with him for more than 20 years. She still loves him, and they have a daughter who's still in the house. Leaving will break all their hearts, but staying seems impossible. The decision she's faced with is a terrible one to have to make."

"And a terrible one to live with until she does make it," I agree. "The sheer uncertainty of it all is perhaps the greatest pain. The not knowing what to do."

"Exactly," Lifen sighs.

"And so the problem, you see, is the decision," I say. "What if there were no decision?"

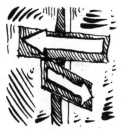

"But there is a decision."

"Describe the decision again."

"She stays, and risks being hit by her husband. She goes, and their daughter loses her parents."

"But what if she *knew* what was going to happen—what if the decision were *made?*"

"Still a tragedy," says Lifen. "Someone gets hurt either way."

"I mean, what if she *knew* that a decision would be made—a decision that wouldn't hurt anybody?"

"If it could happen," she says, "then alright. She would feel alright. The fear would be gone, the anxiety would stop."

"Okay then, let's set up a decision that can't hurt anyone. Say it with the Four Starbucks Steps." I know she knows the four, because we just finished talking about them with a group of businesswomen, up in a financial-services office on the 30th floor of one of those smart new Shenzen skyscrapers. I also know that she knows Starbucks, because the week before we had a staff meeting at the one in Shanghai, after giving a talk in the offices of the Shanghai Stock Exchange nearby.

"Step One," she recites. "What she wants is to no longer be faced with this impossible decision, of whether to stay or whether to go."

"And Step Two?" I ask.

"She would have to find someone else in her life who was faced with an impossible decision—perhaps the same decision."

"Right. Anything else?"

Lifen frowns for a second, and then comes out with one of those fantastic leaps of intuition that I've learned to expect in China.

"But her problem," she says deliberately, "isn't just a question of a decision. The decision is a terrible thing, a terrible suffering to have to face. Behind it though is the violence—at the same time that she works on the decision, she must also work on the violence."

"Good," I say. "Let's continue with the decision, and then go on to the violence."

"Okay then—in Step Two she's found a person who is faced with a similar, very difficult decision. What next?"

"Step Three always happens at Starbucks; she'll sit with this other person, and try to help them resolve their decision."

"Does she have to *succeed* in resolving it?" I ask.

Lifen considers for a second. "She may succeed, or she may not; that depends on her friend's seeds. But in either case she plants seeds for her own decision to be made, just by offering whatever suggestions she can."

"Or maybe she plants seeds for her decision to disappear," I say. "What if there were no more violence?"

"Well that would be the best; in that case, yes, there would be no more decision to be made."

"And how to stop the violence? Where is it coming from?" I'm twiddling a pen in my hand, but Lifen doesn't need the hint.

"It's like the pen," she says. "It's like her husband, her daughter, her entire life: all coming from her own mind, from the seeds there."

Let's pause here and allow me to say something. Spousal abuse is a very sensitive subject, and the last thing that people want to hear is that somehow it's the fault of the person being abused. If I wanted to be politically correct, it would be best to avoid this question altogether; but it wouldn't be the truth.

The truth is that *everything* around us, good or bad, is coming from *us,* from how we ourselves have treated others in the past. You just can't go around saying that some *percentage* of what happens to us in life is coming from us, and some other percentage is coming from others. We need to hold this line in our thinking: I am responsible for everything in my life, even abuse, and that equally means that I am empowered to stop it, simply by changing myself, by changing my own seeds. Accepting responsibility brings the power to change things.

"So if it's like the pen," I continue, "then how to change it?"

"Remove the seeds inside of me that make me see it," she says easily. "If I *want* something, like a decision that resolves itself, then I have to provide the same thing to others, first. If I *don't want* something, then I have to stop doing the same thing to others."

"The exact same thing?" I ask.

Lifen knows where I'm going. "Not exactly," she says. "Ongoing violence from a spouse could—or I should say, certainly does—come from smaller acts of violence which I have done myself. And to stop those seeds, I have to look into my own life and try to find something small that I'm inflicting on others."

"Perfect," I say. "A two-pronged approach. Make new good seeds to see decisions decided before they even come up; remove old bad seeds for seeing violence in your life. What happens then?"

"The hitting stops," she says, "and at the very same time the decision melts away—along with the terrible anxiety she feels about the decision."

"Go to it," I say simply.

Question 52

After many years with my wife, I've come to see that abuse can be emotional, and not just physical: I've become afraid to be myself, because she might not like it; and now I feel like I'm getting smaller and smaller, just shrinking into a corner. How can I stop this subtle abuse, and get my life back?

I get this question, or some variation of it, from a great many people. At the moment I'm at a weekend business retreat just outside of Tel Aviv; Moishe is asking it this time. He's a good man; you know the kind: he'll do anything for you. And he's trying to do anything for Erit, and it seems she is taking advantage of it—a kind of abuse as sure as the physical, and just as debilitating. Here, about halfway through the 100 questions, it's time to start introducing the other three sets of four formally, as we answer.

"So do you do the same?"

"What same?" he replies.

"Do you take people over, dominate them, slowly turn them into nothing of their own?"

We both know the answer. It's the last thing that Moishe would wish on someone. He is one of the most self-effacing, humble individuals I have ever met. If the Diamond Cutter Principles are an expression of perfect justice in this universe—if we always get exactly what we give—then to be dominated is the last thing Moishe should be.

Or not? I decide to challenge him.

"Moishe, you know the Four Laws, right?"

The Four Laws of Karma

1) Like makes like: If you plant a watermelon, you get a watermelon

2) What you get back is always much, much bigger than what you did

3) If you don't do anything, you're not going to get anything back

4) If you do do something, you *must* get something back

He nods. "The Four Laws of Karma…yes, I know them."

"Okay then. Let's go at it backwards. What's the last of the four?"

"Nothing can happen to you if you haven't planted a seed for it."

"And the third law?"

"If you *have* planted a seed, then something *will* happen."

"Right. Now tell me; is something happening?"

"Yes!" he answers. "Moishe is disappearing! He's being taken over by Erit, very slowly, very surely. The things he used to be—thoughtful, responsible, serving—are all slowly fading; and now he does only what she directs him to, even if it is the opposite of what was good about him before."

"So Law Four says…"

"It can't be coming from nothing."

"And Law Three says…"

"I *must* be doing something to plant what's happening to me."

"And Law One says…"

Moishe thinks for a second, but I can see he's been working on building an understanding of the four, because his answer is full of certainty. "It must be the same," he says. "Whatever I'm doing must be the same as what's happening to me."

But then he looks confused, as well he should. He's definitely *not* a domineering personality. Quite the opposite, and we both know it.

"It doesn't make sense," he says it out loud. "I'm just not that kind of person. I don't go around overwhelming people emotionally, until there's only me and none of them."

"But the Second Law of Karma?" I ask quietly.

"Seeds grow," he says. "In the moment after a seed is planted in the mind, it begins to grow, exponentially. While it waits deep within the subconscious, the seed doubles in power every single day."

I nod. "You're at work; a decision has to be made by your team. You really want it to go a certain way, so you push a bit. It only takes a few minutes."

Moishe picks up the thread. "In 3 minutes spent imposing my viewpoints on my team at work, I plant, what—a couple of hundred seeds? And let's say I do the pushing on Monday. By payday, two weeks from then, these 200 have split into…" he pulls out his cell phone and does the math, then sucks in his breath. "Over a million seeds."

He does a few more calculations. "These million open up and produce Erit in front of me, controlling who I am, again at the rate of 65 seeds per second. Which means that 3 minutes of controlling someone on my team at work has turned into 3 or 4 hours of Erit not letting me be myself.

"It doesn't matter then," he concludes, "if I'm not trying to impose my way on people very often. If I do it once or twice a week, *even in a very tiny way,* then according to the Second Law of Karma…and the fourth…and the first and the third," he looks a little dazed, "I will have a wife who prevents me from being my own person, every time we're around each other."

I look him in the eyes with pride. I can see he's thought it out, right there. The Second Law of Karma says that—even if he's preventing others from being themselves for just 3 minutes a day—then these will be sufficient seeds for total control by his wife. The fourth law says that if he hadn't been controlling with his team at work, none of this would be happening.

The First Law of Karma states that being controlled must come from the same *kind* of thing: controlling someone else. And the third law assures that it's going to keep happening, until he stops trying to wipe out the individuality of every person on his team at work.

"So who will it be?" I ask.

Moishe nods. He knows that now I'm moving from the Four Laws of Karma to the Four Starbucks Steps, which we've already covered so often here, in the first 50 questions or so. The second of those steps is for Moishe to think of someone on his team at work whom he is domineering. He thinks for a minute—which really counts as a meditation, because he's purposely grabbing his mind and forcing it to consider a certain thought: who at work is less themselves, because of Moishe's actions?

"There's Shimone," he nods. "He keeps mentioning that he would like to be working more on the creative side of the business, but he's good at the accounting and it fits my needs much better if he stays there. So in a way I'm forcing him into the mold of a much less interesting role, just because it suits what I want."

Now that Moishe's got what's going on, let's look at a solution. Back in Question 34, we talked about the idea of switching names with someone else, so that we could learn to pay attention to others' needs with the same intensity that we watch out for our own needs. That is, if your name is John and my name is Mike and I want to learn how to be a better person, I just glue my name on you, and glue your name on me, and go from there—with my usual prejudice for taking care of what Mike wants. Except that now you are Mike, and so you get a lot more attention to your needs from me than you used to.

That particular spiritual method is credited to a lama whom we met a while back: Master Shantideva, who lived about 13 centuries ago. He called it "Switching You & Me." He also said that to prepare for this we could first do a practice called "Equal Rights for You & Me."

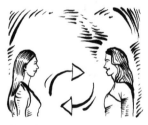

This just means that we try to be very democratic in how we treat others: We recognize that they have just as much a right to stay themselves— in their interactions on the team at work—as we have to stay ourselves, in our interactions with our partner.

So "Right," I say. "You make sure that you let Shimone approach tasks in his own way on the job, and then by the time you get home you've got some new seeds to see Erit respect your right to be yourself. It's not that you don't learn things from Erit; that's one of the most important goals of any relationship. But you do get equal rights to your own personality, and to your own way of doing things—even as you and she do things together."

Moishe breathes a little sigh of relief; we stand up and head back to the auditorium. Even a shy person wants to be a person.

EMOTIONAL SUPPORT

Question 53

I've had several serious problems at work this year, as well as a couple of major personal challenges. Whenever I seek my wife's help and support I don't seem to get much, and it's hard to go it on my own. What's the seed I need to plant to feel like we're in this together?

I got this question from a friend by the name of Terry; he and his wife Lee had recently been on a little side trip to see some tourist sites in southern Arizona. In the middle of the trip, Terry got a call from work with some pretty bad news; he told Lee about it right away, hoping for some consolation, but she was in the middle of texting on her phone and didn't even seem to hear him. Apparently this has been going on for a while.

"You know the Four Flowers, right?" I ask.

Terry thinks for a second and says, "I do—they got covered in the second level of the Diamond Cutter Institute training that we took."

"Tell me why it's good to know about them."

"For me," says Terry, "they are one of the most important parts of the training. I mean, we grow up with a certain idea about the word *karma:* 'Don't step on a bug, Johnny, or one day someone will hurt you.' And we hear about it in the Bible too: 'You reap what you sow.'

"But most of us don't really follow it, because just *how* karma, or sowing, really works isn't all that clear. I mean, where is what I do recorded? When I yell at my wife, it feels like I've done something bad—but what makes it bad? How does it come back to me?

"Do the words that I've spoken to her somehow fly off into the air somewhere, like a boomerang, and circle out around Pluto; then circle back somehow and hit me in the head a couple of months later? Or is it true what they say about Saint Peter, that's he sitting at the Pearly Gates of Heaven, taking notes about everything I do all day long, all life long? And then at the end he shows me the book and decides what happens to me?

"I mean, you can think of it in either one of those ways, I guess, but for me the Four Flowers gives me a model that fits how I was taught about everything else—it makes sense to me."

Four Flowers Review

1) You get back the same thing that you gave

2) Doing it becomes a habit

3) What you do creates the people & the world around you

4) It also creates the world that you step into next

"Why do you think they call them 'flowers'?" I ask.

"It took me a while to figure that one out. I mean, what the Four Flowers really explain is exactly how karma comes back to me: how the seeds open. In this case—yelling at my partner—the seeds are planted as I watch and hear and *feel* myself get mad: impressions of what I'm doing come in through the doorways of my eyes and ears and general awareness.

"Those impressions are 'pressed' into my mind, into my deep subconscious, and they sit there below my conscious thoughts, like seeds beneath the surface of the soil. Somehow they 'cook' there—that's a real mystery, what goes on inside a seed as it's getting ready to split open—and then when the time and the conditions are right they crack open and send up a sprout.

"Except that a mental sprout is made of light—not light reflected off of it, but itself made of light, like the inside of a light bulb or the flame on top of a candle. It's a tiny little picture made of light. It doesn't have a size—we can't say that it's this big or this small—but a person who is very sensitive, someone who's been meditating a lot, can actually see the seed open and the image come out, and it *feels* to them about a half an inch high, and it *feels* as though it's floating somewhere towards the back of their head.

"And then—this is what I like most about the Four Flowers—that little luminous image comes out say through my eyes, and glues itself on top of the colors and shapes in front of me."

"Why colors and shapes?" I ask. "Why not a thing or a person?"

"That's the cool part," says Terry. "I mean, think about it. Your physical eyes—your eye*balls*—can only detect shades of colors, and the outlines of shapes. There is some very sensitive tissue at the back of the eyes—made of rods and cones—and these change according to the image placed in front of them, like old-fashioned camera film.

"An oval shape of reddish color appears before my eyes, and there's another roundish shape inside that oval which is opening and closing. The first is the face of my boss yelling at me, and the second is his mouth moving as he does the yelling. But my eyes aren't what interprets the roundish shapes as being an angry boss. That decision can't be made by the rods and cones at the back of the eyeball; they don't have that capacity.

"What's really happening is that *seeds* are opening in the back of my mind, and luminous pictures are flying out to the two roundish shapes, overlaying them, lending sense to them. The shape that these pictures take—whether I see my boss yelling at me, or telling me that I'm doing a good job—is all coming from the seeds in my mind. And those seeds were planted there the week before, when I was talking to my partner.

"So in a way," Terry wraps it up, "the seeds and those little pictures of light explain very perfectly *why* what I do comes back to me. I don't have to *believe* in them blindly, I just have to *understand* them. Which makes it a lot easier to be a good person—to stop myself when I'm about to yell at Lee.

"The seeds and the pictures—the guts of the Four Flowers—explain exactly *why* there is a perfect justice to the universe. And that's just a gosh-darned *comforting* thing for me."

I smile at Terry with affection; "Just right!" I exclaim. There is a place in the Heart Sutra—perhaps the most famous Buddhist book of all time—where the Buddha has been listening to one of his students explain the thing about the pen. The student does a good job, and the Buddha basically blurts out, "Right on! Right on!" I really like that part.

"Okay," I breathe. "So let's get down to the answer to your question. Of the four ways in which our mental seeds flower inside the mind, what is the third?"

Terry counts mentally for a moment and then replies, "Environment—the things and the people we see around us as we go through our day. It's not just that yelling at my wife at home will create a boss who yells at me at work. I will see people in stores and on TV, and just walking down the sidewalk, who are yelling at each other."

He thinks for a moment and asks, "Are you saying that if I go at it from Flower Three then I will see a different Lee? That she's a part of the world around me, and if I change my own seeds she'll change along with everybody else I ever run into?"

"There's that," I agree, "but I was actually thinking about those other people. I mean, I was thinking about it as sort of a feedback loop—like when you're talking into a microphone but you're standing in the wrong place and everything you say doubles back from the speaker into the mike, over and over really quick, and creates that huge screeching sound.

"I mean, there's been this big shift in our culture just recently. Everybody has a cell phone, and when they get a call or a text they just pull it out and—even if they're in the middle of a sentence during a conversation with somebody—they suddenly ignore the person they're talking to and switch to the one who wants to communicate with them on the phone. And the person across the table from them, the one they were just talking to, 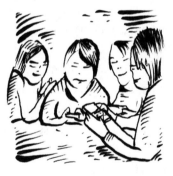 just sort of retreats into silence for a minute or two, because they know they have to wait.

"According to Flower Three, this suddenly ignoring someone that you're having a conversation with is going to create lots of people around you who are ignoring each other. I mean, look. I was in central China recently—a city called Hangzhou. There were four teenage girls sitting around a table in a coffee shop, all of them texting on their phones, completely ignoring each other for like 45 minutes.

"On the way out, my Chinese teacher made a joke to them about ignoring each other, but then they all giggled and told her that they were texting *each other,* around the table. Go figure.

"Anyway, Buddhism has a special word for this idea of a feedback loop. It's called *sansara,* and it basically refers to a huge, self-perpetuating, downward cycle. You yell at your wife, so your boss yells at you. You yell back at him, and this plants a seed to see him yell back at you many more times—and the wheel goes round one more time. Those of us who have heard about the seeds are pretty familiar with this kind of loop.

"But there are a lot of other loops going on, and Flower Three really helps us with one of them. So suppose that you bring your laptop on a vacation trip and at some point you sit down on the bed in the hotel and you stick your nose in it, ignoring Lee..."

Break bad cycles in your life by planting seeds

Terry gets it immediately; his face starts to get a little bit red.

"...and you see this email from the office with some bad news in it. Now we all know that ignoring Lee for the time it takes to check the email could very well plant a seed for her to ignore you for weeks, while you are trying to get some empathy from her for something hard that's happening in your life.

"But Flower Three says that the very same seed will also create people all around you who are ignoring each other—like the girls around the table in the coffee shop seemed to be doing. And that's another feedback loop. You see other people check out in the middle of a conversation to look at an incoming text, and you start to think that's an okay thing to do. And so you do it with Lee, and with a lot of other people.

"Each time you act this way, you create another seed to see people ignoring each other. And maybe—for them—*you've* been created by their seeds, so you also ignore people in front of them. And then *they* get the idea that it's alright socially to do that, and pretty soon the whole society is ignoring each other, and creating seeds which will guarantee that Acceptable Ignoring continues for a really long time: a whole culture of ignoring.

"You can turn Flower Three around though, and that's how I want you to try to deal with what's happening between you and Lee. Instead of buying into ignoring because you see others around you ignoring each other, approach people that you see ignoring each other—gently and skillfully—and encourage them to interact with each other more warmly, to listen and to empathize more.

"This attempt will create another loop, one which is positive. It will plant seeds for you to see a different world around you: one in which people who get a text or a call when they're relating to someone else face-to-face just wait to check it, until their 'real' conversation is sweetly finished."

"And then Lee will be there to support me when I really need it," smiles Terry. Still, his eyes wander down to his laptop case, and I know his email addiction has just touched him. Oh well, it will take some time.

Question 54

I've always been really healthy, and my relationship with my partner is very active—whether in bed or out biking together. Recently though I got sick for a few weeks, and instead of showing me concern he just acted really inconvenienced, which made me feel terrible. What's the karma for a partner who's more compassionate?

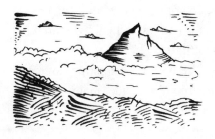

I got this question one day at Diamond Mountain, our free university in the southwestern US. I could see from her face that the situation was really causing Sam (who's a woman) deep concern—you could almost say anguish. Perhaps it's one of the most painful situations we can ever encounter in our life, when a partner doesn't do something to help us when we're sick; maybe doesn't even bother to ask how we feel.

"So Sam, you know about the Pen Thing, right?" (Which by the way we covered back in Question 1, because…well…it's the most important thing of all.)

"I do," she says. "You hold up a pen, and a human sees it as a pen, and a dog sees it as a chew-toy. Which proves that the pen must be coming from me—which proves that *everything* is coming from me."

"Good. And you've heard about the Five Paths?"

She nods again. "I have, and I like the very idea of them—milestones on the spiritual journey of every person who takes to the way. I mean, when you're driving from Phoenix to Los Angeles, there are signs practically the whole way, telling you how many miles you've got left to go.

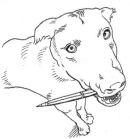

"With spiritual things, it's not so easy. What percentage of your old anger do you still have left? On a scale from 1 to 10, how loving are you? And how long left to go, before you reach enlightenment? I like the Five Paths because they give you an idea of how far you've come, and how far you've left to go."

"Okay then," I say. "Let's see how the Five Paths relate to the Pen Thing. What's the first of the five?"

Sam thinks for a moment. "It's called the Path of Collecting; basically, it's the period in our spiritual evolution when we are collecting enough good seeds to have our big breakthrough, which happens at the third path."

"Good. But what it is that gets you onto this first path, in the very beginning?"

Sam smiles wryly. "I like that part of the Five Paths too, because it just seems so true to me. According to the ancient Tibetans, what gets you on the first path is a good healthy disaster in your life. Losing a loved one; breaking up with a longtime partner; listening to the doctor tell you you've got a really serious disease—that kind of thing. This is what it takes to get you thinking about the real purpose of life, and how to fulfill it."

We sit quiet for a moment, because we're both remembering how Sam herself got started on the spiritual way: her mom's suicide, many years before. She shakes herself out of it and we go on.

"Second path?" I ask.

"Path of Preparation," Sam answers. "The second milestone. Somebody appears in your life and shows you the Pen Thing—how the pen is coming from you, from your mind, and not from its own side. Which sort of means that nothing is itself, at least in the way we've always thought it was.

"Huh," she says suddenly. "I never thought of it, but I guess you could say that working to plant a lot of good seeds on the first path—basically, taking care of people more than we ever did before that—is what *creates* a person who shows up in your life and explains the Pen Thing to you."

I try to nod wisely, but to be honest I hadn't really thought of it that way before. The seeds from attempting to answer other people's questions sometimes flower as their answering some of your own.

"And how is this path a preparation?" I ask.

"You need this path to get to the next one, the third, which is the big breakthrough: You *see* a certain thing, something you could call Ultimate Reality, or maybe even God. And so the third is called the Path of Seeing."

"Right," I agree. "But I think you could also express it just in every-day terms, without the religious connotations—although they're fine if that's what calls to you. I mean, the whole Path of Seeing doesn't last longer than a single day, although it might take you years to get through the first two paths to reach it.

"And the Path of Seeing has two parts. The first part is what you were talking about: some kind of communion with a higher place. And it only takes say 20 minutes for the whole thing, although when you're in the middle of it you might not be exactly aware of how much time is passing.

"The deeper point, when someone tells us about The Pen, isn't that the dog sees one thing and you see something else. It really comes down to how much the pen is a pen, by itself. I mean, when it's just me, a human, sitting in the kitchen on a chair looking at a pen, I can say that right now it's a pen—a pen that's coming from me.

"But when the dog steps through the door and approaches the table, things get a little more complicated. The little stick has to be a pen and a chew-toy at the same time. Technically...

"Do you really want all this?" I ask Sam. It suddenly occurs to me that she might not.

"Don't be condescending, Geshe Michael," she grins. "People *want* the gritty detail, and they grasp it, and it helps them a lot to put all this stuff into practice, in real life."

I look down for a moment, chastised. "Okay then. Technically, you've got two realities going on right there, in the same kitchen at the same time. The dog is validly experiencing a world where there's a chew-toy in the human's hand—and it's real, because it's making the dog slobber just thinking about chewing on it, and he *can* chew on it.

"In the other reality—in my reality, the human's reality—the stick really is a pen, because I can pick it up and write with it.

"But now suppose I take the dog out for a walk, and we leave the stick alone on the kitchen table. *At that time,* which one is it? A pen or a chew-toy?"

Sam laughs. "I know the answer to that one, I've heard you do it a dozen times. *At that time,* it's neither a pen nor a chew-toy—it's just...nothing, waiting to be something, available to be something. What the Buddhists call 'emptiness,' or maybe better to call it 'potential.' If the dog walks back into the kitchen, the stick *becomes* a chew-toy. If the human walks back in, the stick *becomes* a pen. But by itself, alone, it's just...nothing yet."

"Okay," I smile. "Hold on to that thought. On the second of the five paths, we're getting used to the idea that the pen is coming from us, from one of those tiny luminous pictures that popped out of a karmic seed in our mind—a seed which perhaps we planted last week, by being nice to someone, loaning them a pen maybe.

"But on the third path—on the Path of Seeing—it's infinitely more intense. I mean, Sam, right now…right this instant…I want you to point to one thing in this room which is coming from itself, and not from you."

Sam raises her hand and straightens out her first finger and looks around the room and suddenly just laughs again and shrugs. "There's nothing," she chuckles. "Nothing to point to."

"Okay—now hold that thought. Hold your mind on the nothing-to-point-to which is all around us both right now. That's what you see—but in a much deeper way—at the Path of Seeing. That's what Ultimate Reality is, and maybe in one way that's what God is too. The fact that nothing is anything by itself, which means that—with the right seeds—it could be anything. The world could *become* heaven, the way the stick in the kitchen *becomes* a pen."

I can see the excitement in Sam's eyes, but then she gives a tiny bit of a frown. "So…how is all this going to get Phil" (that's her husband) "to give me some tender lovin' whenever I'm under the weather?"

"Oh…yeah," I stumble a bit, forced back to the subject. "Well okay, that's just the first part of the Path of Seeing, the Ultimate Reality part. After the 20 minutes are over, and for the rest of the day, you start seeing all this other amazing stuff. One of the things you see is how selfish you've always been—how selfish we all are, all of the time. How self-interested every single thing we ever do or say or think really is. Even when we're praying, even as we are helping someone else with a task, even as we sit and explain the seeds to someone, it is always infected with self-interest: What can I get out of this?"

For at least 20 minutes in your life, you *must* see ultimate reality

I pause and Sam looks up at the ceiling, pensive. "So I guess you could connect that part too to the part that came before. I mean, maybe seeing God, or whatever you want to call it, is what it takes to see who you really are yourself."

That insight dumbfounds me, and we're quiet for another bit. "So about Phil," Sam prompts me.

"About Phil, you've got to realize what's really going on when he's so selfish that he doesn't even really acknowledge that you're sick, much less help you. You've got to look into your own heart and identify the seed that's creating this level of selfishness, not just in Phil, but in yourself, and in all of us—in an entire planet full of people. Why are we all so caught up in ourselves?"

Sam works it out slowly, step by step. "If what we've just said is true, then it's only at the third path—at the Path of Seeing—that we finally become fully aware of just how self-interested everything we ever do is. And the essence of the third path is that we can't point to a single thing around us which is *not* coming from us."

A light comes on in her eyes. "It's *knowing* where the world comes from that starts to shake us out of the planetary disease of selfishness. And it's *not knowing* where it comes from that plants the seeds to be and to see selfishness.

"Phil doesn't give me the attention I need when I'm sick because..." her eyes open wide, "...because *I* don't completely appreciate that he's coming from me, and only from me."

"How to fix that?" I ask, quickly.

"Well, I guess that's pretty easy. Next time he seems selfish, I could like go into the bathroom for a minute or two and think about *anything* else that's going on in my life, and try to see what I'm doing to create it and perpetuate it. Because although *not* thinking about that isn't selfishness in itself, it is the root of selfishness: and it's why I have to see selfishness around me."

I give Sam one more good look and decide to push a little further. "Great; we have a plan! But if we want to take this one more step..."

"Ready," she says gladly.

"I mean, it's one thing to fix Phil's selfishness by using the seeds. But from what we've just said, it seems like the problem is a lot bigger than that. The whole world is selfish—the whole world is acting pretty much the whole day out of self-interest. How do we tackle that?"

Sam gives it a thought. "I guess you could have a big education campaign...I mean, travel all over the world and try to teach people where things are really coming from. Then selfishness would become obsolete, because everybody would realize that everything comes from them; and if they want something good to happen they need to plant the seeds for that; and the only way to plant these seeds is to provide other people with the thing you want for yourself. And that's the complete absence of selfishness."

I smile indulgently, since we both know that this kind of campaign is how I spend a good part of my life.

"On the other hand," she says with a mischievous smile, "the campaign would work a lot better if you just thought about Flower Three—the way that seeds create the people around you. In that case, the best way to see selfishness stamped out in the world around you would be to become a good example yourself: deal with every problem in your life by using seeds, and it will just rub off on—_as_—everyone around you." She looks at me significantly.

"I'll try," I say.

We stand up and move towards the door. "Uh, didn't you forget something?" she says.

I look back to see if I've left something behind.

"No, no," she laughs. "We never talked about the fourth and the fifth paths."

"Oh yeah," I do the walk-and-talk. "Path Four is called the Path of Getting Used To. Which just means that you get used to your new insights into the essence of seeds, and use that understanding to wipe out—forever—the last of your negative emotions: anger, jealousy, desire, and anything else of the like."

"So then somehow those emotions must be based on ignorant self-interest"—Sam does that seeing-a-connection thing again, which I'm really starting to appreciate. "And I suppose that the fifth path isn't really a path at all—it's just the place you reach when you're completely unselfish, because by that point you're never _not_ using the seeds to make things happen in your life."

I nod. "They call it the Path of No More Learning, or sometimes simply Nirvana."

Sam nods. "Sounds good to me."

Question 55

When I look back on our relationship, I feel as though my wife has always been critical of me—constantly complaining, and almost never acknowledging the good things that I do. What is the karma for having someone be more appreciative of you?

Okay, this question was also asked in Paris. But to make it clear, I'm a Paris wanna-be, not a Paris regular. We make up excuses to hold Diamond Cutter Institute programs there even if it doesn't exactly make sense financially. I just want a little bit of that grace and elegance to rub off on me.

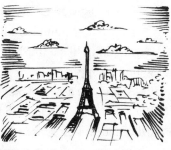

So anyway I'm sitting with Marie-Elise and her husband Georges on a balcony in the Montmartre district, watching the sun go down in a glowing russet gold, surrounded by that unique pale-blue sky. The Eiffel Tower is down to our left—an impossibly perfect Hollywood scene of the city playing itself out.

"As usual," I begin, "it all has to do with The Pen; and with diamonds. Let's start with the diamonds." Georges gives me a quizzical look, but settles down to listen.

"Okay, so when our diamond company in New York got big," I say, "we're making maybe 3,000 pieces of jewelry on a really good day. We were dealing mostly with tiny little diamonds, so there might be an average of 10 stones in each piece of jewelry.

"Which means that we would need to buy 30,000 diamonds to fill the orders for that day. You purchase these diamonds in bags, which also means that buying 30,000 diamonds of the exact sizes you need might require picking up another 20,000 diamonds in sizes that you don't need that day.

"Okay, so you have to buy 50,000 diamonds today. To get the 50,000 you might buy bags (actually we call them 'parcels') of 10,000 diamonds each from 5 different suppliers.

"Except that nobody keeps parcels full of 10,000 diamonds of exactly the same color. When a group of diamonds is used in a ring, the color of the stones has to be the same, so to get your 10,000 diamonds you're typically going to have to ask for a parcel of 12,000 diamonds.

"A lot of the 12,000 stones are going to have chips or holes or black spots in them, so say we need to ask for 3,000 more stones on top of that: 15,000 total in each of the 5 parcels. Then somebody has to sit down and pick up every tiny diamond—one by one—and decide whether the color and clarity are right or not.

"So to fill your orders for the day, a whole skyscraper floor full of people is going to have to pick up and examine nearly 75,000 tiny diamonds, holding a sharp pair of tweezers in one hand and a jeweler's lens in the other."

This gets a "Mon Dieu!" out of Marie-Elise.

"So say that the number of off-quality diamonds in any given parcel tends to be something like a third of the stones. The buyer who negotiates the parcel with the supplier takes a sample and decides just what percentage of off-quality stones we are allowed to reject and return. Then the buyer goes to the sorting supervisor and asks them to tell the diamond sorting staff to take out a third of the stones, those with a yellowish tint or a black spot or a chip.

"A big group of sorters sits with the pile of 75,000 diamonds for most of the day, picking them up one by one, rejecting 25,000 stones. The 25,000 go into separate parcel papers to be given back to the suppliers; and the 50,000 go into a parcel paper headed for the selected stock, and from there to the jewelry factory downstairs.

"Except sometimes a person whose eyes are all bleary from having stared at thousands of stones for the last few hours accidentally puts the Good Diamonds parcel back into the Diamonds To Sort box. The sorting supervisor gives this parcel of all-white, unchipped stones back to the same team of sorters by mistake, and instructs them to take out a third of the stones—those that are yellow or chipped.

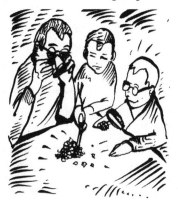

"And you know what happens?" I conclude.

Georges waves his hand. "Obviously! The sorters look at the first few stones and immediately notice that they're all good quality, and they alert the supervisor to the mistake."

"Not so," I say. "The sorters will go through the whole 50,000 stones that they just certified as perfect, and they will take out another third as yellow or chipped. And if you give them all *those* stones again, they will again reject another third."

Marie-Elise is getting a little impatient—perhaps we could say, complaining, in her mind. "So what's that got to do with Georges' supposed problem?"

"Okay. So in the diamond company we made up a name for this phenomenon: we called it 'relativization.' You can find the same idea in the ancient Tibetan scriptures."

"How's that?" asks Georges.

"These holy books say that if a human being walks into a room with 10 people in it, they will within an hour like 3 of these people; they will dislike another 3; and they will feel neutral about the remaining 4.

You will always dislike 3 out 10 people that you ever meet; so it's not them

"But then if you take 10 people that they like and you put those 10 people in another room and this same person enters the second room, they will again like 3 of the people that they liked before; they will *dislike* 3 of the people that they liked before; and they will decide that 4 of the people that they liked before are neither here nor there."

Marie-Elise gets it first. "That makes sense," she says, "if how you see all 10 of the people in the room—in *either* room—is actually coming from you. It's just like the diamond sorter. It's not that a third of the diamonds in the parcel are inferior; it's that there's something in the sorter's mind that is going to see a third of the diamonds in *any* parcel as being inferior, even if they just got through deciding that all the stones were fine."

"Good," I jump on it. "And that's what's happening as we go through a day with our partner. If we have the seeds in our mind to see a third of what they do or say as irritating, then we will—and we'll complain about it, with good reason. And if suddenly they agree to stop doing or saying whatever we find irritating, then by tomorrow we'll find something wrong with another third. And it's not that the complaining is wrong; we do, validly, see 33% of everything about them as something worthy of complaint."

Marie-Elise throws a little self-satisfied glance at Georges, but he's not falling for it. "But *why* does she continue to see 33% of me as irritating?"

"Ah," I smile. "That's easy. Some percentage—say, what? 5%?—of what *she's* been doing or saying is irritating to somebody else. That plants seeds that grow into seeing 33% of everything *you* do as irritating."

This time it's Georges' turn to glance at his wife. I have to redirect this train of thought quickly, or we're going to have the Cheese Casserole problem.

The Cheese Casserole goes back to a story I heard from one of my younger colleagues. When she was born, her mom was in some kind of new-age group—which already makes me feel old, because I knew about the group at the time, and here's a full-grown woman standing in front of me who was just a gleam in her parents' eyes at the time.

Anyway, Mom used to help with the cooking, in the house of their Master, who came from India. As can often happen, there was some competition going on between the students, everybody wanting to be the one to cook the dish that the Master liked the most.

So Mom comes down some stairs holding a steaming-hot platter of cheese casserole for the Master, and she trips on the last stair and dumps the whole thing on the floor.

"That's your karma!" smiles a competing student with satisfaction.

The Master walks over to this woman, lifts up his foot, stomps on her big toe, and smiles. "That's your karma!" he says.

So just a little warning here. Once you start learning about the seeds, don't let it take you into Karma Games. "Karma Games" is where Georges is telling his wife—either in his words, or just in his thoughts—that because everything she sees in him is actually coming from her, it's all her problem, and he doesn't have to listen to any suggestions she gives him for improving. Marie-Elise can play the same game, telling Georges that at any given time there really is 33% about him which warrants the complaints.

So I jump in with The Pen. "Now how are we going to shut down this cycle, this particular little feedback loop? Georges isn't 33% irritating, or 90% irritating or 10% irritating, any more than the parcel of all-white diamonds has any yellowish stones at all. We've got to find a practical way that Marie-Elise can stop planting these 33%-irritating seeds.

"We could go at it through the first of the Four Flowers," I suggest...

"Meaning," she says, "that I could stop doing to others what Georges is doing to me. That is, I could be really careful not to do or say anything irritating at all, and that would shut down the seeds for seeing irritating things in Georges."

"Right," I agree, "and that's an option. Is there any other option? What about the second of the Four Flowers?"

"That's the habit thing," pipes up Georges. "Start seeing anything as 33% percent irritating, and you're going to keep seeing other things as 33% irritating, whether they really are or not."

With the word *really,* both Marie-Elise and I roll our eyes at Georges. But you can figure that out on your own.

"Good," I agree. "I mean, once we realize it's our own mind that's forcing us to see *everything* as 33% irritating, we can just try to counter that habit with another one."

"How so?" she asks.

"It's pretty simple," I say. "I mean, when I was a kid, I used to sing in a chorus. The director was a sweet grandfatherly type who would pull out ancient songs and make us learn them—like the whole of Handel's *Messiah.* But there was also a song that Judy Garland made famous..."

"You mean the little girl in the old *Wizard of Oz,*" smiles Marie-Elise.

"Right. So anyway, the song is called *Look for the Silver Lining,* and it's terribly corny; but it's also pretty profound. Here's the main verse:

I have found a point of view
To ease the daily grind;
So I'll keep repeating, in my mind,
'Look for the silver lining'."

Looking into two blank stares I realize that I have to do some explaining, English-Frenchwise. "The idea is that you can get caught out in a rainstorm, and the sky can be covered with dark and ominous clouds, but if you look closely you can always see one of the black clouds edged with a lovely border of gold or silver, where the sun still shining over the clouds is starting to break through them.

"There's always something about Georges, and about any other situation, which is actually extremely beautiful. We just have to get into the habit of concentrating on the 67% of pure white diamonds, and not the 33% of the yellow."

"Doesn't sound like a planting-seeds approach," grumbles Georges.

"Sounds more like a 'Just think positive' approach. I thought we were trying to get away from learning to cope with the bad, instead of just making sure that it never happens in the first place."

I think for a moment. "Yes I admit, it does sound like that. But what I'm talking about is Flower Two. We are already seeing a certain percentage of what our partner does or says as irritating. Even if they stop doing whatever we find irritating, by tomorrow we will see the same percentage of irritating things in them, because that's the percentage of bad seeds we have in our own mind.

"But even on a terrible day with our partner, there are some really nice things about them that we're still really attracted to—that's why we chose them as a partner in the first place."

Georges and Marie-Elise exchange a little glance of yearning that only the French know how to do. Things are looking up already.

"So we just grab hold of our mind—which can be like grabbing hold of a wild elephant—and wrestle with it for a few moments, and force it to focus on some of the things that are beautiful about our partner, rather than on the things we find irritating right now. In fact, this kind of wrestling is exactly what the word 'meditation' means: learning to *direct* our thoughts to where *we* want them to go, rather than having them wander off to where *they* want to go.

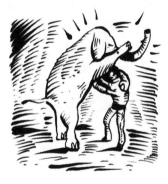

"Now for the first few days, this is going to be a pretty artificial exercise. The third of our partner which is doing and saying irritating things is still really strong, and calling to us. But every time we see something negative we use it as a reminder to think about the positive—the silver lining; and there really is a lot of it there.

"Every time we just glance at something we like about our partner, it plants a seed in our mind, even if it's small and weak compared to the power of what's being planted when we're feeling some healthy irritation.

"The Second Flower says though that even this weak seed is going to bloom as a habit. Within a few days, every irritating thought we have about our partner triggers a second thought, of looking for something to appreciate about them. Each good seed contributes to a habit of planting more good seeds. And pretty soon we're back to the first days of our relationship, when we were—*really*—seeing only beauty in our partner."

By now Georges has his arm around Marie-Elise's shoulders, and they're both looking pretty dreamy. But she has one last issue.

"Okay, but aren't the irritated seeds also creating a habit of being more irritated? Why should the weaker admiring seeds make more of a habit than the stronger irritated seeds?"

"Because they are founded in truth," I say, and stand up. But Georges grabs my arm and pulls me back down.

"How's that work, exactly?" he asks. I nod.

"Okay, well that's one of the most moving moments in the entire career of a monk in a Tibetan monastery. We spend like 25 years in intense study and meditation and debate, and then finally we go through several weeks of really tough oral exams, in front of all the monks in our monastery. And in my monastery at the time, there were over a thousand of them.

"If you pass the final exam, then you get one of those big yellow geshe hats, looks like an old Greek warrior's helmet. In fact, on the day of the final they pass out those hats to everybody, even to the smallest little monk in the monastery.

"Everybody puts on a hat and then somebody gets up to ask you the final, final question in your 25 years or study. And that question is always the same."

"Well, what is it?" asks Marie-Elise.

"They ask you, 'Will there ever be an end to suffering in this entire world?'"

"And what's the answer?" says Georges.

"The answer is 'Yes'!"

"And then they ask you, 'Why?' And you always say, 'Because truth is stronger than a lie'—that is, sooner or later everyone in the world will figure out that the only way to get what they want is to help others get it first. And then the lie of selfishness, which never works, will be overthrown.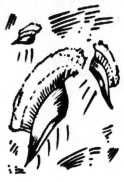

"And then everybody grabs the geshe hat off their head, and throws it in the air, like a Frisbee, and yells at the top of their lungs in celebration! So cool!"

"So cool!" they agree.

Question 56

Our relationship has been struggling for quite some time, getting more and more tense every month. But we really love each other and we want to make it work. I was thinking maybe some professional counseling might help—what do you think?

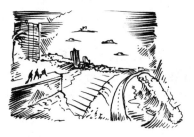

This question came during a stroll along some cliffs overlooking a long line of unruly waves off of Lima, Peru. I'm walking with Estrella on one side, and her partner Carlos on the other. I can feel Carlos tense up when Estrella speaks; as often happens with this question, I can tell it's been a sore point between them for a while.

"But like," objects Carlos immediately, "how are we going to know if the counselor is a good one or not? All the ones that I've ever met are just getting over their own recent divorces. How do we know they're not just going to take our money, and make things worse than they already are?"

This gets into something I like to call "The Magic of Empty Teachers." And it's another good chance to talk about the third of the Four Flowers, which is a really important one.

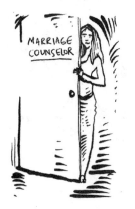

"So you go to find a marriage counselor," I begin, "On the internet, or by asking around. Except...do you really *find* them?"

Carlos and Estrella have attended enough of the classes I've been giving at the nearby Universidad del Pacifico to know the answer. "Not really," says Estrella. "Because there's nobody there to find."

"How so?"

Carlos picks it up. "They're coming from you,

from the seeds in your mind. It's not like the marriage counselor is standing there at the door of their office, and you walk up and start talking to them. From the end of the corridor outside their office, a small picture of a counselor is coming out of your mind. By the time you walk down the same corridor and stand at the door, a much bigger picture of a counselor is coming out of your mind.

"There's an illusion of walking down the corridor, but really your mind is just pumping out bigger and bigger counselors, until you're right up next to them, shaking their hand.

"So can we say that you don't *find* a marriage counselor? You *create* a marriage counselor. Same as a partner."

"Right," they respond, in unison.

"So you create the person; but do you also create what they say?"

"I suppose so," says Estrella, obviously thinking on it. But then a little frown appears on her forehead.

"You go to a marriage counselor so they can help you with your marriage," she says.

"Right."

"And if they're going to *counsel* the two of us, then by definition they have to know something that we don't already know."

"Right again."

Carlos sees the problem too. "So...how can I create a counselor or a teacher who knows more than I know, if they're coming from me?"

"Second Law of Karma," I answer.

Estrella remembers. "Seeds always expand, hugely, by the time they open."

"Right. So say that I plant a seed for a teacher, by sharing a skill which I know with a coworker in my office—maybe I help them learn how to use a certain computer program, or a certain app on my phone. The seed I plant multiplies deep down in my mind, until it finally splits open and flowers—into a teacher, or a marriage counselor."

"So we *do* need to go to a marriage counselor," concludes Estrella, with a smile.

But Carlos is a step ahead of her. "I don't see why. I mean, if the seed of trying to share what we know with somebody else is strong enough, couldn't it just flower in our own mind as some sudden understanding about what we need to do to fix our relationship by ourselves? Why does it have to come back to us *through* a marriage counselor?"

I nod. "That's a really good question, and it gets into the idea of a Pattern, and an Instrument. It's true that the seeds we plant by sharing something we know how to do with someone else can—more often than we imagine—come back simply as a new idea inside our own head: a new insight into how we could get along with our partner.

"But the way in which a seed from sharing is planted means that very often there is a Pattern to how it opens up and flowers. In the case of learning something we need to know, the Pattern is often that it comes back to us through another person—through a teacher.

"It is true that we are creating the teacher, and that the vast expansion of the original seed is creating ideas they share with us which we never could have thought of on our own. But this particular Pattern is so typical that what we learn will most often be coming back to us through an Instrument—the Instrument of a teacher.

"Think of the Instrument as a delivery system, the package that holds the thing that we purchased online, from the store to our door."

Carlos smiles. "But the Instrument—the teacher through whom the seed flowers—is also coming from a seed."

"That's true too," I admit. "Which gets us into Flower Three. We don't just want a marriage counselor; we want a marriage counselor who knows what they are talking about. We're creating the person, to appear in the world around us: that's Flower Three. But another part of Flower Three is that we are also creating what they say to us—the words that come to our ears from the outer world.

"And so whether the marriage counselor is really *helpful* or not is also coming from us. It's that thing about the car and the extra features."

A moment of silence. "Uh, I don't remember that from your talk," says Estrella finally.

I cast about for an example. "So if you don't have a partner," I ask, "how do you find one? I mean, according to the Diamond Cutter system?"

"Well you don't find them," says Carlos. "You *create* them."

"Right," I correct myself. "And how do you *create* them?"

"Well, you might plant a seed, by 'adopting' an elderly person in a nursing home—by going to visit them on a regular basis, every week or two. Being there to provide them companionship plants a seed for a partner who shows up in your own life, bringing you companionship."

"Right. So that's like ordering a new car, you see. But then you have to figure out the features that you want in the car: do you want the car painted red, or blue; what kind of stereo would you like; are you going to order the hands-free phone or not?

"Same with your partner; you use Flower Three to create all the qualities you want them to have: loyal, sensitive, helpful. Each one of these qualities has its own seed, which is separate from the seed which creates just the basic partner, the basic car model.

Carlos ties it back to their marriage: "So it's one thing to create a counselor who's going to give us suggestions, and it's another thing to create one who is going to give us *good* suggestions."

"Right. Sharing the knowledge that you have with others—teaching someone else at work what you know how to do, even if they might compete with you later—is the seed for the teacher. And making sure that the person at work knows how to do your job *as well as you do* is the seed to have a marriage counselor with all the frills: one who gives you good advice.

"So now you tell me," I conclude. "Should you guys go to a marriage counselor or not?"

They answer me together. "If it's a counselor that we plant, okay. If not, not okay."

Okay.

FIDELITY

Question 57

I recently found out that my partner was cheating on me. I feel crushed, and unsure what to do—should I leave, or believe him when he says he loves me and will stop? I feel torn either choice I make.

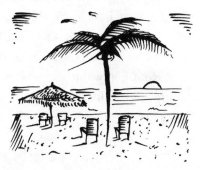

This question, or some variation on it, is sadly one of the most common that I ever get. It raises a lot of issues, but since we're on the subject of the Four Flowers, let's look at it that way. I think especially with Flower Four, which we haven't had a chance to talk about yet.

So I'm walking across a green lawn at a small resort in Malaysia near a place called Johor Bahru, which is a city on one of the routes from Malaysia to Singapore. Singaporeans often come here to take a beach vacation, and we're having a weekend retreat about finding your passion in life. Yiling is asking the question; we can see her husband Lee sitting at a table in the outdoor restaurant nearby—he knows we are trying to work this issue out.

"So there are crucial moments in a person's life," I begin. "Decisive moments, where something can go either way and determine the entire rest of our life."

"It does feel like this is one of those," agrees Yiling.

"But there are even more crucial moments," I add, "like the one at the very end of this life. I think if we look at those critical few minutes, we can get some insight into where you should go with Lee in the coming weeks."

"Sounds a bit strange," says Yiling, "but I'm desperate. So yes, let's go there."

"Okay. You know about the Four Flowers, right?"

"Yes," she says. "You talked about that in Singapore last year. These are the four ways in which a single seed splits open, to give forth its flowers in our life."

"Right. So I would like to go through Flower Four with you, and see how we can use it to decide which way you go at the crossroads you face this month, with Lee."

"Great, thank you."

"Okay, so Flower Four is perhaps the most difficult to really understand; let's start from the beginning. Right now, as we walk across this lawn, are we planting any seeds?"

"I think so," says Yiling. "I mean, we are trying to work out a pretty serious problem. If we succeed, then it will mean a lot for the lives of two people, for years to come. Definitely some powerful seeds, good seeds."

"Right. Now, in the last 10 steps across the lawn, already talking about this problem, how many seeds have we planted?"

"Well, I know that it's 65 seeds per second; so if we say a second for each step, we've planted over 600 seeds already."

"Right. Now the Second Law of Karma says that those seeds are going to multiply for as long as they sit within the 'soil' of our mind—until they open up and ripen. They will double, every 24 hours."

"Got that," says Yiling.

"And when they are ready to come out," I ask, "how many come out, every moment?"

"Also 65," she answers. "Our life is like a film, seeds opening at 65 frames a second, so we have the illusion that the world and time are moving around us."

"So...do you see any problem with the math?"

"There *is* a problem," she nods. "If seeds are being created at a rate of 65 a second, but those seeds that are created are constantly multiplying until they ripen into my life—which passes at only 65 seeds a second—then I'm always piling up thousands and thousands of extra seeds, every day of my life."

"Exactly," I agree. "And what happens to these extra seeds?"

"Well," says Yiling, "the Fourth Law of Karma says that—once a seed is planted—it never just goes away. Every single seed we ever plant is stored, indelibly, in the mind; and it will stay there for many years, if necessary, until it flowers into some experience in our life. But that's a problem," she says, mentally doing the math.

"Right," I agree. "There will always be a backlog of seeds building up in our mind. Now what happens when we reach the end of our life—when the automobile of the body breaks down?"

"I know what you mean when you talk about the body as an automobile," says Yiling. "We've talked about it before.

"That is, we see a car pull over on the side of the high-way—and there's obviously something wrong with it, and it's not moving forward any more. But none of us would assume, when we see a car pull over to the side of the road and come to a stop, that the driver inside the car must have died. Just because the car can't move any more doesn't prove that the driver can't move any more."

Just because a car breaks down doesn't mean the driver is dead

"Exactly. So the body can break down, and come to a stop, but that doesn't necessarily tell us anything about the mind. We can't be sure that the mind has stopped, just because it no longer has any way to communicate with us through talking lips or moving hands. It could be that the living mind is stuck inside a broken body, like a driver locked inside a car which has broken down.

"Alright then. Now what about the seeds at this point?"

"Well, I think that is one of the most interesting things about the whole idea of the Four Flowers," she says. "Flower Four is describing this very moment. I have spent an entire lifetime storing up extra seeds, seeds which cannot be destroyed, in the storehouse of my own mind. They don't just disappear when my body stops working; they are still there, and they will still open and throw a new world ahead of me."

"Example?" I ask, simply.

"Like the last movie you went to," she says. "We tend to think that there's a whole movie up there in the projection booth somehow; and that in each passing moment, the projector grabs the next bit of the movie and sends it to the screen.

"But what's really happening is that seeds are opening in my mind, at their usual rate—65 per second. They throw ahead of us the next minute of the movie, like stepping stones crossing a garden."

Here Yiling is talking about an example that I often give which—like so many other examples that I use—comes from the 25 years that I spent living in the same house with my teacher from Tibet, serving and learning from him.

For many years, even as I lived with him, I had the idea that everything I needed to know was contained in those exquisite, ancient books from Tibet that lined the walls of his room—and I would spend every possible moment curled up with one of these scriptures in front of my nose. And just as I got settled and comfortable he would call out from the kitchen: "Hey Mike! Can you come outside and help me with something, just for a minute?"

And of course it would never be just a minute, but more often like an hour, or an entire day. On this particular day, Rinpoche has decided that he wants a little path, of flagstones.

He stands on the front porch. "Look, Mike," he points out to the lawn. "Every time it rains" (and where we lived it was almost always raining) "we have to walk across the lawn and get our feet all muddy and wet. Wouldn't it be great if we had a path out to the driveway?"

I wince, remembering the recent project to build a sidewalk around the entire house and adjacent temple. Dancing around a cement truck with a trowel, and finding out the hard way why you always wear gloves when you work with cement.

"Oh no, not cement," says Rinpoche cheerfully. "I was thinking we could use flagstones."

Now that sounds more reasonable. Buy like 20 flagstones, then just flop them down on the lawn between the porch and the driveway, and I can get back to my old Tibetan books. From Lama I get the specs that he wants— what color, what kind of stone—and head off to the garden supply store.

Within the hour I'm leaning off the porch with the first flagstone; I aim it out in front of the stairs and drop it. Then I step on that flagstone and lean out over the lawn and drop the next one. Within 10 minutes I'm standing in the driveway, looking back at the new path with satisfaction. All I need to do now is just walk back over the same stones and into the kitchen door and into my bedroom and back to the 15th-century author I had been reading before Rinpoche suddenly decided he couldn't live without a flagstone path.

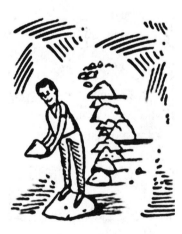

In fact I can see him over at the house now, stepping off the porch onto the first flagstone. He doesn't stroll across the lawn on the stones but freezes there on the first one, shifting his weight from foot to foot, looking down and frowning a bit.

We've been together so many years that I can pretty much read his mind. "Is there something wrong, Rinpoche?"

"Well Mike, this stone wobbles back and forth. I mean—I saw on the TV, there was this show about Italy, and those guys were laying sand underneath the flagstones, so they wouldn't wobble." He looks at me expectantly, and without another word I'm into the house and on the phone to a gravel company, ordering a load of sand.

And so a big part of the day melts away as I pine for my scriptures, tearing up flagstones, laying down sand, and setting the flagstones again, one by one: Step on a stone, lean over to smooth the sand ahead and drop the next one, step on that one, a tiny wobble, Rinpoche scowling, pick it up again, adjust the sand to the contour of the stone. It's like half an hour per stone to get it up to Rinpoche Standards.

Finally I'm out to the end, stepping off the last flagstone onto the driveway, with an undeniable feeling of satisfaction. It's *good* to do things right, and now I can run back to my books. Except that it's getting dusk already, and time to cook Rinpoche's supper. But that's okay—I will have some quiet time afterwards.

Rinpoche comes out on the porch in the darkening shadows and steps off onto the first flagstone. Shifts his weight from side to side and smiles with satisfaction. "No wobble!" he yells to me, across the yard.

But then he leans down and stares closely at the stone, steps off to the side, and squats down, like a golfer trying to judge the angle of a shot. "Hey Mike!" he yells, and I have this bad feeling about how I'm going to spend tomorrow.

He points to the first stone. "Big problem!" he says.

"What's that, Rinpoche?" I try not to groan.

"The sand raised the stone up!" he exclaims.

"Well yes, Rinpoche," I try not to show my irritation—very bad manners in the Tibetan tradition, when relating to your lama.

"The lawnmower blade will hit it when you cross this part of the lawn."

I lean down and take a look. As usual, he's completely correct.

"Well, tomorrow morning you can dig out the path a bit, and lay down the sand again," he declares. Lama's word is law, and that's how I spend the next morning.

This went on for I think four days. I must have crossed that lawn a hundred times, stepping onto one flagstone and dropping down the next one, adjusting it, and then stepping onto it to drop the next.

At some point it dawned on me that this exercise, like so much else which passed between Rinpoche and myself, was a lesson. Our whole life consists of laying down the next flagstone, stepping onto it, and laying down the next one. Seeds ripen in the mind, and throw ahead the next moment of our day, and then we step into it, into the next moment of the physical world around us, into the people around us in that next moment. And more seeds ripen in that moment, and they throw forth the next piece of our life. This is what Yiling is talking about with the car that's broken down on the highway.

"So can seeds still be opening after the body dies; after the car breaks down?" I ask her.

Yiling ponders for a moment. "We've said that millions and millions of seeds have piled up in your mind by that point. And we've said that they never just fade away; that they must, sooner or later, open and flower and create the things around us. Except that..."

A light comes on, and her face takes on that look of excited discovery. "We all know that seeds in your mind create the place and the people around you, at any given moment. But what creates the *mind* with which I see these places and people?"

I always have a pen handy in my pocket, for just such questions. I draw it out and wave it around. Open my mouth wide and pretend to gnaw on it.

"Oh," she says simply. "My mind as well is coming from seeds."

I nod.

"So...even after the body dies, the seeds in my mind are...throwing ahead of me the next moment of my mind, of *me*..."

I nod again.

"And then all those excess seeds in my mind start opening, and my mind starts seeing...new things: new places, new people, a new world."

One more nod. "And that's the Fourth Flower," I finish. I've got her mind where I want it, and now I wait for her next question.

"So...what's that got to do with deciding whether to stay with Lee, or leave him, because he's cheated on me—whether or not I should believe him when he says he won't do it again?"

"*Why* are you seeing him cheat on you?"

Yiling blushes. "Because I have a seed that opens up in my mind to see him cheat on me. Which means I must have *planted* that seed. Which means that at some time in the past I must have cheated on *someone else.*

"But I *haven't,"* she exclaims.

"And what's the Second Law of Karma?" I ask.

"Seeds multiply...oh," she says, and remembers. "I mean, we were just sending a few emails back and forth...nothing happened, really.

"But it *grew*..." she sighs.

"So what do I do now?"

"So there are lots of thing you can do: clean the seed, help others patch up their relationships. But I want to go a little deeper with you on this. The essence of what you want right now is to figure out what's going to happen in the next few weeks and months.

"You stand at a crossroads in your relationship with your husband. It could go either way. Maybe he will keep his promise to stop messing around, and maybe he won't. We want to make sure that he will.

"This moment in your life, you see, it is very similar to the moment of death that we've been talking about. This is a special moment too, a cross-roads. All the millions of seeds—the backlog of seeds—in your mind are especially potent at the moment of death. One of them is going to crack open at the one moment of decision and determine which world, and which people, you see around you next—and even what kind of body you will look down and see as you step into this new world.

"The ancient books say that we have to be extremely careful at this one moment, because—even more than the seeds that decide our moment-to-moment flagstones in this current life—the seeds in the mind in the moment that the body finally breaks down will decide much of an entire lifetime to come. At this moment we cannot—we *must* not—cause a bad seed to crack open."

"And the same for me," she understands. "I'm at a very crucial moment with Lee. I absolutely *cannot* have a seed open that will cause me to see him cheating again. Because that would be the end."

"Right." And I wait for her last question. Then it will all be alright.

"Assuming," she says, "that out of millions of seeds in my mental store-house there might be some more that will cause me to see him cheating on me again...is there some method I can use to make sure that one of them doesn't open?"

"Now you're asking the right question," I smile. "You're at the threshold of a new life, a new life with Lee, and we want to make sure that no bad seeds open.

"We know the general rule that the seed is there; and that it cannot be destroyed. But is there sort of a special way that we can rob it of its power to create a Lee who is cheating?"

Yiling nods, hopefully.

"There is such a way. The ancient books call it 'scorching the seed.' Personally I like to think of it like the nyjer seed that I feed to the wild birds that visit my house."

"Never heard of it."

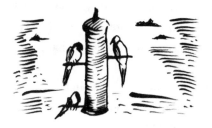

"It's a special seed that they import into the US from India. The little yellow finches love it. Except that it grows into a really nasty thistle bush. So there's a law that you have to sterilize the seed with a special treatment if you're going to ship it into the US. The whole seed is still there, and just as yummy to the birds, but it will never start growing by accident and take over your whole front yard.

"And that's what we're going to do with any seeds that you possess to see Lee cheating again. We're going to sterilize them."

"Okay," Yiling says with determination, "just tell me how." I can see that somehow she's thinking this will involve brain surgery, or something similarly drastic.

"In a moment of life-changing decision, in a moment of the crossroads in a relationship for the rest of your life, and even in the moment of death, when seeds are being selected for the next world you step into it, there is one special way to make sure that bad seeds don't crack open.

"And that is simply—in as many moments of your day as you can— **you just think about how the people and things and events around you are coming from the seeds in your own mind.** It's absolutely, completely, weird; or maybe just what you might expect if you really thought about it carefully.

"The way to sterilize your bad seeds—the way to make sure that you never see your husband cheat again—is simply to stop and pause, over and over throughout the day, to think about how everything around you is coming from you.

"The sun that came up this morning is coming from seeds I planted by trying to bring happiness and light into other people's lives. The breakfast I had this morning came from seeds I planted by helping others have enough. The very eyes with which I read these words came from seeds which I planted by helping others to see, to understand the things that they must.

"And so what stops your husband's cheating is just this: constant, joyful, grateful understanding, in frequent pauses throughout the day.

Yiling feels the truth of it, the rightness of it. I see a plan from in her sparkling eyes

SELFISHNESS

Question 58

In our conversations especially, but also in just about everything else we do together, my partner is so self-absorbed and selfish that she seems to be totally unaware of what I would like, or what I need. How can I get her to think about others once in a while?

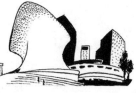

I'm sitting with some DCI Mexico staff in a little white alcove just outside the theater of the Soumaya Art Museum in Mexico City. This is a new museum built just recently by Carlos Slim, in memory of his wife; it has a truly awesome collection of Rodin pieces. Mr. Slim is, by the way, at present the richest man in the world, topping Bill Gates and Warren Buffett.

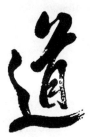

I'm about to give an evening talk there, when Rodrigo turns and asks me this question. We've already covered the same thing a couple of ways so far here in the book, but let's go at it this time from the Dao (which is sometimes written as "Tao").

"If it were me," I say, "I would just try getting her to think about the Dao."

"Dao…I've heard of that," says Rodrigo, "but I can't say that I'm really clear on what it is."

"It's Chinese for *path*," I reply, "but it has a special meaning in the classic Chinese book on the subject, the *Dao De Jing*—which is sometimes written as *Tao Te Ching*. The word *jing* means 'an ancient book of wisdom,' while *de* means 'virtue.' So the idea is that virtue becomes a path."

"Sounds nice," says Rodrigo, "but how does this Dao apply to fixing Fernanda's selfishness?"

"Okay," I reply. "Let's start with the snake and the rope."

"I know about that," he says. "You're walking through your Arizona garden in the evening; suddenly you look down and there's a rattlesnake stretched across the path ahead. You jump and give a little yelp but then you realize it was just an old piece of rope all along. You calm down and feel a little dumb for getting so excited."

"Right. The point is that things weren't at all the way you thought they were. And not knowing this could actually hurt you if, for example, you stumbled and fell when you jumped out of the way of the rattlesnake-that-wasn't.

"Being selfish—watching out for Number One—is the same basic mistake. It doesn't work, it *can't* work, because it assumes that the world works in a certain way, when the world doesn't work that way at all. When you are selfish, you are working against how the world really works—you are working against the Dao.

Being selfish never works

"When you work against the Dao, you always fail. Get Fernanda—get any normal, thinking person—to see that they're hurting themselves by being selfish, and they'll just stop it, on their own."

"So how do I teach her the Dao?" he asks.

"There's this beautiful verse about it in Tibetan," I reply. "It says:

May I always cherish each living creature,
Understanding that—for reaching the ultimate goal—
They are more precious than a jewel
Which grants your every wish.

"They're talking about a mythical gemstone from ancient India; it was like an Aladdin's lamp. You asked the jewel for anything you wanted, and that thing would suddenly appear.

"The people around us are just the same. If we are selfish—if we ignore what other people want, if we ignore their needs—then we have no soil in which to plant our seeds, and everything we ever try to do will fail.

"Teach Fernanda about the seeds; this is the Dao, this is the Way of Virtue. 'Virtue' here just means being nice to other people, trying to be aware of what they need, and helping them to get it. When you do, then you plant the seeds for everything which you want.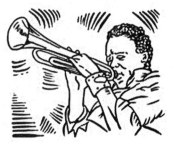

"It's not possible to continue being a selfish person if you know how to get the things you want."

Rodrigo looks up; he wants more, but as Miles Davis once said, "Less is more." I stand up and head for the theater.

FOOD & WEIGHT

Question 59

My husband never helps with the cooking; left to himself for dinner, he just eats a bag of potato chips in front of the TV. How do I plant a seed to see him be more interested in cooking, and sitting down to a nice meal with me?

This question came while I was in Los Angeles giving some business talks near Wilshire and the 405. A private dinner was arranged for six or seven of the partici-, pants, at a lovely house on Venice Beach. We are settling down to coffee afterwards, gazing out to the beach through a window which is pretty much the front of the entire house.

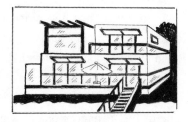

William looks a bit grumpy that his wife Laurie is attacking his eating habits—I'll have to find an answer that brings them back together.

"I've thought about this one a lot," I say, "because I have much the same habit. I find myself snacking all day—and sometimes I have the presence of mind to pause and check myself to see if I'm actually hungry.

"Often I discover that I'm *not* hungry. And then I check to see *why* I'm eating right now, and it turns out that it's just some kind of nervous habit; like tapping your foot, or checking your emails again when you just checked them a few minutes ago. It's not that I'm under any special anxiety or stress, but just that I need to be doing something. So I go over to the fridge and take out something almost at random, and start eating.

"Sometimes I'm the opposite: I eat a nice healthy little salad for a late lunch, and then I feel happy and contented and I just don't even think about the refrigerator again.

"So I've come to identify this contented state of mind—I've learned to recognize when it's there, and when it's not there. What I've figured out is that this is not just some random place that my mind goes to once in a while;

rather, it's actually a truly meditative state of mind. And so I've started to call it Meditation Mind. I think it's a very practical solution to a lot of our problems around food.

William's ears prick up; he's not particularly interested about their family eating habits, but he is curious about meditation. "So…what is 'Meditation Mind'? And how do you get into it?"

"You can think of the whole exercise of meditation," I begin, "as learning to drive a car. Except the car is your mind.

"Look. One day while I was studying in the Tibetan monastery, my main teacher decided that he wanted to go visit Ganden Monastery. At the time this was like a 12-hour drive, some of it through lush green countryside, and some of it fighting through knots of people and pigs and cows choking the streets in little Indian towns.

"In those days, the monastery had one ancient Hindustan Ambassador. This is a car model that was swiped from the British in the late 1950's and hasn't changed at all since then—for most of the period that I was spending a lot of time in India, it was the only car you could buy there.

"So somehow a bunch of the elders in my particular college decided that one of the teenage monks—a particularly naughty one—was the reincarnation of a famous lama who had passed away about the time the boy was born. They tried to push the child into becoming a religious scholar but he just wasn't interested, and finally he got out of it by learning to drive the monastery car, which was almost as prestigious.

"So he's driving—which is scary enough, especially in a country with almost no street signs: one time trying to find the Bangalore City Airport we ended up hopelessly mired in mud in the middle of a cornfield. But now my teacher gets it into his head that his attendant Nawang should also learn to drive; so the two monks switch up front.

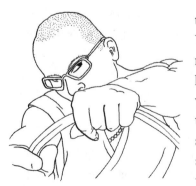

"Within a few minutes we discover that Nawang has this special spatial sense. Whenever he turns to look at the other monk telling him how to drive the car, he spins his whole upper body too, along with his arms and hands. Which means that every couple of seconds he's rocketing straight towards one of the ditches on the side of the road, as the rest of us scream in terror."

Laurie looks over from the coffee service at the side of the living room, stirring in some sugar and obviously wondering what this has to do with William stuffing his face with potato chips.

"Oh…so meditation, you see, it's exactly like driving down a ragged Indian road and trying to stay out of the ditches on either side."

"How so?" asks William.

"Well, you can pretty much *define* meditation as weaving a middle path through two states of mind which most of us find ourselves in most of the day. And both of these two states of mind ruin our Meditation Mind. When we don't have Meditation Mind, we feel like going to the fridge and eating—not because we're hungry but because, in a very fundamental way, our mind is slightly nervous, or bored.

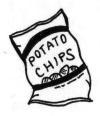

"If you just keep your mind clear of the two ditches, then you have Meditation Mind. And then you feel happy, contented, and clear. When your mind is particularly clear, you relate to food in a different way. You don't have this urge to grab a plastic potato-chip bag between your teeth and tear it open mindlessly.

"Instead," and here I give Laurie a significant look, "you might actually start finding it sort of meditative to focus your mind on preparing and eating a beautiful meal: carefully selecting a recipe which you would both enjoy and find interesting to prepare; gently walking through the vegetable section of a nice grocery to explore the freshest ingredients; and then working shoulder-to-shoulder in the kitchen, wrapped in an affectionate silence.

Meditation enemies: Busy Mind & Dead Mind

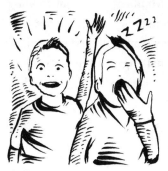

"But to get there, you need to get to Meditation Mind; and to get there, you need to avoid the two ditches. And for that you need to know what these two are, and how to recognize them in your own head."

"So what's the first one?" asks William.

"The first ditch you can call Busy Mind. We all have Busy Mind, and the sad thing is that we don't know we have it. Even if we did know, we probably wouldn't think it was much of a problem. I think that with the advent of many new electronic diversions—cell phones, games, texts, web surfing, this minute's latest songs—the old problem of Busy Mind is about 100 times worse than it ever was before.

"Busy Mind is restless. You sit down to eat breakfast, and suddenly you think of something else you have to do. You pull out your phone to text somebody, and maybe grab a bite of cereal inbetween that and the next text. While you're texting, you decide you have to look if you have any new emails, so then you're walking through the living room with a piece of toast in your hand.

"When you do open up your laptop to check your emails, a news service pops up a list of the ten worst movies of the year so far, and you dutifully read through something you never needed to know—something you will forget within half an hour.

"Where does Busy Mind get you? Slowly you lose your ability to concentrate on anything at all, and somehow you convince yourself that you're more informed and more 'linked in' with other people on the internet, when really you're just losing the ability to have any meaningful interaction with anybody—or, in our example here, with the food that you're eating.

"You lose the ability to taste the food, and you lose the ability to discriminate between something which is good to eat and something which is not—it all begins to taste the same. Slowly this tears down your body, and your health.

"And when you lose your ability to concentrate, or to relate to other people in any meaningful way, then you begin to avoid other parts of life. Instead of facing challenges head-on, with gusto and decisiveness, you start retreating from life. All the days spent in Busy Mind then push you into Dead Mind—and that's the second ditch we need to avoid.

"Dead Mind is easier to identify than Busy Mind. If you want to know what Dead Mind feels like, then eat a huge meal and then try to concentrate on some task at home, or at your office. You feel sleepy and dull and uninspired; even if you are able to force your mind to face a challenge, you quickly retreat and leave it unresolved. Another easy way to get to Dead Mind is just to sleep one or two hours less than you personally need to feel refreshed."

"So how do you keep out of the ditches?" asks Laurie, who is also beginning to get interested now and has come to sit on the edge of the couch, next to William.

"Well, as I said, the first job is just to realize that you *have* Busy Mind or Dead Mind at any given moment. This is not such a challenge if someone just tells you what these two are like, and you pause from time to time during the day to see if you've slipped into either one.

"For Busy Mind, you need to cut down on stimulus. Download a timer for your computer that automatically keeps track of how long you've been on, and try to limit yourself to sessions of an hour and a half, with at least half an hour between sessions doing something else—especially anything which gets you out of doors, or moving somehow.

"Choose a specific time of day for dealing with most of your emails and texts; try to control them, and don't let them control you. When you are interacting with someone in person, have the courtesy to give them your full attention; if a text or call comes in on your phone, take it later.

"Try to limit the amount of time you spend listening to or watching the news. It's good to have a basic awareness of local and international events, especially if there's something going on which might provide us with a chance for serving others. But a great deal of the news is meant only to get your attention and take up your time, so that advertisers will have more opportunity to sell you something. Learn to glance at the news to catch major trends which might actually affect your life, and then let the rest go. Your mind will be much more calm and peaceful.

"Possessions are a great contributor to Busy Mind. Again, think of your bedroom closet: gaze around the floor and mark the shapes and colors of the shoes there.

"But of course you're really looking at these shoes in your mind—in your memory, because in your memory you have a little inventory of all the possessions that you own, like a file folder on your laptop. Every time you buy another thing, another picture gets added to your memory.

"And the space in the mind is limited, just the same as the space on the hard disk inside your computer. The best way to ruin a good computer is to fill it up all the way to capacity; the same applies to your mind. So if you want to stop Busy Mind, evaluate all the stuff in your house frequently. If you find things that you're not really using—things that are just taking up house space and mind space—then get rid of them, give them away. Local charities are happy to take them and turn them over to people who don't have enough.

"Finally, try not to overschedule your life. Only take on the amount of activities that you can give peaceful, clear attention to. And you know what that attention feels like—like the quiet joy of reading a good book, or listening to some of your favorite music, or losing yourself in a great movie.

"But don't go to the other extreme," I warn.

"How's that?" asks William.

"It really is just like driving a car. Think of how a person's hands move back and forth unconsciously on the steering wheel, as they drive and talk to a friend sitting next to them. Meditation Mind is the same. You find yourself on the edge of the Busy Mind ditch on one side of the road, so you make a correction in your course, and cut back on all the promises you're making to do things for people.

"But then there's a danger that you'll go too far and just sit at home doing nothing—which is driving on the edge of the other ditch, Dead Mind. Once you learn to *feel* where your mind is at any given moment, you'll discover that we all tend to alternate between Busy Mind and Dead Mind.

"You get too busy, so you cut back; and then you feel dull because you don't have enough interesting work to do. The trick is to keep correcting and then counter-correcting, like hands on the steering wheel. Life rarely stands still, and well-considered correction is an important skill to learn."

"So suppose you do find yourself coming up on the ditch of Dead Mind," says Laurie. "What do you do then?"

"There are certain signs that you're falling off into Dead Mind. You feel a lack of purpose; you procrastinate a lot, or prioritize your life in a way that you know isn't realistic—avoiding the tasks that you need to get done, as you while away hours on things that aren't so important.

"To get yourself back on track, it helps to sit down and draw up a list of things you need to get done, and then try to get yourself on a schedule. Find a friend who is interested in helping you get out of your funk, and ask if you can send them one email a day describing just one task you've worked on today—one step towards your big hopes and goals—even if it's only for a few minutes.

"Friends are one of the most important ways of keeping your mental car out of the two ditches on opposite sides of the road. Choose them carefully; the ancient Tibetans say that your friends are like the molds used to make little Buddhist statues: as you interact with your friends—as you are pushed up against them like soft plaster inside a mold—your own personality will be shaped by theirs.

Stick to the middle

"That is, find friends who seem to have discovered how to avoid falling into Busy Mind or Dead Mind, and try to be around them. Ask them to help."

I pause and think for a moment. "So…do you remember *why* we are talking about driving down the middle of the road, trying to maintain Meditation Mind?"

William nods. He gets it.

"I guess the idea is that we can try to live our whole life in a way which promotes a peaceful, attentive state of mind—where we really enjoy the people and things around us, and not in any superficial way. This will spill over into our eating habits: we'll begin to take more care and pleasure in what we eat, rather than just eating out of nervousness or boredom."

He gives Laurie a shy look. "There's this recipe I know for crème brûlée," he smiles.

"*After* a good Caesar salad that I've been playing with," she laughs, and slaps him on the arm.

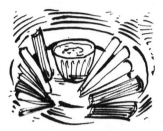

Question 60

When I met her, my wife was really trim; now she eats practically all day, terrible junk food, and she looks terrible too. I'm also worried about her health. What's the seed to save her from her appetite?

This question is very similar to the one we just had; so you should go back and read that answer before going on to this one. I want you to notice that, up to now, we've been approaching this food problem in conventional terms: reach a place of engaged calm—keep your mind on a middle course, without falling into the extreme of being too busy, or of not being busy enough. A centered, focused mind is not interested in eating in an unfocused way.

Problem is, there will be days—or months—when you want to follow this perfectly reasonable advice, but you just can't do it. It's easy for me to sit here and tell you that you're too busy or too bored, and that's why you're eating poorly; but you probably know that already, and you've probably already tried to change, and found it difficult.

So now let's go at it not in conventional terms, but in terms of the seeds: this new Diamond Cutter system, which is going to give you the power to make changes in your life that you haven't been able to manage so far, in an entire lifetime of trying.

The first of the Four Flowers says that what you want to happen to you will happen if you just make it happen for someone else. In our case here, this means that if I want to stop my bad eating habits, I need to do something to help someone else stop their bad eating habits.

This doesn't mean that I personally need to end the junk food addiction of my whole country. The First Law of Karma says that I just have to make some efforts to help others who have the same general problem: like begets like. The Second Law of Karma says that seeds multiply wildly. I don't have to solve everybody's eating problems; I just have to take some modest, focused actions to help support one or two other people in their effort to eat better. Those seeds, once planted in my subconscious, will start to reproduce on their own, and create a whole lifetime of healthy eating for myself.

Flower Two says that if I can just get a small start on practicing this unique method of dealing with a food problem, then that will be enough to trigger a small habit, which will automatically grow into a bigger habit. So I just have to get started on something small to help other people eat better.

Deep down, every one of us enjoys taking care of others. Sharing food is one of the most basic forms that this enjoyment takes. And so a very simple but very powerful practice to help me with my bad eating habits is, for example, to bring some healthy snacks to work and set them out on the counter next to the coffee machine. Every day I try to put out some fresh sliced carrots or celery or fruit, and whenever I see people congregating there I make it a point to see if they'll try some. I'm careful to observe which of these healthy snacks seems to be more popular, and I bring more of those the next day.

I may not be able to eat well myself right now, but that doesn't mean I can't facilitate others' doing so. And when I do, it plants seeds and it plants habits which will inevitably grow into seeing big changes in how I myself relate to food.

But how is all of this going to change your wife? The urge to take care of others is so deep inside each of us that it's not going to be difficult to get her involved in the carrot-giving too. Catch your wife in the kitchen on a day when you have friends coming over, and give her a sales pitch like this:

"Honey, you know Sam and Jane are visiting today."

"Wednesday—right. They always come over on Wednesday."

"Well you know, I was thinking about how Sam seems to have lost so much of his energy in the last year or two. He doesn't want to do anything except watch TV. And I heard this thing on the news, that eating more fresh veggies can really boost your energy.

"So I was thinking, what if we cut up some carrots or other vegetables and put them on a few plates and spread them around the living room before Sam and Jane come over? And then you and I can make it a point to eat some of the veggies in front of them, and maybe get them to try some too."

Your suggestion may not be greeted with wild enthusiasm, but she probably won't stop you either. Get your Mrs to pitch in as much as she wants to—this will plant some seeds for a regular habit of putting out healthy snack plates. In a while she'll be out looking for new veggies for Sam and Jane, and gradually that will change her own way of eating. Keep going until it happens; find lots of ways to help your wife help others to eat well, and then she will eat well too.

Question 61

I recently became a vegetarian, which doesn't interest my husband at all, and now I often have to cook separate meals for us. That's a lot of extra work, and eating separate dishes also seems to create distance between us. What to do, karmically?

I got this question from a woman named Meiling after a talk I gave in Tai-

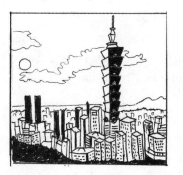

wan at a building named Taipei 101, a beautiful, highly "green" skyscraper with 101 floors located in the middle of downtown. We're going down in the elevator, which is super-fast but hey, it still takes a while.

Chinese people following Buddhism have always considered eating vegetarian to be a spiritual practice; they say that eating the flesh of an animal which has been kept its whole life in captivity—and then slaughtered in mental terror—has an effect on our mind, making us more likely to feel anger or fear.

From personal experience, I think I would agree; and to be honest I don't think I could take a knife from the dinner table and slit the throat of some warm fuzzy creature sitting next to me, so I could eat it then and there—which is I guess what we are asking someone else to do for us, when we buy a piece of meat at the grocery store.

The purpose of this particular section isn't to talk you into becoming a vegetarian, but just as a side note, it is pretty obvious that if you want your spouse to be more loving and gentle, then the best thing seed-wise would be to avoid animal food products as far as you can; in America, they result in the violent deaths of 8 billion farm creatures each year.

As far as health, it's becoming pretty obvious that a vegetarian diet is the best. You can get plenty of protein from vegetable sources, and stay trim and strong as well: I've been vegetarian for over 25 years and do fine in a yoga class filled with people who are all young enough to be my kids.

As far as the question of whether animals can *feel* it or not when we kill or confine them, I do have a few personal observations. My father was an avid hunter and fisher, and from a young age my brothers and I were trained to use high-powered hunting rifles, and deep-sea fishing gear. When the hook is set in the jaw of a fish, they go absolutely crazy with pain: they run, and it can break a fiberglass fishing pole in half—they leap out of the water, to a place where they can no longer breathe, because they are driven mad by the pain.

The last time I killed an animal it was a deer that I had shot; my dad had me slitting it open to clean out the guts while it was still breathing. I will never forget the look that the deer gave me with those soft brown eyes at the moment. I handed the rifle to my father and told him I would never kill an animal again. And every animal that we eat for meat is killed and gutted in the very same way.

One last story. Not to belabor the point, but just so you know—about how the animals feel. From 2000 to 2003, I did a 3-year silent meditation retreat in a tiny Mongolian yurt, out in the middle of the Arizona desert. There was a high wooden fence around the yurt, with a box built into it. Friends came and left food there for me, every day.

A local rancher allowed us to put the yurt on his land, which was about 5,000 acres of pristine desert. He had maybe a hundred head of cattle grazing there—the idea is that you just release the cows into the desert, to eat anything they might be able to find. A lot of them simply die. The survivors you try to catch, and sell to the slaughterhouse.

Every cow has a hole punched in its ear with a special gun, and a yellow plastic tag attached, with a number on it. So anyway the cows were curious about me and used to come to the fence to try to peek in. Number 23 was especially friendly, and I started to push my leftover Cheerios out to her on a big platter every morning. We got to be pretty close, and she would let me scratch her nose under the fence.

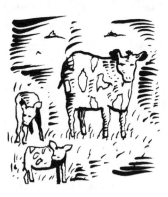

One day she showed up with two baby calves. They were obviously her own kids, and in the silence of a long retreat I could clearly sense the pride she felt for them. Mom would nurse the children in front of me, and nuzzle them with obvious affection.

One day the kids showed up with their own plastic ear tags on. These tags were a different color—bright orange. I was curious and climbed to the top of the fence to look at the tags up close. They didn't have a number, they just had a single word, in big black letters: TERMINATE.

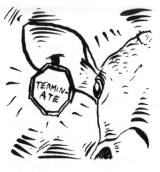

What I learned later on is something that I guess is pretty obvious, but growing up in America we are never taught to think about it. The girl cows are milked, so that we humans can have milk and cheese and butter. To give milk, the girls have to be kept pregnant, and nursing afterwards. To keep them pregnant, you only need one or two boy cows, bulls.

But otherwise bulls just eat a lot and are useless for milk, so when baby bulls are born you let them grow just a bit and then you kill them as calves. This is why veal was invented: it's almost all baby cows who had the bad luck to be born as boys. Number 23's two kids were both boys.

I only saw the kids a few times, and then the whole family disappeared for a week or two. One morning Number 23 came back alone. She looked haggard, almost crazy. She came up to the fence and I pushed a bowl of Cheerios under, but she ignored it. She stared at me through the slats of wood. And then she went to one of the thick posts that held the fence together, and started to bash her head against it, wailing. It's a sound I will never forget.

Animals feel pain too

So I know from my own experience that animals do have feelings, and emotions as well. If everything we do plants a seed, then to cause them pain and terror can only make us unhappy. I strongly believe that eating the flesh of animals and forcing them to produce milk for us *creates* the fat and cholesterol in these products, and *causes* the diseases we get from these products: high blood pressure, blocked arteries, heart problems, and cancer—especially breast cancer.

But that's just my own opinion, something I want to share. Let's get back to Meiling's question, and whether she's going to cook separate meals for her and her husband, whose name is Jianhong.

"Well," I begin, "do you think it would help to just talk to him, convince him to become a vegetarian too?"

"Well," Meiling says, "Of course I did try that at first. I gave him lots of good reasons why he should become a vegetarian, but he just didn't listen. To put it very simply, sometimes he's just really in the mood for the taste of a good steak, and he doesn't care about all those other reasons."

"That's not at all uncommon," I assure her. "The whole point of the Diamond Cutter approach is that we give up bad choices—which means we give up trying to choose between two courses of action when neither one of them is going to work for sure.

"That is, you can argue with Jianhong and try to convince him to be a vegetarian. That might work, and it might not work.

"Or, you can go the other way, and just let him eat his meat—you can cook two separate meals every night. But you're already tired enough when you come home from work, and it is strange for a husband and wife to eat different dishes at the same table, instead of sharing."

"So what am I supposed to do?" says Meiling with exasperation.

"You know the Four Laws of Karma, right?" I ask.

"Sure, you've spoken about them all week, up there." She points to the top of the Taipei 101 building; by now of course the two of us are standing out in the square built around its base.

"And what is the third of those laws?" I ask.

She thinks for a moment. "If I don't plant a seed, then I can't expect a result."

"Right. You can talk at Jianhong all day about becoming a vegetarian, but that's not sure to convince him, and you know that. If you *plant the necessary seeds* and then talk to him, the words will have the power to change his mind; if you *don't* plant the necessary seeds, then the words won't work. It's not the words that do anything, it's the seeds behind the words.

"If you don't know about the seeds, then you struggle between two possible solutions. Each of them may or may not work: trying to convince him, or cooking him his meat. The Diamond Cutter says that we should just go for the root cause, and then the situation will work itself out beautifully, without the struggle."

"You mean, if I plant the right seeds, he'll decide to become a vegetarian?"

"It could be that, or it could be that some other solution will suddenly appear, something that neither of you has thought of yet. Maybe the seeds will create a person next door who loves to cook soy protein into duck shapes that

Jianhong decides he's crazy about …who knows?

"Now tell me the Fourth Law of Karma."

Meiling nods. "If I do plant a seed, then the result I want will come. I can't stop it from coming, even if I wanted to." She smiles; I feel like she's imagining Jianhong attacking a big brown juicy soybean duck right there in the middle of the dining room table.

"So what will this particular seed be?" I ask. "What is the first of the Four Starbucks Steps, for making this little duck miracle happen fast?"

What is the essence of the thing you want?

"I have to decide what it is that I want," she replies.

"The very *essence* of what you want," I add. "Is it really that you want Jianhong to become a vegetarian? Is your main intention that he eats in a way which will help him live longer? Or is it that you don't want the tension between you as you eat your separate meals? Or is it the extra work that you don't want? Be honest; all of these are okay as intentions. But to pick the right seed, you need to pick the right goal—because you'll need to match the seed to the goal."

Meiling thinks for a minute and then breaks out into a grin. "Geshe Michael, you're always telling people that they shouldn't settle for just a part of what they want. I want Jianhong to become a vegetarian, and I want it for all three reasons: I want him to stay trim and strong, and not get chubby and have a heart attack from all the fat and cholesterol in the meat. I *also* want us to sit down in harmony to the same dish every night. *And* I want to avoid all the extra time and cleanup that cooking two different meals always requires."

"You got me," I smile. "So real quick then—tell me what the seeds would be for each of the three. I still think though that you should start with one, concentrate on that one until it starts to flower in your life, and then go on to the others."

"Okay. Number one, I want him to become a vegetarian. I'm thinking I could use Flower Three to make that happen: if I were a *really good* vegetarian, a vegetarian for the right reasons, then I would start to see more vegetarians around me—including my husband. So I'll be a lot more careful about not eating any food which has caused pain and suffering to any living creature.

"And then I'll use Starbucks Step Four to send this seed to Jianhong. That is, as I drift off to sleep at night, I'll think about all the dear little animals I've saved, and send the energy of their life to my husband."

"Number two: I want to sit down with him every night and eat in harmony. For that, I'm going to use the second and third of the Four Powers for removing old bad seeds. That is, I'm going to try to remember anything I have said or done in the past in my office which caused a lack of harmony between me and the two women who work closely with me. And then I'm going to be super careful not to repeat the same mistake—I might even keep a little diary to track how well I'm doing, each day."

"Third: I want to avoid the extra cooking and cleaning. For this I'll concentrate on the second of the Four Laws of Karma. That is, I'll stay very aware of how even the smallest things I do expand hugely as they come back to me. I'll think carefully before I give work to the employees whom I supervise at my job; I'll be very sure not to give anybody even the smallest task that will waste their time, or cost them more time. I'll be super-careful with respecting other people's time, and then my own time will be saved. Somehow, no matter what else happens, I will plant little seeds that will save me from ever having to cook two separate meals again, for my whole lifetime."

"I do think it's the lady next door, with the soybean duck," I smile.

"I can see her now," says Meiling. "She not only has a passion for cooking soy ducks and giving them to her neighbors, but she also cleans her neighbors' apartments, just for fun."

"Uh, that's gonna take its own seeds," I warn. But I can already see the wheels turning inside her head.

Question 62

This question may sound somewhat petty, but it really matters to me. Basically, my wife never cooks any of the foods that I really like—just the ones that she prefers. What seed do I have to plant to see her consider my tastes too?

I got this question on a long drive back to the city from a retreat we held outside of Moscow, for members of a large Russian banking corporation. Yuri is a BIG guy, and from sitting next to him last night at dinner, I know that he loves to eat. It seems a pity then that he rarely gets to eat what he really wants; he is a quiet, unassuming, wonderful bear of a man who is trying to make his marriage work by constantly capitulating to whatever his wife wants.

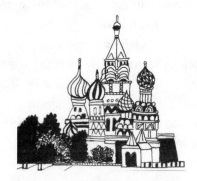

"Personally, I think you need to work it out a different way," I begin.

"What do you mean?" he asks.

"I mean, right now, you're just trying to keep the peace in your family. You especially don't want the kids to see you fighting, so you think you're doing the right thing when you let Eugenia make all the decisions, for example in the kitchen.

"But—I was reading something in a book recently, a book about an idea called non-violent communication. The author was talking about how oftentimes—when we let someone else have their way about something, even if don't really want to—then in our mind we start to keep score. 'I've let you have your way three times this week about what we should eat for dinner; so now tonight I get to decide what we have.'

"I think you're letting Eugenia decide what's for dinner a lot of the time, but deep down you're not doing it freely—inside, you're keeping score. And the score is so unbalanced by now that you're really starting to feel bitter."

Yuri's huge hands shift on the steering wheel, and he stares out at the snow-covered landscape. "I guess you're right," he admits. "I am keeping score, and the score is really unfair by now. If she let me choose what's for dinner every night for the next ten years, we would still never be even."

He gives that characteristic Russian shrug. "So I guess I should really be more spiritual about the whole thing, right? I should just let her have her way, and not expect anything back, not expect to get my way on the dinner once in a while. That would be the noble thing to do."

Now he's got me irritated. "Pull over," I yell. "Here, at this gas station."

His eyes go big and round but he pulls over. We walk silently side by side into the convenience store at the station, and sit down in two rickety wooden chairs to drink a couple of Buratinos—sort of a caramel soft drink. Yuri looks worried, but eventually I calm down enough to go on.

"That whole idea—that it's noble to suffer in silence, that it's wrong to tell your wife what you really want for dinner—absolutely irritates me," I admit. "That's all wrapped up in the very, very wrong idea that either she gets what *she* wants for dinner, or you get what *you* want for dinner; but that it could never work out that you both get exactly what *you both* want for dinner, with the same single dinner.

It is not a virtue to suffer in silence

"This whole game of giving in bitterly to what the other person wants, or giving in because if you give in enough times then the score will be in your favor and you can rightfully demand what you really want, never works out. Eventually the relationship falls apart—people are in a relationship because it fulfills some need that they have, and if staying in the relationship requires that you *don't* get what you need often enough, then something bad is going to happen to the relationship. You'll never want to stay together, or if you do then you'll hate each other."

"So *shto delat?*" Yuri asks, in that very Russian way: What to do?

"Just plant seeds," I say. "Plant seeds, and then sit back and relax. Fourth Law of Karma: If you plant the right seed, she will start cooking what you like for dinner, and *she'll* like the food too. *Every* situation is a win/win situation if you approach it with the seeds. And if you don't approach it with the seeds, then somebody's going to lose, and you'll be stuck in an unhappy marriage."

"So what to do?" Yuri muses again. "Maybe I should start being more careful in my company, to give people jobs that they like!" He owns a successful shipping firm.

"You could do that," I agree, "and in time it would work. But I think you should *teach.*"

"Teach?" I can feel him tighten up already. He may own a big company, but I know he's mortified standing up in front of a crowd and speaking.

Teaching is one of the greatest seeds of all

"Look," I say. "It's one thing to approach situations with seeds—with the Diamond Cutter Principles. You want Eugenia to pay more attention to what *you* enjoy for dinner, you pay more attention to what your employees enjoy doing. Observing the laws of karma is one thing, and it's a very necessary thing.

"But as you do observe these laws, I want you to be especially aware that you're an example for other people. Do try a lot harder to accommodate, as far as you can, what each of your workers enjoys doing, as you hand out tasks in your company.

"At the same time though, the seeds you plant while observing the laws of karma will be infinitely more powerful if—in a way which is appropriate given the circumstances that surround you in your life—you share with people what's going on, what you're trying to do, the new system that you're following. It'll bring you, much faster, magic dinners that are exactly what you want, and exactly what Eugenia wants, at the same time.

"Hand a supervisor a list of people's tasks for the week, and then say something like, 'Well, I hope that gets me some *vareniki* for dinner this week!' A few people will ask you what the heck you're talking about, and then you can explain—maybe almost as if it were just a joke—how you're trying to get what you want by planting seeds: by helping others get what *they* want." (*Vareniki,* by the way, are unbelievably addicting sweet cherry dumplings that the Russians picked up from the Ukrainians.)

"And then when you *do* get your dumplings—when Eugenia starts cooking exactly what *you* want for dinner, because miraculously it's exactly what *she* wants for dinner too—then be sure to brag about it at work. Be an ex-

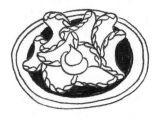

ample of someone who's found a new way to make things happen in their life; because being an example is, quite simply, the best way to teach people.

"Setting up opportunities where other people can have what they want is the seed to get what you want, for dinner. But being a living example of the truth—the truth that the way to make your own dreams come true is to make other people's dreams come true—is the single fastest way to plant and grow a seed."

Soon we're sitting in heavy Moscow traffic, but Yuri's face is as calm as usual, and now it has hope as well: he has a plan. And I have a feeling that every car in front of him looks like a cherry dumpling.

FINANCES

Question 63

I love my partner, but he can't hold a steady job, which makes it hard to keep up with the family bills. What's the karma to see him take some financial responsibility here?

I get this question in a tiny chapel on the campus of Javeriana University, in the Colombian city of Cali, where I'm about to give a talk to about 300 of the students. It's pouring rain outside, and I've ducked into a pew in the back to tune my sitar—sort of a big guitar from India

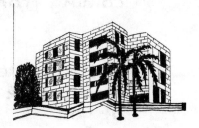

with a real pumpkin shell attached to the neck of the instrument. I often like to start my talks with one or two short classical songs from ancient India.

I pull the sitar out of its cloth bag, and suddenly little pieces of dried pumpkin spill out all over the church floor, compliments of Avianca Airlines. In the middle of all this, Angelica—one of the organizers of the talk—needs to know *right now* how to get her husband Andres to help with the bills. I try to focus on her while one of my erstwhile assistants runs to try to find some duct tape to fix the pumpkin, within the 6 minutes left before we're scheduled to start the talk.

"So...I want to go at your problem by using the Four Powers," I begin, and wait.

Review—

The Four Powers for stopping old bad seeds

1) Think about the pen: Remember where everything is coming from

2) Strong decision to stop this seed before it multiplies inside of you

3) Make a promise not to make the same mistake again

4) Do something positive to balance the karma

"Oh yeah…you covered those at the Intercontinental Hotel last night," she says. That was a wild talk, over a thousand amazing people and an air conditioning system that wasn't quite working.

"I'd like you to try using the third and fourth of the Four Powers," I say. "Now tell me how you think you might do that."

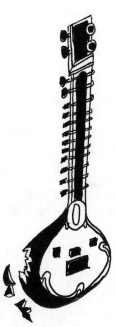

Angelica thinks for a minute. "If we're using the Four Powers," she starts, "then we're trying to short-circuit the bad seeds that I have in my mind which cause me to see Andres refusing to take any responsibility at all for helping with the bills.

"Power Three is the one, they say, which does the most to defuse these bad seeds. It says that I should make a commitment myself not to repeat the same actions which are planting the seeds to see Andres this way in the first place."

"And what kind of actions are those?"

"Well, what I'm doing must be—in its essence—something very similar to what Andres is doing to me now; except that the Second Law of Karma says that it must be a lot smaller than what he's doing."

"Right. So now we have to be like a detective: We have to figure out some small thing that you've been doing which is similar to how Andres is avoiding the bills."

Angelica looks up at the ceiling and thinks, while I start figuring out how the pieces of the pumpkin should be taped back together. It's kind of like a jigsaw puzzle, but a lot more nerve-wracking, since I've only got a few minutes left to solve it.

"Okay," she says then. "I've got it."

"Give it to me," I say, still distracted with trying to fit pumpkin shards together.

"So like…there are little jobs that I'm supposed to be doing for work, all the time; stuff like answering not-so-important emails about a new plan for getting online classes going at the University, or fundraising to fix the air conditioners in the registration office. And lately I find that I just avoid these little emails altogether. Nobody's going to be on my case if I avoid answering them, but it does put subtle pressure on all the people who are waiting for me to respond.

"It's just a little example where I'm avoiding a responsibility that I know is rightfully mine. A good way to bring in the third power right here would be to make a commitment not to continue avoiding the small email responsibilities that I have at work."

"Good. Now what about Power Four?"

"If Power Three is negative—a commitment not to continue doing something—then Power Four is positive: a promise to undertake some action in order to make up for the bad seeds I've been planting."

"Which would be...like what?" I ask.

Angelica thinks for a minute. "My supervisor at work has been trying to get me to answer a survey that he sent out a couple of weeks ago, to see how all the employees in the company are interacting with each other in tough situations. He's asked me a couple of times if I had any ideas about it, and I've just been blowing him off, because it doesn't really affect me that much.

"What I mean is, if I wanted a nice Power Four, I could not just answer his survey, but actually go to him and offer to take responsibility for getting all the surveys filled in and collected: I could take responsibility for something that's not exactly my problem, and then maybe it would occur to Andres to help me out with paying our bills."

"Good," I say. "And just to make sure, what's an approach that *isn't* sure to work with Andres and the bills?"

"Oh that's easy," says Angelica. "It's everything I ever tried before to get him to help with paying the bills. Arguing with him; letting them shut the electricity off, to get his attention; sitting down and making elaborate plans with him about who pays what. All that's ever gotten me was irritated," she huffs.

"So maybe we take responsibility," I muse, "to stop doing things that don't work."

"I'll work on that one," she says. The duct tape arrives, and we bend to the task before us.

Question 64

My husband and I are buried under a mountain of credit card debt: almost every penny of our income is used up just to make the monthly interest payments, and we never seem to be able to get ahead. This puts a lot of strain on our relationship. Any karmic suggestions?

This question comes up in the basement kitchen of a mosque in Montreal, where I've been invited to speak about the idea of achieving financial independence through using the Diamond Cutter Principles. The talk is over; it was followed by some beautiful prayers led by the imam and an assistant, Mahmood, who looks like a Bollywood movie star: tall, dark, and handsome. And now we're sitting down to a bountiful lunch together.

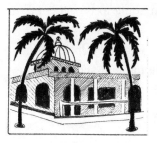

Mahmood comes and seats himself next to me. Turns out he's a successful international banker who speaks a whole pile of languages.

"You know, this idea that you're talking about," he begins, "the idea that generosity towards others is the root of our own financial success, is very much a part of Islam. In Pakistan we speak about the Five Pillars of our Muslim faith—and one of them is *zakat*. This is an offering that we make annually to the poor, based on a certain percentage of our income; it starts at around 2.5% of what we have made for the year, and goes up in certain cases, for example when we've experienced an unexpected windfall. Anyway, I was thinking that we've always been taught to plant the seeds that you're talking about; it's just that there's not much detail on how those seeds work."

"I get the same comment from Christian friends," I nod. "They feel really happy to learn exactly how we reap what we sow—how it actually comes back to us, through seeds opening in the mind."

A woman named Malika has sat down next to us and is listening closely; she's from the Maldives, a tiny Muslim country of islands off the coast of

India. The islands only barely rise above the level of the sea, and there's great concern that they will not survive the rise of the water caused by global warming in the coming decades. It's actually Malika who asks the question about her family's mounting credit-card debt.

"So basically, what you're telling us is that the answer is a sort of educated *zakat:* we keep helping others financially the way that Islam has always told us to, except with a greater appreciation of how it all works on a subconscious level. The best way for my husband and I to deal with our credit-card debt is to keep following our own *zakat:* to help others get out of their debt."

"Which is really hard when you're already in debt," I point out. "It's very difficult to keep a generous state of mind when you don't have any money at all."

Malika jumps on it. "Yes, that's the whole problem—and for me it has two parts. I can understand what a big part intention plays in all this: I understand that the main thing is for me not to let go of my desire to give, even when I don't have much to give. I can see that this will still make big seeds.

"But what I'm wondering about is the Four Starbucks Steps that you were describing. I mean, as I understand it, Step Two is mostly intention and planning: I choose the person that I'm going to help deal with their credit-card problems, and I decide on the coffee shop that I'm going to take them to in order to start on this work together.

"But Step Three is bothering me. This is where I actually do something: I actually go with them to the coffee shop, and talk to them about strategies for working out their debts. At this point it's probably really powerful if I can give them some financial help directly, or for example help them pay to get into a school where they can learn a new job.

"My question is this: If the First Law of Karma is true, and if like always leads to like, then how am I ever going to get out of debt? I need to help my friend financially, if I want my own finances to improve. But the *reason* I'm helping them is that I *don't* have the means to help them financially—I don't have any money to plant, in order to get more money back."

I smile. I'm ready for this one.

"I call this the Patagonia question."

"What's Patagonia?" asks Mahmood.

"A very beautiful area of mountains and lakes in South America, far down towards the southern tip; it includes parts of both Argentina and Chile. So a few years ago I was approached in Buenos Aires by a friend named Matias; his hope was to start a real-estate business and sell land in Patagonia. He wanted to know what he had to do, in order to plant the right seed. So I told him…"

Mahmood jumps on it. "To help somebody else start a business."

"Right. And then he tells me…"

Malika's ready. "He tells you that he doesn't *have* any money to help somebody else start a business. Because if he did, then he wouldn't be coming to you to ask how to get some money of his own, to start his own business."

"Right. So I told him there was something really important that he needed to know. It is true that like breeds like: if you want *your* credit-card debt to disappear, you have to help somebody else make *their* credit-card debt disappear. But that doesn't mean you have to give them money to get money. You can give them something else you have which helps them, and then re-direct the seed to come back to you as money.

"In the case of Matias, I encouraged him to find somebody who was just starting their own business, and who could use some physical help with the place—painting, basic carpentry or plumbing, stuff like that. And then he could just re-direct the seeds to the financial success of his own business.

"So he looked around and found a woman named Florencia who was trying to start a yoga studio for kids living in the sections of Buenos Aires that they call *villas miserias:* the 'neighborhoods of misery.' He pounded nails and painted walls for about a month, and they got a good program going for the poor kids.

"On the day they wrapped up the finishing touches of the center, he came home and opened up his laptop on his bed (he didn't have an extra room to use as an office). And there's an email telling him he's invited to help with a $1.5 million-dollar real-estate deal in Patagonia.

"Moral of the story: To get out of your own credit-card debt, you're going to have to find someone else who's also underwater with their credit card. You may not be able to actually give them money to help pay their card off, but remember: 'Time is Money.' You can keep giving them freely of your time, help them in other ways to save them from more debt—watch the kids, pick up groceries, plant a vegetable garden at their house, get them into some kind of job training program.

"At night, you're going to have to work to re-direct the seed. Use the fourth of the Starbucks Steps: stick to your Coffee Meditation, as you lie down on your bed to go to sleep. Think to yourself, 'Today, I spent some of my own time to help my friend get one more tiny step out of their credit-card debt. I send those seeds to the debt that my husband and I are struggling with.'"

Malika smiles. You can see that—perhaps for the first time—she's able to picture life without credit-card debt. And she has a way to make it happen.

"By the way," I add, "they fell in love, and later on they got married—Matias and Florencia, I mean."

Malika smiles. Everyone likes a happy ending.

The Four Starbucks Steps, one more time!

1) Say what it is you want in your life, in a single short sentence.

2) Plan who it is you're going to help get the same thing, and which Starbucks you're going to take them to, to talk about it.

3) Actually do something to help them.

4) Do your Coffee Meditation: as you go to sleep, think of the good things you're doing to help them.

Question 65

My husband is so cheap sometimes that it really embarrasses me—we'll be out to dinner and he spends half an hour going over the bill, then gets into a fight with waiter about 50 cents here or there. How can I make him more generous?

Eva's asking me this question in a noisy diner on Manhattan's Upper West Side. I'm meeting with her and her husband about a project we're working on together to help refugees in South Asia—he's off at another table talking to some friends, and she kind of sneaks the question in while the server is getting the bill ready.

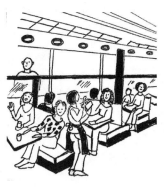

"First of all, let me ask you a question," I say.

"What's that?"

"Is it even *possible* to make another person generous?"

"Well," she says, "there is Flower Three: If I'm generous, with a good understanding of *why* I'm generous, then I'll see more generous people around me."

And then she pauses. "But I can't figure out why I'm seeing someone so close to me in my life showing so little generosity. It's not like I give away every penny I ever earn, but on the whole I do enjoy sharing what I have

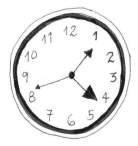

with others, whether it's giving an extra-big tip to a waiter at a restaurant, or cooking a big dinner for all my friends."

I pause and think for a moment. This has been on my mind too.

"I was thinking recently how time has changed, even just in my lifetime. When I was studying in the monastery, I might make a date with a monk from another cloister to come visit him 'Sometime next spring.' And then when you feel like it you just hop on one of those antique Indian buses and ride a couple of days and show up whenever you like, and it's all okay.

"Now someone tells me we'll have an internet call at 7pm and I'm sitting at my laptop and watching the seconds count down, and I get really irritated if they're 80 or 90 seconds late. We've come to measure time more and more minutely, and I honestly think that seconds have come to mean more to us than money.

"So let's go to the first of the Four Starbucks Steps and see exactly what it is that you want—what's the *essence* of what you want?"

Eva thinks for a moment. "I see what you're getting at. It's not that I really care about the money—about how Joseph looks at money. It's more the counting of the pennies: the habit of being so caught up in the tiny, unimportant details. I mean, who *cares* if the bill for dinner was 50 cents over or under? Especially when it was a really wonderful dinner."

"That's the feeling I was getting from you. When you say you want Joseph to be more generous, it's not like you're putting a certain dollar amount on it. You want him to be more generous in his thinking; more open, more spacious.

"We both know that—if he feels tight or nitpicky at any given moment— it's coming from you, just like we see with The Pen Thing. Now if you're not being nitpicky with money, what is it that you *are* being nitpicky with?"

Eva nods. "It's like you said, I think. I don't bust people's heads over a few dollars here or there. But I am a stickler on time—I do count minutes, I count seconds. I do get upset if a person shows up at ten after four, rather than four on the dot; I do stand in front of the oven grumbling at the person who wrote the recipe, if a cake takes five minutes longer to rise than they said it would."

"I like that," I agree. "So what we're saying, I think, is that the main place where most of us have a problem being generous is with time, and not with money. We all really resist giving each other a few minutes of space, as we rocket through the day we have planned for ourselves.

"I had to take a driver's test recently, which meant that I had to read the driver's manual, something that I haven't done for decades. I expected it to be pretty boring, but I found this wonderful suggestion there. They said that a great many car accidents—and a lot of serious injuries—are caused by people in a hurry. Much more than drunk drivers; more than bad weather, or tires blowing out on the highway.

"And the solution they suggested, it was so simple: When you're going someplace in your car, plan for it to take 10 minutes longer than usual. Then you'll never be in a hurry, and you'll never have an accident because you were in a hurry."

Eva nods. "So in my case, I just learn to live with a little more of a buffer, timewise, in everything I do. I'm generous with my scheduling: I stand up to leave after tea with my friend ten minutes before I really need to go, just in case she wants to say one last thing as we're walking out. And then I can give her my full attention, which breeds a sort of generosity in my life—a kind of feeling which is almost…luxurious.

"I can feel it," she says.

"I can see that you do." The waiter has finished with the bill and is headed towards our table; Joseph is walking over from the other direction. I can see that he's reaching into his pocket. What's the fastest a seed can ripen?

OUT WITH FRIENDS

Question 66

When we're around other people, my husband just doesn't know how to keep his mouth shut—and he always spills a lot of stuff about us that I consider very personal. What seed do I need to plant to see him be more discreet?

I don't know about you, but I find this one of the most irritating things that a person can do. I'm working with a participant in a DCI program on ways to improve a difficult situation with their partner, and then someone else barges in to report something very personal that the partner said the day before, which is only going to make matters worse.

Anyway, I want to point out two very simple facts here.

One: The things that most irritate us about other people are, without question, the most irritating things that we do personally. If we are surrounded by people who don't know when not to say something, then it's certain that we ourselves are also saying these kinds of things all the time.

At any given point in our life, we have a certain amount of challenges going on. These challenges change from day to day, year to year. But at the moment they always seem like the most important challenges that we've ever had, because it's hard to remember exactly the pain of the past, and we haven't hit the future challenges yet.

Our life is a mirror

Remember though the idea that our life is a mirror. The challenges which we're having today are a direct reflection of how we've been leading our life in the past few weeks and months.

Which leads us to the second point. The more that a person around us is similar to us, the more difficulty we will have in recognizing that they are coming from us.

If having one of my employees blurt out inappropriate statements to a client is the thing I personally find most irritating, it's going to be that much more difficult for me to acknowledge that what I'm really seeing is my own habitual behavior, reflected in the people around me—*as* the people around me.

The solution here is easy, if cruel in its honesty. When you feel really upset by something that someone is doing around you, get away by yourself for a few minutes, sit and think. They are coming from me—and if it really irritates me, then it must be something that I'm doing myself, all the time.

Instead of criticizing the other person, even mentally, push your mind in a different direction: What is a single thing that I've done in the last day

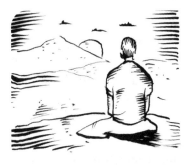

or two which is almost exactly the same as what upsets me so much in this other person? What will I do to stop acting this way myself?

This is the third of the Four Powers, and it kills the seeds that are making you see your husband spill his guts out to everyone he sees, about things that are personal between the two of you.

The nice thing is that you don't have to say anything to him. No arguments, no discussions, no ultimatums. Just the quiet, peaceful correction of your own heart.

Question 67

My wife has this way of flaunting her femininity in all kinds of situations—flirting with everyone from the parking attendant to a bank officer, and it really makes me uncomfortable. What's the karma to see her be a little more sensitive to my feelings on this?

I'm walking with Mark up Fifth Avenue in Manhattan, which seems like an appropriate place for this question; we are surrounded by the window displays of Saks Fifth Avenue, Prada, Harry Winston and Tiffany's—and his wife Toni is eating them up, which gives us a chance to talk, standing off towards St Patrick's Cathedral.

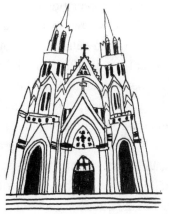

"It's a tough question, in the modern world," I start. "I mean, there's this paradox..."

Mark frowns, he knows what I'm talking about. "Yeah...we want our partners to be beautiful or handsome, and we want them to dress sexy—we want them to look good next to us, as we walk down the street."

"Right. And we want other people to look at them, but only in a certain way. We don't want them looking in a suggestive way—we don't want them actually doing anything. It's a fine line between admiring and flirting, isn't it?"

"Right," he replies. "So what...you think I'm just being jealous? That she's just being like, vivacious, and not flirting?"

"That's something important in the Diamond Cutter system," I answer. "If it feels to you like she's flirting, then that's real: the feeling is real. If it's making you uncomfortable, then that's real. Everything in the situation— how she's acting towards a guy on the street, how he's responding to her, and how you feel about it—is real. And that means that it's coming from you, and you can change it. I mean, what would be ideal for you? What do you want?"

"I want her to be beautiful, and I really enjoy buying her things to be beautiful in," he smiles, giving a nod to Toni across the street, who is pointing to something in a window over at Rockefeller Center. "I want her to look great when we walk down the street together. I want people—even other guys—to appreciate how beautiful she is. But I want to feel secure about the whole thing; I don't want to think she might be coming on to some guy, flirting with them, you know, like serious."

"So can we say it like this? That you are in favor of beauty, but not in favor of being disloyal?"

"Exactly," he sighs.

"That there is an appropriate appreciation of her good looks, and an inappropriate appreciation of her good looks?"

"Exactly," he says. "You've got it."

"So look, can we agree on one thing? I mean, a partner can just be very sociable—which is a good thing; or they can be seriously flirting with other people—which is a bad thing. Our partner can say or do things, the very same things, and sometimes we feel proud that we have someone who knows how to be warm to others, and sometimes we feel that they're flirting."

"I know where you're going," says Mark. "I've been around when you teach. She's talking to someone else on the street, someone who's stopped to tell her they like her dress, and my mind is filtering the whole thing. Sometimes the filter is a good one, and I admire how she's reaching out to a stranger. Sometimes the filter is a bad one, and I get upset that she's flirting with someone. She could be doing the very same thing in each case, and I see it according to my own filters."

"Where do the filters come from?"

"I know," he says. "They come from seeds."

"And what kind of seed would create the bad filter? The one that makes you perceive her as flirting, instead of perceiving that she is reaching out to a stranger with a moment of warmth?

"Why are you seeing an inappropriate appreciation of beauty?" I add quickly.

"Well, I guess...I guess, according to the Diamond Cutter ideas, I must be engaging in some kind of inappropriate appreciation of beauty myself," he blurts out, without really thinking about it.

"Now we're talking. Any ideas how you're doing that?"

Mark blushes immediately. "Well, you know...sometimes, like, I do look at stuff on the internet…girls…"

"Is it beautiful?" I ask.

"Well, it's attractive…it attracts me."

"Is it appropriate?"

"Well, do you mean…would Toni approve? No, I don't think so."

"Is it appropriate in the way we're talking about here, though? When you look at porn on the web, are you hurting someone else's relationship, in the way that it would hurt your relationship if Toni were really flirting with somebody?"

"I never thought about it that way," Mark muses. "I mean…it's just girls, pretty girls."

"Do they have partners?"

"How would I know?"

"Do you *think* they have partners? I mean, a *pretty* girl?"

"Well…I guess they probably do, I guess a lot of them do have partners."

"And how do you think the partners feel about them taking their clothes off so you can watch them on the internet?"

"Well, I mean…nobody's forcing them."

"What you mean is, they get paid to do it. They get paid a lot, and they probably need the money. And the partner might not know at the beginning, but he'll probably find out—it's all on the internet. And then he might complain and he might not, because they might need the money for a place to stay, or for the kids if they have some. Then they're both forced into a place where they don't really want to be—and *you're* forcing them.

"It seems pretty inappropriate to me. And it seems like it would plant a seed for a bad filter. Toni might just be trying to reach out to someone, and you're going to see it as flirting, every time."

"So a beautiful body is a bad thing?" he says sharply.

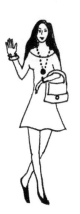

"I didn't say that. It can be the most beautiful thing in the world. But there's an appropriate way to appreciate the beauty—one that doesn't hurt anyone; and an inappropriate way to appreciate it. Ask your partner, she'll probably have a pretty clear idea of which is which. If you want a partner, and you want a partner who doesn't flirt around, then listen to her."

Toni is running back across Fifth Avenue to the corner where we're standing. She's laughing and her dress is flowing with the wind. She looks great. We appreciate it. Mark nods, with conviction.

COMMUNICATING,
PART TWO

Question 68

Sometimes I just feel like being comfortably quiet together with my partner, but she often takes this the wrong way, and thinks I'm not interested in what she has to say. How do I get her to appreciate companionable silence?

This question came in Guadalajara, Mexico, at a late-night dinner in a *really* hard-to-find balcony restaurant that specializes in the cuisine of Durango, which lies a little farther north. We've been driving around the few blocks below for like an hour scrutinizing storefronts on the bottom floor without looking up and seeing the restaurant was here. My Tibetan teacher used to say that you could put a dog on the roof but he'll still look down.

Enrique is asking the question; Elsa is up on the balcony above us, ne-

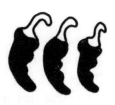

gotiating caldillo and relleno and maybe some mostachote with the waiter. Enrique has been teaching the 4x4 for a while, and I figure he's ready for some mental gymnastics.

"So give me the names of the 4x4; just the names of the four sets of four, and tell me what they do," I say, looking out over the city as dusk begins to descend.

"Four Flowers—four ways that seeds open. Four Starbucks Steps—four ways to speed them up. Four Laws of Karma—four rules which govern all seeds; and the Four Powers—four things you have to do to shut down an old bad seed."

"Okay. So let's play a game, and by the end of it we'll have the answer for how to get Elsa to enjoy companionable silence once in a while, without accusing you of being grumpy. Starbucks Step Number One…"

"Say it in one sentence: I want her to see that I enjoy being quiet sometimes, in a pleasant way, and not because I'm upset or something."

"Flower Number Three."

"Generally speaking, people have to plant their own seeds. I can't change her, she has to change herself. But my seeds do create the world and the people that I see around me. Flower Three says that if I plant some *really good* seeds, I will see her change, as all the rest of my whole world changes, to appreciate quiet a little more."

"Power Number One."

Enrique has to think on that one for a few seconds. "I guess...it's understanding why I'm seeing something negative in front of me. She misinterprets my desire for silence; she thinks it's because I'm upset in some way, because at some earlier point I myself planted the seeds, by mistakenly judging someone else's motives. That is, the problem's coming from me, and not her. And that means I can change it, by changing myself."

"Karmic Law Number Two."

Again, he considers for a minute. "Well, I guess really there are two parts to that here. I mean, I have to go looking for whatever I did—and am probably still doing—to see what I'm seeing in Elsa. But really there must be two different things that I did. One makes me see a person who's not that interested in quiet; and the other makes me see a person who misunderstands my desire for quiet.

"In either case, Karmic Law Number Two says that when I go looking for what I must be doing to make her this way, I should look for something which is a lot smaller than what I'm seeing in her. Because between the time that seeds are planted and the time that they flower, they multiply wildly, deep down in the subconscious."

"Okay, good job on the 4x4," I say. "So let's go looking for our two seeds. How are you yourself *not quiet* in your daily life?"

Enrique frowns. "Well, I don't see that I have a big problem with that. I never bother the neighbors; I do play rowdy music now and again, but mostly I try to use my earphones. Our office at work has a tile floor, and it drives me crazy when people push their chairs across it and make screeching sounds— so I'm really careful not to do that myself. I'm *not* a noisy person."

"Tennis balls," I muse.

"Huh?"

"Tennis balls. Get a bunch of old tennis balls, punch a little hole in one side of them, and stick them on the ends of the legs of all the chairs. Amazingly quiet then when people push the chairs around."

Enrique nods, and then smiles at me. "Hey; that's not a karmic solution, it's a normal solution."

I smile back. "Right you are. And according to the Diamond Cutter, normal solutions are lousy, because…"

"They might work, and they might not work," recites Enrique.

"Exactly. Which draws into question whether they are even solutions at all. Which is itself the cause of the pain and confusion of the entire world. I mean—unless you take care of the real causes—you might get a really bad reaction to the tennis balls."

"Yeah," muses Enrique. "Like how professional does our office look to a wealthy client, if everybody's sitting in a chair perched on fluorescent green balls?"

"Right. That's the problem with the 'normal' solutions to things. Okay then, let's get back to your search for the seeds. Is there anyplace in your life where you're *not* quiet?"

Enrique thinks for a moment. Then, as I watch, a light goes off in his head.

"Inside my own mind," he breathes, with a little sense of wonder. "I mean, I'm talking to myself in my head *all day long:* constant chatter, constant planning, never asking my own mind to *just be quiet* for a few minutes. I bet that's what's planting the seeds for me to see Elsa show so little interest in occasional moments of silence."

"Okay, so watch that one—start by setting aside a few purposeful moments of quiet inside your own mind, maybe when you're driving home from work sometimes. Don't plan, don't review the day. Just try to be super-alert and quiet inside—be in the moment. Watch the patterns in how the cars move around you, appreciate the sky and the clouds, feel the touch of the steering wheel in your hands. *Be quiet."*

"Got it," he says. "Now about the second seed…"

"She misinterprets your need for friendly silence now and then. It means that she's judging you, and she's not aware that her judgments are mistaken.

"So how are we doing in the judging category?" I ask. It's kind of a mean question, I think to myself—it seems to me that all of us are misjudging each other, all the time.

Enrique thinks for a minute. "It's not so much the people I'm around all the time; I mean, I get enough feedback from them, and I see them often enough, that I think I can safely guess where they're at, in general. I guess it's more that I judge people whom I don't know: people I see on the street, people that walk past me in the grocery store."

We talked about this back in Question 20, and you might want to go re-read the solution we proposed there. It was about the power of fantasy: rather than making assumptions that what we see around us is just normal stuff, we create epic stories that help life be more magical, and which eventually come true. But I take a different tack with Enrique today.

"So let's go back to the 4x4. Second of the Four Powers."

"True regret—not guilt—that I've planted a bad seed."

"And what's the difference between regret and guilt?"

"Regret, intelligent regret, is looking for a way to fix the problem. Guilt is more likely to sit and mope about *how bad I am.*"

"And how to come to a *healthy* state of regret?"

"That's all tied up in the Second Law of Karma: I feel sorry about judging people lightly all day long, because I'm very aware that this small judging will come back to me as some very heavy judging."

"As, for example, when someone close to you misunderstands, almost constantly, why you want to stay quiet sometimes."

Enrique smiles. He's got it, he's got a plan. We watch as a tough-looking guy gets out of a car under a streetlight down on the street. He starts strolling around, as if he's looking for something.

"What do you think he does for a living?" I ask.

"Dunno," says Enrique. "Maybe some kind of mafioso. A guy from the Zeta gang maybe."

I stand up. "He's a filmmaker, one of the best in Guadalajara. Just finished a movie starring his little kids as superheroes who save the world. He's coming to dinner with us. I better tell him we're up here."

Enrique looks down, chastened. "Okay, I'll try harder," he says.

4 x 4

The Four Starbucks Steps (Make seeds grow fast and big!)	The Four Laws of Karma (Understand how seeds work!)
The Four Powers (Stop your old bad seeds!)	The Four Flowers (How seeds become your reality)

Question 69

My wife, for some reason, prefers to communicate by yelling. Like I can be sitting in a room on the other side of the house, and if she wants to ask me a question she'll try to yell at me through 6 walls, rather than getting up off the couch and coming over to the door of the room I'm in. What's the karma to see her speak a little more pleasantly?

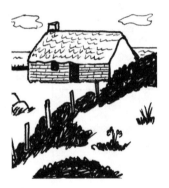

This question comes in the living room of a pleasant Irish cottage outside of Galway. We're all sitting in the back, looking out the sliding glass window at miles of rolling impossibly green hills, with the sweet smell of the peat burning somewhere near. It's the week that the rowan trees blossom—pure white dotting Irish green, like a reflection of the puffy clouds scattered overhead in the pale blue.

"I mean," says Liam, "and we're talkin' *stone* walls here, walls of good Irish stone, and not your cheap American plasterboard walls."

Luckily, his wife Eire (whose name means "Ireland") is in the kitchen, buttering up a pile of fresh-baked scones. There's no question who's the boss in this family.

"It doesn't seem to me a question of volume control," I begin, being careful to keep my own voice down. "But more of *style*. Basically, what you want is for Eire to be more graceful in her delivery."

Liam thinks for a moment. "Yes, that's it," he nods. "In fact, that's how she used to be, when we first got married. She would sidle over to the door of my study, all sexy like, and ask me her question in the sweetest way."

So that's what we're really dealing with here, I think to myself. We covered this back in Question 26. Why do things change? What happened that made Eire slowly shift from a crooner to a yeller?

"So the seeds got old," I say. "Where do you think that fits into the 4x4?"

I can see Liam working through 16 possibilities in his mind. And then he makes a wonderful leap in his thinking. He shifts his pipe to the side of his mouth, and his bright blue eyes light up.

"Well, I think that the last of the Four Starbucks Steps might play a part here," he says earnestly.

"How's that?" I ask.

"Well now, Step Four, as you know, is the Coffee Meditation. Of course here in Ireland that would be a stiff cup of black tea," he adds.

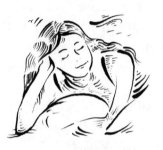

"And how does that relate to yelling through walls?"

"Well, the thing is, when we first got married, I obviously had a lot of seeds going off to see Eire doing the most wonderful things. Like *wanting* an excuse to get up off the couch and come see me in my study, so she could say something sweet to me.

"But every time she did come to see me, I used up a bunch of those seeds. And after a while the seeds were all finished, and she started yelling at me through the walls when she wanted something."

"So how is Coffee—or Tea—Meditation going to help that?"

"Well, I was thinking, you know. Usually we do Coffee Meditation about something good that we've done in the last day or two, you see."

"Right."

"Well now, you're always saying that there's no expiration date on a Coffee Meditation."

"Right—as you drift off to sleep, or if you wake up too early in the morning, or in the middle of the night—you can purposely turn your thoughts to good things that you've done, whether they were yesterday or last year, or ten years ago. And when you do that, you still get tons of fresh new good seeds.

"In fact," I say mostly to myself, "I guess you could even define meditation as *purposely turning your thoughts* to whatever you want to."

"Okay," nods Liam. And then he turns the tables on me. "But then there's the third of the Four Powers…"

"Uh," I scramble. "You promise not to do a negative thing again?"

"Yes," he replies, "but I was thinking more how you need to figure out what negative thing it is that you promise to stop. That means that you have to do a little detective work, figure out what you must have been doing before.

"So why can't we turn that around? I mean, I must have planted some great seeds just before I first met Eire, way back before we were married. That's what made her so attractive and sweet.

"So if there's no expiration date on good karma, can I do Tea Meditation on some good seeds that I planted a really long time ago? Even if I don't remember exactly what I did to plant them, but just remember how they flowered? As Eire, standing sultry there at the door of my study, asking me something?"

I think about it. "I don't see why not. I mean, in principle, it's the same thing as Power Three. We can clean an old bad seed that we don't remember planting, just by figuring out logically what we must have done to plant it. I don't see why we can't do Tea Meditation in the same way—be happy about whatever you must have done to plant that beautiful Eire that you first met, even if you can't recall exactly what it was."

"Right," says Liam excitedly. "And *if, before I fall off to sleep, I'm happy about old good seeds that I must have planted to make Eire speak sweetly way back when, then that should plant more of the same kinds of seeds.*"

"And she'll stop yelling through the walls, and get up off the couch to come and ask you her questions in a very nice way."

But Liam's already past that. Huge clouds of blue smoke are rising from his pipe as he puffs furiously and stares at the ceiling in thought. He mumbles something about what used to happen on the couch in the study *after* Eire asked her questions sweetly—but I leave him to his own plans on re-planting that.

Question 70

My husband and I rarely have big arguments—shouting matches—but it does seem like we are bickering at each other almost constantly: small unkind words to each other, again and again throughout the day. What's the karma to get a little sweetness into our exchanges?

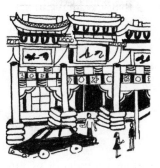

I got this question in Vancouver, before a talk to members of the substantial Chinese business community there. We're sitting on blue plastic chairs in the dining room of a vocational center downtown, watching through windows as people file in to the attached auditorium. There won't be much time for the answer, so I'm thinking how to make it quick.

Qinglan is looking at me intensely across the table; it means a lot to her, I know, as do all the questions that people ask about their partners. We can see her husband Zhiwei on the other side of the window, handing out programs to the participants as they walk in.

"This gets back into the subject of cycles," I begin.

We've covered these kinds of cycles, or feedback loops, in Questions 26 and 53; you may want to check those first and then return to our conversation here.

"Even I can see that," says Qinglan ruefully. "He says some small unkind thing to me; then I say something a little sharper back to him; and then he responds with more and walks away. But we both keep some kind of bitterness about it inside, and the next time we talk I just pick it back up where I left it, before he walked away. I understand that it's a cycle; I just don't know how to break it."

Understanding how a cycle works breaks it

"Well, there are temporary ways to interrupt a cycle, and there are ultimate ways, which stop a cycle permanently. I guess you know some of the temporary ways."

"Yes, yes—we've got a pile of them from our parents, who've had a long, supposedly successful marriage: there's peace in the family; or rather, I would call it a long-standing truce, but no joy. Our parents have stayed together, to keep the family going, and they give us suggestions for that—but they just don't seem that happy with each other.

"They tell us never to go to bed angry with each other, which works a lot of the time, but if we kept to that there would be times that we'd have to stay up all night. Or our parents tell us to think about the effect that our constant bickering has on our kids, and we appreciate that, and we try not to do it in front of them. But then it feels like we're just bottling up our feelings, and they fester inside of us, and it just gets worse later on.

"So what I'm asking for is some kind of permanent solution. Is there a way to break this cycle that we're stuck in: constant, escalating tension as we bicker with each other across the whole day."

I nod. "There is a way, and it doesn't take more than a minute or two to share it." That better be true, I think to myself, because I can see the head of the local Chinese chamber of commerce getting up to introduce me.

"Okay, listen, Qinglan. It's short, and it's simple.

"The only thing that can really break a cycle of bickering is to understand exactly what's going on. The ancient scriptures call this the Perfection of Wisdom." From somewhere back in the cobwebs of my mind comes the Chinese word for it. "*Bo-re bo-luo mi-duo,*" I squeeze it out.

"I've heard of that, but what's it mean here?" she asks.

"Very simple. You have to know exactly what keeps this cycle of bickering going. It's not psychological, it's karmic. And they're not at all the same thing.

"You get up in the morning and you're trying to make the bed and Zhiwei says something about how bad the dinner was last night. Instead of getting mad, you've *got* to think about why he said that.

"It's *not* something that he decided to say. It's something that he *had* to say. He was *forced* to say it.

"Why?" I ask.

"Well if what you said last night at UBC was right, he's complaining about dinner this evening because I was complaining maybe to somebody at work about our boss, the week before."

"Right. He's coming from you. His bickering is coming from you.

"Now what's the *stupidest* thing you can do when he complains about dinner?"

Qinglan looks down, sheepishly. "Well, the stupidest thing to do would be to bicker back at him, when he bickers at me."

"Why?"

"Because then I plant more seeds to see him bicker at me."

"Right. And then he bickers with you more, and you bicker back, and you plant more seeds to see him bicker again next week. And the cycle just keeps going."

"So what are you saying? Just *knowing* how the cycle works is the only way to break it?"

"Exactly. And that's the Perfection of Wisdom: that's the *smartest* thing you can do. You refuse to bicker back. And it's not because he didn't say something mean to you; he did. But if you respond with the same, then you plant seeds to see him continue saying mean things.

"Look," I say, getting up and straightening my tie. The introduction outside is done, and the audience is looking around, wondering where I am. "You're not going to be able to do it right away. The first time you think to apply this Perfection of Wisdom—this knowledge of what keeps the cycle going—it will be half an hour *after* you already bickered back to Zhiwei. It will take you that long to remember that you just planted a lot of bad seeds to hear him bicker at you again, next week.

"Next week, when he bickers, you'll still say something back, but maybe it will only take 15 minutes for you to realize that you just created more future bickering from Zhiwei.

"The time gap gets shorter—your awareness of what you're saying becomes better and better—and then *one day you will stop yourself before you bicker back,* just because *you don't want to see him start some bickering next week.*

"And then the cycle is broken," I smile, and run for the door.

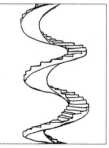

ADDICTIONS

Question 71

My partner seems more interested in pictures of girls on the internet than he is in me. What seed do I need to plant to get his attention?

As you can see by now, I have the good fortune to travel the world, and to enjoy being with people from many countries, who teach me while I supposedly teach them. Here's what I'm seeing nowadays.

We're all painfully familiar with the addictions that people have to alcohol, or drugs. But I think the addiction to computers has become even more serious, perhaps because computers do contribute in a huge way to feeding and clothing and housing the ever-increasing population of our world. I don't think that we could have done it in recent decades, if it weren't for the computer.

At the same time, computers are hurting us, and perhaps it will take another generation or two before we really appreciate how bad it is. So when we answer this question about a person who's addicted to porn on the web, it can apply just as well to someone who's addicted to internet video games; or Facebook; or just email.

I think the nature of an addiction is that we know it's hurting us, but we don't have the strength to stop. Our addiction can hurt our family or friends, damage our reputation, harm our bodies and minds—and in moments of clarity we understand that. But we still can't stop ourselves. That's when we call it an "addiction."

The beauty of the Diamond Cutter system is that it gives us the power to stop, when we don't have the power to stop.

So anyway this question, in many different forms, has come to me all over the world—because the many different forms of computer addiction are a global problem. Why don't we pick up the conversation with Ivana, as we walk together across the Charles Bridge—one of the most beautiful sites of Prague, in the Czech Republic.

"Yes then, it's an addiction: to me it fits the definition of an addiction. He wants to do it, he knows it hurts him, and he can't stop," I say.

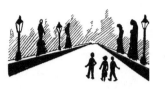

"I mean, it's worse than you think," she replies. "There are more and more days when he can't get it up, or can't keep it up, and I have this strong feeling that it's because of all the time he spends with porn on the internet. On top of that he gets all flustered whenever I walk in the room and catch him by accident."

Branislav is walking ahead of us, showing some friends one of the many famous statues on the bridge. It does seem to me that in recent years he's become a little nervous, not as grounded as he used to be.

"Does he really *want* to stop?" I ask.

"I think he does. I know it sounds like a contradiction: he's addicted to porn because he likes it, but he wants to stop. I think somehow it makes him feel cheap—that somehow it's demeaning, and he would rather get his mind back, be able to focus on other things again."

"Good. Then we can just help him work on his own seeds. What you have to keep in mind is that, when we work on an addiction using the Diamond Cutter, we're not appealing to a person's reason, or their willpower, to get them to stop. Because if they could stop the addiction that way, they would have done so a long time ago."

"I understand," agrees Ivana. "We've been through that already, a thousand times. Stopping this addiction is obviously going to take something different, something new."

"Okay. So you and I should talk about what seeds Branislav has to plant; and then at home you guys work on it together, in a slow and comfortable way." She nods.

"Look, you know what a serious problem alcohol is in the US, right?"

"Here too," she says.

"And people have spent billions and billions of dollars to try to stop their drinking. I mean, there are rehab centers where you can pay a thousand dollars a day, you know what I mean?" Ivana nods. Crowds of sightseers are flowing around us on the bridge, but she's focused, and it feels like there's just the two of us.

"But you know what? They found out that the most effective treatment is free. It's called Alcoholics Anonymous."

"I've heard about that. How does it work?"

"You just get together informally with other people who have a drinking problem, and each of you talks, and you support each other. The key of the program is something called a 'sponsor.'

"A sponsor is most often a person who's been going to AA meetings for a while, and who has been able to avoid taking that 'first drink' for a year or more. When a new person starts attending the meetings, they have the option at some point to ask someone else to be their sponsor. The sponsor agrees to help them learn the AA principles, and might also allow the new person to phone them, for example, when they feel tempted to take a drink.

"One of the co-founders of AA said that there were a number of reasons why he himself took on the role of sponsor for other alcoholics. First, he felt that it was his duty; and he also found that it was a great pleasure to help others. So too it seemed a great way to repay his debt to the person who had first helped him.

"But I think the most important reason he mentions is that every time he helps someone else as a sponsor, he 'takes out a little insurance for myself against a possible slip'—that is, it helps him avoid a relapse into drinking himself.

"And that's the key; that's the reason why AA works so well. When you take responsibility to help another person who has an addiction, you plant seeds to see your own addiction stop."

"So the best way Branislav can help himself is to help someone else."

"As usual! And then, you see, it's not a matter of willpower or being reasonable, because we *can't* be reasonable when we're addicted. He simply plants the seeds, keeps planting the seeds, and then when they start growing inside of him they take over, and he just automatically stops."

"But how is he going to help somebody else if he can't even help himself?"

"It's in the trying. Just trying to help somebody else plants the seeds. Trying the best he knows how—that's enough. You know the Four Starbucks Steps, right? You know what he has to do."

"Just let me run them by you," says Ivana. We are near the end of the bridge, and Branislav is heading back towards us. "First, he needs to decide what he wants: he has to say, 'I want to overcome this addiction to porn on the web.' Secondly, he needs to find someone else with the same problem, and make a plan for helping them."

"Or just someone with a similar problem," I add. "It's good if they have the same addiction as he does, but if it's some other kind of addiction—alcohol, eating, whatever—that will also work. It's just that then he'll have to 'redirect' the seed during his Coffee Meditation time."

"Got it," she says. "Third, he has to actually help this other person; say, by taking them out to a Starbucks or someplace like that, and sharing ideas on how to stop their mutual addiction.

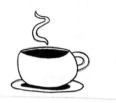

"And then fourth, before Branislav goes to bed he should think about the good job he did while he was choosing the person; and planning how to help them; and actually talking to them.

"Coffee Meditation!" she smiles.

"Coffee?" says Branislav, as he walks up to us.

"Sounds great! There's a place back near the other side of the bridge, on the water."

Okay, well maybe this time I'll get to look at the statues. We turn around to repeat the walk.

Question 72

For a long time in our relationship, I was completely unaware that my wife had a serious addiction to alcohol. On many days now it seems to take her over completely; it feels like she has more of a relationship with her bottle than she does with me. What's the seed for overcoming this addiction?

This question comes up at a break in a talk I'm giving in the Hong Kong Convention Centre, with its exquisite view of Hong Kong Harbor. William asks the question on the stage inbetween times as I sign some books; he points to 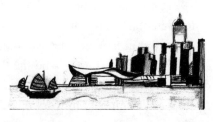 Sue, still sitting in the audience, who with a nod tells me that she's alright with him asking the question. Both are Chinese, and both are Buddhist.

"You want me to give you some Buddhist mantra or charm, that will make her suddenly stop drinking," I say first.

William's look tells me I'm right.

"Well, I don't do that," I tell him. "And even if I did, it would only work because of your own seeds. So we need to talk about seeds, planting seeds."

"Should I ask Sue to come up?" he asks.

"Not necessary. There are two ways to work on an addiction. One is for the person with the drinking problem to plant the seeds to see their desire for alcohol simply stop." This is the approach that we just covered, in Question 71, and you may want to re-read that one before going on to this one.

"But there's another approach which you might also find helpful, depending on the situation. Here we use a combination of Flower Three, and the Second Law of Karma, and the third of the Four Powers."

"Flower Three," says William. "I do something myself which changes the world around me, and then Sue changes along with all the rest of the people and places in my life."

"Right. And now I know it may be difficult to hear, and it's certainly not something that most people want to face, but you're a friend and I want you to try something. In the end, it's actually very empowering."

"Okay," says William, with that Hong Kong mixture of Chinese patience and British stiff-upper-lip.

"The point is that Sue is *already* part of the world around you; and that world is indeed coming from the seeds which you are planting, even now. If you see someone close to you struggling with an addiction, Flower Three says that you must have the seeds to see it. And to have the seeds, you must have done—and at some level you must still be doing—something similar, yourself.

"You mean I must be engaged in some kind of addictive behavior myself, and that makes me see Sue with her addiction to alcohol?"

"Right. And the Second Law of Karma says that the seeds—your own little addictions—are a lot smaller than Sue's, since seeds in the mind multiply even faster than the ones we find in nature."

William picks it up. "And the third of the Four Powers states that I can disable the seed of my own addiction, just by recognizing that I have it, and making a commitment to work on it."

"Exactly. The whole Diamond Cutter approach is based on acknowledging that your own seeds are creating all the people and all the situations around you—which is not something that most of us want to hear, when something is going wrong. A person in our family with a serious addiction, whatever addiction it is, almost always puts a tremendous strain on everyone else in the family. Even the best people can begin to resent the time and trouble that caring for an addicted family member demands, sometimes over a period of many years.

"And so there is a resistance to the idea that this person's behavior is coming from me; nobody in the family wants to hear it. Working with this idea though immediately makes us more humble, and more sympathetic. It also brings us tremendous joy, because we suddenly realize that not only are we responsible for the situation we're in, but we are also empowered to change it, just by working on ourselves.

"So we begin with some detective work: what do you think the seed might be? What small addictive behavior might be planting a seed in you to see Sue the way that you do?"

William does the gaze-at-the-ceiling: natural meditation. "Coffee?" he says simply.

"Is it an addiction for you?"

"Well, it's not that I like to think of myself as being addicted to coffee, but I do think it fits the definition of an addiction. I need to have it every day; I know that it hurts me; and I can't stop drinking it, even though I know it hurts me."

"How exactly does it hurt you?"

"I've thought about that," says William. "I mean, it definitely makes me nervous. If I drink a cup of coffee after 2 o'clock in the afternoon, I'll have trouble sleeping that night. So even if I drink a cup earlier in the day, I have to believe that it's not great for me—I think the caffeine must linger in my bloodstream, perhaps even for days.

"Even when I have trouble admitting what the coffee does to me, I can see the effect that it has on the people around me. It does honestly seem that people who constantly have a cup of coffee in their hands are different from other people: less focused, less able to keep their mind on things."

"So how do you apply Power Three?"

"Think about the effect that the coffee has on me, and on the people around me...and maybe make a commitment to limit myself to one cup a day, or to drink it only before noon. That commitment, as I continue to honor it, damages the old seeds that I've accumulated over the years with my little coffee addiction. Fewer addiction seeds open, and I see less addiction in my life around me. Including Sue's drinking. Gradually, but steadily, her focus shifts—from her bottle back to me."

"Sounds like a plan," I smile.

KIDS

Question 73

I want to have kids, but my husband doesn't. What's the karma to get him interested in having a family?

This question came to me during a break in a talk in Kuala Lumpur, the capital of Malaysia. It was our first visit there; I'm overwhelmed both by the size of the crowd (over 1500 people) and by the warmth of everyone I've met. Even the business people seem to get choked up when we broach the subject of how the Diamond Cutter ideas bring people together, across borders.

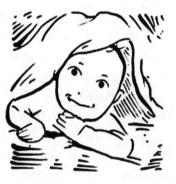

I look down off the stage and see that the line of people waiting to ask a question stretches back almost to the back of the huge auditorium. That's okay; this particular answer is an easy one, and we'll be on to the next person in a minute.

Farah leans over to catch my answer in the murmur of the crowd; her husband Amir is over on the other side, wrestling with their camera.

"Why do you want to have a baby? What is the very essence of having a child?"

Farah thinks for a moment. "I think it is the chance to give yourself completely to another person."

"So you want to see Amir support this idea, of giving both your lives over completely, to another person."

"Exactly."

"And to see that in Amir, you're going to have to plant a seed."

"Yes."

"And what would that seed be?"

"I don't know…I suppose it would involve giving *myself* to someone else even before the baby, so I can create the baby to give myself to again."

"Who could you give yourself to more than you do now?"

Farah gets it immediately. "Why, I could give myself more completely to my husband, to Amir."

I nod. "Look, I'll tell you something that maybe you haven't thought much about. A lot of husbands get nervous, deep down inside, when their wives start talking about children, because they've seen what can happen after a child comes. Sometimes the wife gives herself to the child and takes herself from her husband, and he feels left out, sometimes even for the rest of his life. And then he's not as devoted to the child, or to the family, as he might have been. Perhaps he feels that, when the two of you first got married, you already promised to give yourselves to each other, completely. And now somehow you are giving up on that promise."

Farah nods. "I understand. If I want to see my husband happy to make a child with me, I need to keep my first promise, to give myself completely to him. Then he will join me to give ourselves to our child. If I keep giving myself to both him and our child after our baby comes, I will continue to see him giving himself to both me and the baby, for the rest of our lives."

"And they live happily ever after," I smile. As Farah and Amir leave the stage it occurs to me that the translator has probably never heard about American fairy tales and how they always end, but I have a feeling it's going to happen anyway.

Question 74

I'm pregnant and thinking of having an abortion, but I'm not 100% sure. Any advice?

I get this question almost every day, sometimes several times a day. I'm very aware that it's not an easy question to answer, and that as a male—and a monk—I cannot fully feel how a woman would feel the issue. But I do have some experience with it, and some feelings of my own to share. Before you read ahead, you might want to go back and re-read Question 44, which gives some background about where I'm coming from.

This time the question comes to me in a meeting with some friends from Russia's "Golden Triangle," a group of historic cities clustered in the south. Anastasia is almost whispering, even though we're sitting well away from the others.

"That's not a decision I can make for you," I begin. "In fact, I very rarely try to make decisions for others. Culturally, different countries—and different races of people and different societies and religious traditions—each have their own opinion about abortion, and I think it's important for us to respect this difference in our upbringing. But I can tell you two stories that perhaps will help you with your decision." Anastasia's silence tells me that she wants to hear.

"So you know, a while back I did this long silent retreat, closed off in a single space for three years, mostly in meditation. When I came out, friends invited me to different cities, to come and talk about my experience.

"I remember one talk in New York City. It was still a little hard for me to be around a lot of other people; it was a fairly small space and packed with maybe a hundred people. The organizers had offered me a private office off to the side where I could be quiet, and collect my thoughts before the talk.

"The door to the office was cracked open and I could see the people milling around in the front; then they were all called in to sit down, and the foyer was empty. Suddenly another side door opens, and a tiny apparition appears.

"A lovely Asian girl, maybe four years old, in a pink chiffon dress. She prances around the foyer with a natural, innocent grace, entirely unselfconscious. And then the door to the teaching room opens, and someone calls out, and the girl is gone.

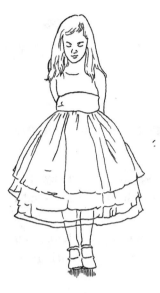

"I stood and went and gave the talk. There was the usual break for refreshments, a chance for people in the audience to come and ask me their private questions while I sit and sip some tea. A Chinese woman approached, and knelt beside me. 'I came to one of your talks before the 3-year retreat,' she says. 'You told us what your lama had told you—that a child's mind enters his or her mother's womb at the very moment of conception. I was way off in the back row, you probably didn't even know I was there; but I was pregnant at the time, and I was considering an abortion.'

"'I went home and thought about what your lama had said, and I thought to myself, my baby is there already, my baby is alive already. And so I decided to have the child.'

"At this point she is weeping openly, tears flowing down her face. 'And it is the best thing that has ever happened in my life, in my whole life, the greatest happiness I could ever have.' She turns and gestures to someone behind her, and the girl in the pink dress steps around her and towards me, shy.

"And then I start to cry too, and I think to myself, 'In all these years of teaching—trying to teach, and as imperfect as I may be—I have at least done this one good thing, I have helped this beautiful child come into this world.'

Anastasia is weeping now too, quietly, as dusk gathers in the woods outside.

"And I'll tell you one more thing," I say. "Just from my heart, apart from all the debate and opinions about abortion—just a practical thing. When I was young, when I was in college, I got a girl pregnant. She was using a contraceptive device—I always made sure that a woman was—but this one time it failed. And she went and got an abortion, because I had made such a fuss about the contraception, and I was overseas at the time and she couldn't ask me.

"My schoolteachers, and many of the adults in my life, had often mentioned in passing that abortions were okay, and so that's what I thought too.

But then after it happened I felt somehow incredibly sad, for years. Later on, one of my lamas taught me how to clean the seed, and I worked on it steadily for some time, and in time it was gone from me.

"In the years since, I've had hundreds of women come up to me in talks and tell me that they've had an abortion, and how terribly sad it made them. I was once even called to a mental hospital to meet a woman who had been coming to my classes regularly, and who had lost her mind after an abortion.

"Those are just my own thoughts," I venture.

Anastasia nods. "Thank you for them." She had the child, and has often thanked me since. What my lama had me do to clean the seed, by the way, was to follow the Four Powers that we talked about back in Question 42—you may want to to back and re-read them there. Here's how I applied them in my case.

For the first power I just thought about The Pen, and how everything and everybody in my life, good or bad, is coming from me, from my seeds. Then, for Power Two, I thought about what this particular seed was going to do to me if I just let it go to multiply and ripen on its own: it was sad and disturbing to think what the karmic retribution would be for scraping someone else out of life.

For Power Three, I made a promise never to be involved in an abortion again, for the rest of my life—and this led in part to my taking the vows of a monk. For Power Four—which is the positive commitment—I organized a children's group in an Asian community, for studying the principles of the Diamond Cutter in a way appropriate for kids.

I kept this up for about five years, and by the end I got some the typical signs that the seed was gone. One of these signs is that you have some small quick disaster in your life—such as a migraine that lasts for two days. This indicates that the bad seed has opened up prematurely; released its energy; and died. Instead of getting into a fatal car accident, I have the headache—this is something that the Buddha taught in fact in the original Diamond Cutter Sutra.

After this sudden experience we have another sign that the seed is finished—which is that we immediately feel very light and happy, as if a heavy burden has been lifted from our shoulders. This is often a burden that we aren't aware we've been carrying, until it's lifted, until we feel what it's like to be freed of it. Suddenly every day is filled with sunshine, and the joy returns to every moment of our life.

Question 75

My husband and I have three children—two of our own and one from my previous marriage. I'm not sure that he's completely aware of it, but he always seems to favor the children we had together, and tends to ignore my first son. What's the seed I need to plant to see him love all the kids equally?

This question came to me somewhere in Texas, on a little "car tour" I once did around the US, speaking in small spaces and trying to get my finger on the pulse of America. Katie and her husband Bob have put us up in their huge suburban home, and the evidence of their three children fills every deeply carpeted inch.

"Why are you asking me this question?" I ask, a little petulantly. "I mean, you never heard me teach the Four Starbucks Steps?" One of my assistants has suggested that I carry a small tape recorder around in my pocket, loaded with an explanation of the Four Steps, and just turn it on when people ask me a question like this.

"I *do* know the Four Steps," replies Katie, sounding a little irritated herself. "Do you want me to show you?" I nod, but in a goofy way so she doesn't stay upset.

The Four Starbucks Steps, one more time!

1) Say what it is you want in your life, <u>in a single short sentence.</u>

2) <u>Plan</u> who it is you're going to help get the same thing, and which Starbucks you're going to take them to, to talk about it.

3) <u>Actually do something</u> to help them.

4) Do your <u>Coffee Meditation</u>: as you go to sleep, think of the good things you're doing to help them.

"Number one: Say what it is I want. I want Bob to treat all the kids equally."

"Step Two: Go through all my friends and family members in my mind, and pick out one who's having a similar problem. I did that—I started asking around, and suddenly I discover that three of my best friends are having the very same issue…"

Here Katie pauses, and a light goes off in her eyes. I suppose that a corresponding light has just gone off in her mind.

"Now that's interesting," she says. "We tend to think that if three of our friends are having the same problem as us, it's because we never paid enough attention to their needs before. But it just occurred to me that we might have some Flower Three working here: that I'm seeing people around me with the same problem as I have because *they're coming from the same seeds as my problem*. And if I work on my own seeds then maybe I help my friends solve their version of the problem too."

She shakes herself out of it. "Anyway, Step Three would be to actually take my friends out to Starbucks and give them some advice to help them with their own husband problem. And that's where I have a problem."

"What's the problem?"

"I mean, when you get to Starbucks Step Three, this system gets a little bit weird. A person who has trouble making money is supposed to plant their seeds by giving advice to somebody else who's having trouble making money; the woman who can't get her husband to treat all their kids equally is supposed to give advice to another woman who can't get her husband to do the same thing.

"But the person who's having trouble making money is the last person to give advice to someone else having the same trouble—and the same with the husband. It seems like a vicious cycle: I don't know what to do to make Bob treat the kids equally; so I'm in no position to give anyone else advice on the same problem; so I will never make new seeds to see Bob change."

I nod my head. "That's exactly the way it is—it's all about vicious cycles. The last person in the mood to share their money is someone who hasn't got enough; the same with a person who doesn't have enough time in the day. In the Diamond Cutter world, we have to work against human nature—the cultural habits of tens of thousands of years in this world.

"You have to break through human nature; and you can do it, just on the strength of understanding. You don't need to solve the problem that your three friends have with how their new spouse treats the children from their first spouse—you just have to provide support for them, reach out, give them someone to talk to. You just need to try, which means that you *want* to try: you have that intention.

"The intention to help someone else is the strongest part of a seed, and seeds planted with strong intention grow like wild. A small attempt to help one of your three friends—to give them the best advice that you can, knowing that you're not in the greatest place to give advice to anybody—is enough of a seed. It will grow, into a whole bunch of happy families."

Katie gives me a mischievous smile. "And now I have something to do my Coffee Meditation on."

"How's that?"

"Tonight—I can just sit on my bed, and be happy that we had this talk, so I could help myself, and help my friends.

"That would be Step Four," she reminds me, as we get up and head back to the meeting.

Question 76

My wife and I have had two miscarriages in the last few years; we're feeling sad and unsure if we'll ever have more children. What karma do we need to plant to have a family?

This question came in Berlin, but not from a Berliner. Alberto has flown in, I learn, not to attend my talk, but to get 5 minutes alone with me in my hotel room, to ask me this burning question. He and Maria already have a beautiful girl—Christina—and they've been trying for another child, without success. The last attempt ended badly, with doctors working without hope over the child, in the local hospital.

"It would be nice," he says, "to have a pair."

"A pair?"

"I mean, one boy and one girl—that would be nice."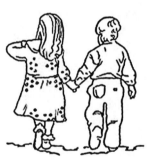

"So you don't just want the seed for a child, you want the seed for a *boy* child," I say.

"Right," says Alberto. He's so sure that I must know the karma for this that I realize I *do* know the karma.

"Well, that would be two seeds," I reply.

"How so?"

"One seed to have a child. Another seed to have the child you want."

"Sounds reasonable."

"Okay then, let's hear the Four Steps for the first."

"One: Maria and I want a child. Two, we need to find someone else who wants to have a child, and make some plan to help them."

"Right. And given how the last one ended, I have a very specific suggestion for the two of you. I want you to find a hospital locally that serves children, small children, with congenital issues—health problems that they've had from birth. And I want you to volunteer to help there, with anything they need: changing diapers, sweeping floors."

"Alright then," says Alberto. "That's our plan. Then we go *do* it, say…"

"…Say just once a week is enough, for a couple of hours. Small seeds make big trees."

"And then the Coffee Meditation, on three things. Happy on our pillows that we planned our service of the hospital in Step Two. Happy that we actually served the babies, in Step Three. And holding that vision of a future, which we've helped create just by our living example: a world where every couple who wants a baby can have one, just by planting the seeds."

"Right," I agree. "Now let's talk about the second thing you want: a boy child specifically, so Christina can have a brother. What's Step One—what's the very essence of what you want here?"

Alberto considers for a moment. "The essence of what we want…why, the essence of what we want here is to have what we want: a boy!"

"That's reasonable. You want to plant a seed that will bring you just what you wish."

"So really then I have to concentrate on helping someone else find their fondest wish."

"Right, and it doesn't really matter so much what it is—the point is in having what you want."

"So I guess find someone, and help them work out what it is they really want the most, and help them to get that."

"Exactly. People are strange. A lot of us are unhappy that we don't have what we want, but we really can't say what it is we want. We're so used to *not* getting what we really want that we don't even dare to think about what it is that we really want.

"And so a good seed for getting exactly what you want—a boy, in this case—would be a Step Three where you take someone out to a coffee shop, and help them work through the question of what they really want in life.

"Encourage them to think big, encourage them to think about what it is they really want, and not to make any compromises. It might actually take them a few meetings to figure out what it is that they most want, deep in their heart, but have been afraid to want. And then give them some support on getting that thing."

Alberto nods, and heads towards the door of my room. "And of course I top it off with some Coffee Meditation," he smiles. By the way, Alberto and Maria did follow this advice—quite carefully and consistently—and I am happy to report that not long back they did have a bright, chubby, baby boy.

RELIGION

Question 77

After many years without a spiritual path, I've found one that I'm really excited about. I try to convince my husband to come to some of the events, but he's not interested and it seems to make him feel resentful. What seed do I have to plant to see him on the path with me? This is something that would really make my life happy.

This question came up at a talk in the town music center of Guelph, outside of Toronto, Canada. Guelph has got to have the highest number of spiritual seekers of any small town in the world: I've run into them in Europe; the Caribbean; and lots of other places. The person asking the question is Missy, and her husband is Eric.

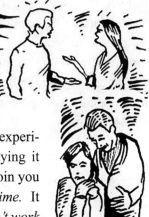

"Missy," I begin, "let's start by getting clear about what *doesn't* work. I mean, you know it from personal experience—the personal experience of an entire lifetime—but it's worth just saying it clearly. It doesn't work to try to convince Eric to join you in your new path, because *it doesn't work all the time*. It doesn't work to argue with him, because *that doesn't work all the time either.* The same with not saying anything: the silent treatment."

If it doesn't work all the time, it doesn't work

"I've got it," she says, with a nod. "You're right on that. I guess it took me a really long time to figure that out—longer than it should have—but I'm there now. I really do understand that arguing with him and all the rest is just not going to work, because it doesn't work all the time."

I nod. "And I could tell you that it's wrong to pressure any member of your family to accept your viewpoints; or else I could tell you that you'll regret it later if you didn't try to share the joy of the spiritual path with Eric.

"But that's all just a diamond deal. You want what you want, and you should have what you want, just the way you want it, so long as it's not something that would hurt someone else. You want Eric to be more open to the path you've found, and you can have it. You just have to plant the seed."

Missy gazes out the window, at the lovely Canadian woods. "When you put it that way, it's pretty clear which seeds I need to plant."

"So what are they?"

"If I want Eric to be more open to my ideas, I need to be more open to other people's ideas. That would plant the seed."

"Right. And the usual rules apply. The Second Law of Karma says that the seed you plant can be much, much smaller than the result you are looking for. That is, to see Eric really open his heart, all the time, to the ideas that you're embracing, then you don't need to invest more than a few hours a week, working on being more open to the ideas and suggestions that people around you express.

"And most important, Step Four: your Coffee Meditation." I watch to catch Missy's reaction to this, and what I see worries me, because I've seen it with hundreds of people before. I can see that she thinks the idea of Coffee Meditation is just something cute—as cute as the name itself—but not exactly crucial. Too cute to be crucial, in fact.

"And it really is most important," I repeat, to get her attention.

"Oh, I know it must be important, or you wouldn't make such a big deal out of it."

"Coffee Meditation really *is* a big deal," I repeat. "And people seem to have a really hard time with it. Either they don't take it so seriously in the first place, or even if they do try to do it regularly as they lay down to sleep, they find that they have a very real problem concentrating on it.

"Somehow, the moment we lay our head down on the pillow we are completely overcome by our worries and neuroses. I can't believe how my boss criticized me at work today; I wish my husband would be more affectionate; I don't know how we're going to pay the bills this month.

"The problem is that—by the time we go to bed—we've been through a whole long day of life, and we're tired. And when they get tired, adults are just as cranky as children. The tiredness tends to exaggerate all our problems, all our worries, way out of proportion.

"And so we fall off to sleep with exaggerated problems on our mind, and as we go through a whole night in bed they grow even more exaggerated. We have trouble falling asleep; we wake up at odd hours during the night; and we find our eyes opening, staring at the ceiling, an hour or two before the alarm goes off.

"All of this changes with Coffee Meditation. We fall off to sleep actively trying to think (that is, *meditating*) about the good things we've been doing for others—we fall asleep happy. And then the mind works on these seeds as we sleep, which causes the seeds to multiply wildly, in the earth below the conscious mind. We wake up joyful, completely refreshed.

"Thousands and thousands of people around the world have sat and listened to teachings on the principles of the Diamond Cutter. A good number of them hear the wisdom, and try to plant some seeds. But whether the seeds grow strong, and fast, depends greatly upon how good our Coffee Meditation is.

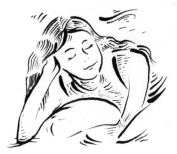

"Coffee Meditation makes all the difference between getting what you want in your life, or not. Don't be deceived by how simple it is, or by the fact that laying down on your bed at night and thinking about all the good things you're doing for people is a mildly pleasant process.

"It's not true that the most powerful karmas you can plant require the most effort or stress. If you think about it, it may actually be the opposite: that if you really find the most powerful spiritual tools of all, the most powerful keys to success, then perhaps by their very nature they are gentle, and simple, and easy.

"Coffee Meditation is one of the most pleasant practices of all; and the most powerful; and the most necessary. Skip your Coffee Meditation, and you are skipping your success, and happiness—and Eric's opinion of your path will never change." I raise an eyebrow.

Missy smiles. "Okay, okay. I get the message. You can plant a seed, but it won't grow without sunlight and water and fertilizer. It sounds like Coffee Meditation is the sunlight."

I nod. The car arrives to whisk me off to Toronto, and I excuse myself. Maybe I can catch some Coffee Meditation in the back seat, on the way.

Question 78

Sometimes I feel that having a relationship—especially one where intimacy is involved—is very worldly, and I feel like I'm missing out on the spiritual side of life. Can I have a physical relationship, and somehow still make it spiritual?

I'm writing the answer to this question in Beijing, where it came up this afternoon. I was sitting in a semi-traditional teashop with Pinglian, and her husband Junlong.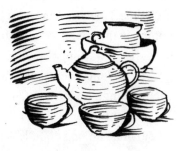

"There's this question about intimacy, isn't there?" I begin. "I mean, it's especially strong in my country, in America. On the one hand, everybody seeks intimacy—it is one of the greatest pleasures and comforts of a human life. On the other hand, the sexual urge is so strong that intimacy with someone can lead to a host of different problems: questions of possession, of control, an entire variety of abuse or manipulation."

"That's true," says Pinglian. "And then among Americans, and also here in China, a sort of schizophrenia has developed: is sex something good, or is sex something bad? We feel that in some way sex is dirty; and so we are careful for example not to expose children to sexually explicit materials."

"And then that very naturally leads to your question," I agree. "It leads to wondering if spirituality and intimacy are somehow opposed to each other: If I want to develop spiritually, should I limit, or even give up, being intimate with another person?"

"Exactly," says Pinglian, and she settles back against the seat of the booth.

I think on it a bit and see a way that the answer should go. "There are two parts to answering this one," I nod. "The first one relates to the story of how the Buddha himself reached enlightenment."

"How's that?" pipes up Junlong.

"Well you see, there are two very different versions of the story. In many of the teachings that he gave, the Buddha described how he became enlightened during his time here on this planet, as he went through twelve different life experiences. To his close disciples though he admitted having become enlightened long before his appearance in this world, saying that he then came here and acted out the process of enlightenment again, simply to show people how it was done.

"He then described how he had actually become enlightened, long before, in another realm. References to this account are found in the ancient writings of Tibet, including those of Je Tsongkapa, the founder of the lineage of the Dalai Lamas, and those of his student Kedrup Je. One of the most detailed records of this enlightenment was passed down by a lama named Jetsun Welmang Konchok Gyeltsen, and is found in the seventh of the 'Secret Books of Gyume Tibetan Monastery,' which is where my own teacher received his training in the advanced teachings of Buddhism. We find additional details in the works of a Mongol sage, Chuje Ngawang Pelden.

"These lamas describe how long ago the Buddha had already reached the level of a high bodhisattva, and was facing the challenge of how to move on into total enlightenment. He was not the first person to become enlightened, but only one among countless holy beings who reached the goal before him.

"A great mass of these enlightened ones cluster around our Buddha as he struggles to make his final breakthrough, and consult among each other (as far as people who can see all time and space need to consult) to decide what will help him the most. In the midnight hour of the final day they call upon an angel named Tilottama, or the 'Lady of the Supreme Drop'.

"They grant our Buddha special permission to take her as his spiritual partner, and the two practice in sacred intimacy. Their combined union creates enough power for them to pass into enlightenment, together, in the final minutes of the dawn: two new Buddhas burst forth with the sunlight of a new day."

Pinglian and Junlong are as engrossed in the story as I am; and so I continue.

"It's no coincidence that their moment of enlightenment coincides with the first moment that the rays of the sun break the horizon. There is a deep connection between changes within our inner body—our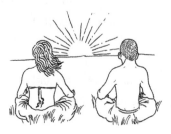

inner, physical network of channels and chakras—and the turning of the seasons in the outer world. Our physical inner energy, which is called *prana*, is making a final breakthrough deep inside, even as our spirit reaches its final liberation."

"What you're saying then," says Junlong, "is that physical intimacy between two people can actually further the process of spiritual development, rather than hinder it."

"That's the idea," I nod. "Sort of like the positive and negative sides of a battery. As soon as there is a deep connection between a man and a woman—physically yes, but also emotionally, and spiritually—then the feminine energy that a man needs to 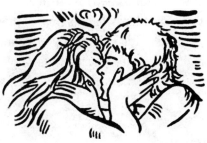 be complete flows from her into him, and vice versa. Thus the story of how our own Buddha became enlightened, together with his partner Tilottama."

Pinglian thinks on this for a moment. "Well it sort of makes sense. As you've said, the sexual urge in human beings is perhaps the most powerful of all instincts; for better or for worse. But we all sense that the urge for enlightenment—the urge to contribute in some way to the happiness of all the living beings there are in the universe—is equally strong, deep down inside. To say that the two are somehow connected seems appropriate."

I nod. "I mean, think of it in terms of seeds. If you reach a point where you've planted a lot of seeds inside you for spiritual evolution, then you're just generally going to have a lot of very good seeds in general.

"That is, we always assume that the process of spiritual evolution is something difficult; something to be achieved through devoted effort and practice, over a long period of time. And that's true. But as you travel further and further along the path, you're going to have to be kinder and kinder to other people, taking more and more care of others.

"And this means more and more good seeds, the farther you progress. There begins a sort of synergy between the good seeds. People with the seeds to be increasingly kinder create seeds to be more and more happy mentally. These seeds affect their subtle, inner body—which then affects their health. They begin to glow, strong and healthy. The seeds for inner peace are automatically creating a powerful outer, physical wellbeing."

Junlong starts to nod. "Oh, and then it would make sense on another level. It's not like in the advanced stages of your spiritual evolution you are suffering somehow—it must be quite the opposite. You must be experiencing more and more physical bliss as you get closer to the goal.

"I mean," he says with a kind of wonder, "it makes perfect sense, in a way, that you would become enlightened in the arms of your wife or husband, in physical happiness as strong as the spiritual one. Because they're both coming from the very same kinds of seeds." He looks over lovingly at Pinglian, who returns the look. It feels very right, and we sit and cherish the moment. Then I see that it's time to move on to the second part of the answer.

"I think it's good that you've mentioned 'the arms of your wife or husband'," I begin. "Because this whole concept of physical intimacy contribut-

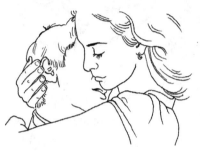

ing to spiritual development is potentially a very dangerous concept, and it needs to be understood correctly. It's an ancient principle, but from ancient times too it has been abused—as the act of sex itself is so often abused.

"Along with the physical intimacy, there must be an intimacy of spirits. And the intimacy of spirits—true love between a man and a woman—is something that can only happen under conditions of great mutual honor and respect. It can only happen where each partner has a completely clear conscience: where each is upholding a very high code of personal integrity."

Pinglian nods. "That makes sense too. It's not just the physical intimacy which creates the bonding of two souls; there would have to be a deep care and kindness for each other."

Junlong picks it up. "Which means that the relationship would need to be stable, and very committed. A commitment that each partner was keeping perfectly. I don't think it could be a casual thing, and especially not the kind of thing where you were fooling around on your partner, by fooling yourself into thinking that you and someone other than your partner were being intimate to get enlightened."

"That's the point," I agree. "It would take a lot of good seeds for intimacy with your husband or wife to further both of you in a spiritual way. If the intimacy were tainted in any way—if either partner was failing to follow a very ethical way of life—then it would only cause trouble for everyone involved. Intimacy can be a great goodness, but it takes great goodness for it to be."

Junlong nods, and gives Pinglian that loving look again. I think all three of us are feeling, at that moment, the real reason why women and men—in every part of the world, and throughout the history of the world—have sought to be in each other's arms and hearts.

SEX, PART THREE

Question 79

My husband just doesn't know how to kiss, and I can't seem to teach him. What's the karma for getting a decent smooch out of this guy?

"Before I answer," I begin, "I think you'll have to tell me what makes a smooch 'decent'."

I'm sitting in Austin, Texas, with Debbie—an old friend. We're waiting in a restaurant next to a yoga studio where I'm supposed to give a talk, in half an hour, about some ancient Buddhist teaching. It's nice once in a while to get questions like this one: nothing terribly life-shaking, because I know that her marriage is going pretty well actually. Her husband Tim ducks his head and smiles, and I think he's just kicked her good-naturedly under the table too.

"I mean," Debbie elaborates, "that in my opinion a kiss should be *gooey*. I'm talking a lot of saliva being swapped." Tim rolls his eyes.

"No kidding," she continues, glaring at him. "I mean, a peck on the cheek—or even on the lips—isn't really a kiss at all, if you ask me." She folds her arms and looks at me with determination, as I scramble to remember if I've ever seen the karma for spit described in one of the ancient sutras.

"I don't think it's the spit," I finally decide. "I think it's the concentration. If it's *gooey* you want, then the kiss is going to have to last a fair amount of time. For a kiss to take time, both of you have to be absorbed in it. Being absorbed means you want him to *concentrate* on the kiss, while he's kissing you."

Tim nods. He looks somehow relieved that we're not going to be spending the next half hour discussing saliva.

"And *concentrating*," I continue, "pretty much means not thinking about anything else during the kiss. You want Tim to be present and content, just standing there kissing you. You want a mutual feeling of total focus, with a sense of enjoyment inside the focus."

At this they both nod. Now we're getting somewhere.

"Which is pretty much the definition of meditation," I add, and sit for a moment to think of what would help them the most…something that my lama always said was the most important place to start.

"Okay then," I say as it comes clear. "This is going to take a moment, but we'll get there." Debbie and Tim nod in unison.

"We're going to have to figure out how to plant the seeds for perfect concentration. I could tell you that you have to practice more meditation every day; or avoid overstimulation like a lot of emails or Facebook; or get enough sleep or eat well or exercise. And it's true that all those things can help your concentration, but only *can*. We're going to have to look deeper, if we want the real secret to a good kiss.

"Let's go at it this way. All day, as we go through our life for a day, we are listening to thoughts being spoken in our mind—am I right?"

"Sure," says Tim. "I mean, we may not notice it very often, but our mind is talking all the time."

Seeds are who is talking in your mind all day

"Good. So I have a question for you. When your mind is talking, and you're listening to it as it talks, are you the one who's talking, or are you the one who's listening? Because you can't be both, at the same time."

Debbie and Tim look a little stumped.

"Well let's put it this way. When you're having a conversation with someone at work, do you first have to think of what you're going to say, before you say it?"

"Sure," says Debbie. "It's a constant process of picking and choosing your words, to get your ideas across."

"Right. So when there's talking going on in your mind, is it that you're going through the same process, picking and choosing the words you want to say?"

"No, not at all," Tim says. "The thoughts just come up, all on their own."

"I think that's right," adds Debbie. "I mean, you can be very depressed and hear sad sentences popping up in your mind, and not be able to stop them at all. It doesn't seem like you have any control over them. Which is why it can be so frustrating trying to give advice to someone who's depressed. It's not like they *want* to hear sad thoughts going through their mind."

"Exactly. And that applies to random thoughts coming up during a kiss as well, you see. Maybe Tim is trying really hard to give you a big, focused, gooey kiss—but these thoughts about other things just keep popping up in his mind. We have to decide *why* those thoughts are popping up in his head, and then we can come to the secret of a great kiss."

I'm twirling a pen around in my fingers as I talk; Tim looks down and smiles. "Okay, okay. I get it. If I see a pen as a pen because of whatever seeds I happen to have in my mind, and the same with how I see anything else or anybody else around me at any given time, then I guess the same applies as well to the thoughts I hear inside my mind. They must also be popping out of seeds."

"Seeds that you planted before," I add. "And the question is, what plants those seeds? More specifically, how do we plant seeds this week, if next week we want to hear thoughts inside our head which are quiet and focused?"

"Well just logically," says Debbie, "we would have to be offering focus and quiet to someone else. That would plant the seed."

"Right again. And there's a way of doing this which can be very helpful. All day long we engage in encounters with other people. We might be walking down the street, and we catch sight of someone we know. We approach them to share a few words.

"As you walk up to talk to a person—any person, any time, and for the rest of your life—pause slightly to observe their face, to see what they're feeling in the moment. Imagine that you can look through their skull into the inside of their mind.

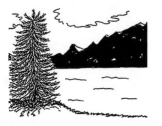

"And imagine that their mind looks like a small lake, a small lake filled to the very brim with crystal-clear water. See how the surface of the water looks today.

"With some people the water is completely still, and calm—which means these people are feeling quiet, focused. The idea then is that, as we close the distance between us, and get ready to say something to them, we need to decide to ourselves that we will respect this quiet: we will not disturb the smooth surface of the crystal lake of their focus.

"We choose our words carefully, and even our gestures, and the expression upon our face. The karma of being considerate this way plants seeds to hear our own minds—a week or whatever from now—as being quiet and focused. And then we can really give someone all of our attention as we kiss."

"And I suppose," Debbie says, as I check my watch, "that we can make even more seeds than that if the other person's lake is all riled up as we approach them. We keep our own crystal lake as calm and unruffled as we can, and then when the two lakes touch and our conversation starts, we get the seeds of helping them feel some peace. We're careful not to be nervous or hyper or demanding."

"It's interesting to think of it that way," Tim agrees. "I mean, anytime two people meet and exchange words, then those words and the body language that go along with them affect both the lakes. And if you want to plant the seeds for good kisses, then you've got to have this intention that the result of every exchange should be a net positive, for both of you. The surface of both lakes, smooth as glass."

"Go for it," I smile, and head off for the talk.

Question 80

I've found some sex magazines that my husband keeps hidden from me in the house, and I think he uses them to masturbate, which makes me feel awful—almost as if he's having sex with another woman. How do I let him know this, and how do I get him to change?

This question came sitting on a bench at a shopping mall in Seattle waiting to start a book signing in a small bookstore across the way. Carol has asked to speak with me privately, and we can see her husband Jimmy through the front window of the store, getting the first arrivals settled, some on the few chairs available, and some on the carpet.

"I think there's a healthy sexual urge," I begin, "and some that are not so healthy. A healthy sexual urge can be very romantic and even strongly physical, but there is an undercurrent of love and respect, a bonding of souls between two open and shining hearts. Both partners are in a healthy state of mind: clear, rested, happy.

"An unhealthy sexual urge, it seems to me, seems to manifest in the opposite conditions. One or both of the partners is tired, or worried, bored or angry. There is a desire for peace or satisfaction then which manifests, mistakenly, as a craving for sexual release. The release never brings the result we were looking for—rather, it leaves us feeling empty and exhausted—but we never quite seem to learn the lesson.

"What I mean to say is that your husband's desire for sexual images, and to masturbate, don't I think reflect a healthy sexuality or libido. It's not that he's not getting enough sex with you, or that he's not attracted to you, or anything like that. Rather, his sexual drive has been derailed somehow by other issues in his life; and it's those issues that we want to look at—then he'll come back to enjoying a healthier sexuality with you. Does that give you any ideas?"

Carol looks up at the lovely clear blue sky; we were joking before about how real estate agents in Seattle choose these once-a-month perfect days to show out-of-state clients around—it's just impossibly beautiful. I let her think for a bit.

"You know, I think you're right," she says finally. "I mean, if I look back and try to guess when he first started with the magazines and all, it corresponds to a period in his life when he began to have some trouble in his career. The company started some downsizing, which is still going on, and there was this combined stress on him: worrying about whether he was going to have a job next week, and dealing with a double workload after so many other people had been laid off.

"So what do you think?" she says then. "Should I encourage him to look for a new job? Or just help him understand why he's having these urges? Which is best for getting him to stop?"

I squeeze my face up into a whacky scowl that I use to make children laugh. "That's a diamond deal, if I ever heard one." I hold up my hands, as though showing two different diamonds to a bewildered customer in a jewelry store. (If you don't remember what a "diamond deal" is, take a look back at Question 34.)

Carol laughs that laugh of a Diamond Cutter enthusiast caught in a wrong-think. "Of course, yes, you're right. No use offering myself lots of different options, none of which is sure to work. I just need to plant some seeds."

"But what kind of seeds?"

Again she's quiet for a bit while she thinks it out. "Jimmy is just off-balance at this point in his life. And I do believe that's what's behind this disruption of his sexuality. To deal with it using the Diamond Cutter Principles, I'd say there are two different ways we could go."

"Which are?"

"Well, first let's assume that the root of the problem is the general stress he's under at work. The Four Starbucks Steps say that he's going to have to find someone else who's under some similar stress of their own—although it doesn't have to be the exact same kind of stress. He needs to take them out for coffee and help them talk their problem out, then follow up with some concrete steps to solve the stress. And then after that, some Coffee Meditation before he goes to sleep, celebrating the good things he's done to help this other person."

"Sounds perfect," I say, checking to see if the bookstore owner is looking for me yet.

"Not really," says Carol. "Jimmy's just not into the Diamond Cutter thing. I think he's sort of watching to see if it works for me, before he tries it for himself. So the Four Steps might work out for him later on, but not right now. That's why I think I'm going to go the second way."

"Which is?"

"The Third Flower." She smiles, and now I know she's showing off; but that's fine, it's great that she understands the options. "If I see Jimmy under this kind of stress, then at some level I must be putting myself under similar stress. That seed spreads from my inside to my outside, past the limits of my own skin, and shapes the people and world around me—including Jimmy. If I can straighten out my own lifestyle, Jimmy puts down the magazines and comes back to my bed."

"So what do you think is going on with your lifestyle, which might be creating this experience of stressed-out people around you?"

Here Carol pauses for a much longer moment; we are both fine with the silence that ensues. Finally she looks up and holds up three fingers.

"I mean, my life *is* stressed, and I think it comes from three different things. Small seeds, but big enough to grow into the stress which I see in Jimmy, and the pictures that he imagines might give him some release.

"First of all I'm just running all day long; somehow I've designed my life so that it needs about 10% more time than I possibly have available. And I get this feeling that if I suddenly dropped half of what I do that keeps me too busy, then in about two weeks I'd find something else to keep keeping me just as busy.

"Second, I have the same nervous habit about eating—I find myself popping little snacks into my mouth all day long, and if I'm really observant of the thoughts running through my own mind at any given moment, I realize that I'm thinking about my next snack almost constantly.

"Third, I have a real problem just sitting still. The other day I was sitting on my bed looking out the window, and for the first time since I moved into my place I realized that I have this really beautiful, green, perfectly shaped tree right there behind the house, and I never took the time to just sit and enjoy it. And then right there in the middle of that thought I started to get up to check my emails, even though I had just checked them less than two minutes before.

"What I mean is, my whole lifestyle is set up to make me nervous and dissatisfied. And it's just a stupendous breakthrough for me to realize that this is very probably the seed that makes me see Jimmy going through this anxiety-induced, unhappy substitute for real and healthy sex. If that's really the case, then I have the power to make him stop: I've always had the power to make him stop."

"I like it," I say, as I stand up to make my way over to the book signing. "And I have a feeling that these lifestyle changes are something that you'd have trouble doing for yourself; but if it's for Jimmy, and for your marriage, then I think you're going to find the strength to pull them off."

Carol answers me with a look of quiet determination, and I can already feel a home with a lot more peace and balance and…real, honest enjoyment… on its way.

Question 81

I sometimes have gentle sexual fantasies that I would like to act out with my wife—where she is wearing some really sexy lingerie, for example—but whenever I try to bring this up I feel like maybe I'm being inappropriate; and she doesn't seem to be that open to it anyway. Are fantasies like this wrong? If not, then how can I get her more interested?

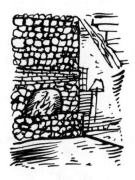

I spend a lot of time teaching in Mexico; a lot of the country is closer to where I live than say Chicago or New York, and the people have an ebullient love of life that you just don't see that often in the States. I'm getting this question sitting on a big comfy sofa in front of a fire in a lodge near Lake Chapala—the largest lake in all of Mexico, wending its way through bright green mountains and at many points stretching out past the horizon. We're halfway through a weekend success training, and dinner is way late, because twice as many people showed up than we expected.

So I have time to tackle Rodrigo's question. Wife Carla is off trying to find futons for the extra participants. I want to get a few things straight first.

"So we're really talking about something gentle; and something that you both agree to; and a lot of mutual love and respect going on the whole time, am I right?"

"I promise," says Rodrigo, touching his palm to his chest.

"Okay. So what's the seed to see someone close to you agree to a suggestion which is very personal?"

"Well obviously; I would have to do the same."

"And do you?"

Rodrigo gazes at the ceiling, checks on that, and comes back to meet my eyes. "Not exactly."

"Example?"

"I mean, look. Like just in the last two weeks Carla has tried to sell me on trying those little loafers that the kids wear—I'm talking kids who are into skateboards, you know? I mean, like, I'm pushing 40, and she wants me to wear skateboard shoes?"

I wave my palm in the air, like…Well then, what do you expect? Rodrigo frowns for a moment, calculating I guess whether seeing Carla in a teddy is worth wearing surfer shoes. The scales seem to tip.

"Well okay then. I'll wear them." And he stands up with finality. I grab his hand and pull him back down.

"It might take a bit more than that," I caution.

"Why more?" he says, looking somehow hurt. "I thought you said that seeds always multiply like wild."

"Exactly so," I agree. "But it doesn't hurt to call in a little more fire-power. We don't know how many old seeds you might still have there in your karmic storehouse, confusing things. Can you think of any other ways to see Carla be a little more open to something new? And I want you to remember another thing: you don't have to plant seeds at home to see things happen at home."

"Okay, I get you. If we look at it that way, then I guess there are a lot more opportunities to plant seeds in my office than at home. I mean, people are constantly coming up to me at work with some new idea about this or that."

"Do any of them relate to making things *more fun?* More creative?"

Rodrigo thinks for a bit. "Well yes, I guess that a good number of the suggestions that people give me would make our work more fun. One person wants to make a training video using all the people in the office, dressed up like…well, chickens. But I thought that was a little weird…" He stops, and looks a little dumbfounded.

"You think Carla thinks lingerie is a little weird? I mean, like dressing up as a chicken?"

I go the safe way—after all, we've already got his mind where we want it. "Well now, I don't think I'd be at all qualified to say. But it doesn't really matter. Just work really hard in your office at staying open new and creative ideas. At night, when you lay down for Coffee Meditation, take those seeds and send them in your mind to Carla. Everything will work out perfect."

Rodrigo flashes a broad smile. "Great," he says. "It's a deal." Then he pauses and says, "Just one more thing. How long do I have to keep this up?"

"How long do you have to keep being open to other people's new and creative and possibly earthshaking suggestions?"

He grins. "No, I know…once I get open to others, I can stay open. I just want to know how long it's going to take before, you know, Carla opens up to my idea, about the lingerie."

"As long as it takes," I say simply.

Keep planting for as long as it takes

"As long as it takes? What do you mean, as long as it takes?"

"Just that," I nod. "Look. You have millions of seeds running around in your little mental seed bank, all waiting to go off. And your seed bank is different from anyone else's, because you've been doing and saying and thinking a specific mix of things that no one else has. So if you ask me how long all this is going to take, all I can say is that it will take whatever time it takes, depending on the unique, overall mix of seeds that you possess inside your own heart."

"So that's it? You're telling me just stay open to people's creative suggestions and then maybe someday Carla will dress up sexy for me?"

"*Someday,* yes; *maybe,* no. There's no *maybe* about it. Plant seeds by being open to ideas, and sooner or later she'll be open to the lingerie.

"But understand two things. One, there's no *other* way that she'll *ever* be open to the lingerie. *Everything* comes from seeds. You can whine, you can persuade, you can yell—but it won't make the least bit of difference, and I think you sense very well that this is true. Until you have the seeds to see her be more open, she won't be: she *can't* be. Plain and simple, you don't have any choice but to get to work and plant the seeds.

"Second, you have to go on planting for as long as it takes. You'll know it's enough planting when she comes out the bathroom door one night dressed exactly the way you always fantasized about."

Rodrigo looks a little frustrated. "I mean…who knows, that could be years!"

"Not years," I shake my head.

"How do you know?" he retorts.

"Because you have a secret weapon. You can speed the whole thing up;

I mean ten times, a hundred times faster than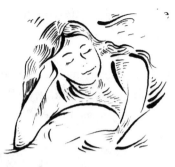
table in front of the sofa. There's a cup of
coffee sitting there, waiting for me, for my
own Coffee Meditation. I was planning to
start as soon as I finished with Rodrigo.

He smiles and goes and pours his own
cup and comes back to sit down next to me.
We relax on the sofa and meditate together
in the firelight, sipping to speed things up.

Question 82

My husband used to be amazing in bed, but for the last few years he's barely been able to get an erection. It makes me feel bad, like something's wrong with me. What's the karma to get him back up?

I don't know when I stopped being shy about getting this kind of question, but it was quite a while ago. You can't guess how many people have this problem, and how many relationships are strained because of it. Nancy is leaning over and asking in a low tone of voice, as we sit in the Joyce Theater in Manhattan. It's intermission time in the middle of 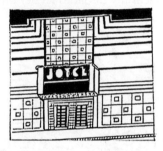 a great modern dance performance, and her husband Stephen is leaning the other way, talking to a friend.

"It's not so much the loss of our intimacy," she continues. "It's more that...well...I can't stop thinking that maybe he just doesn't want me anymore, that he doesn't find me attractive anymore."

"I see what you mean," I nod. "It's not just that you miss the warmth of the intimacy, although I know you do. What hurts more is that you're not sure if he still wants you, if he still values you."

"Exactly," Nancy nods.

"So there's Step One already: I want to feel loved, wanted, valued. Just getting that clear in your mind makes Step Two easy."

"You mean, I need to go look for a person who feels like they're not valued, like no one wants them. And then I have to make a plan for helping them."

"Exactly. And look—I know what you're thinking. You think you don't know anybody who feels like no one wants them, or values them. But I've been through this conversation a dozen times, and I can tell you what's going to happen. If you spend the next 24 hours really checking through all your friends and relatives and coworkers, you're going to come up with 3 or 4 different people who fit the bill exactly.

"It's not that there aren't people around us having the same problem we are; it's just that we're so wrapped up in having that problem ourselves that we haven't noticed them. Start looking, and you'll find people all around you who have the same needs as you do. Maybe it's only when we realize that finding them is the key to ending our own problems that we finally notice how much they're in need as well."

"Okay, so I have to find someone who doesn't feel valued, and make them feel that way—maybe make them feel that I value them." Nancy looks up, and goes inside to try to think of somebody. I let her finish that and then clear my throat to let her know there's more.

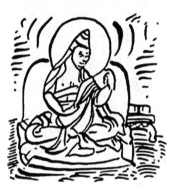

"And look, Nancy, there's something about what you said just now…that you want to make them feel that you value them. This goes back to one of the greatest explanations of seeds ever written: the *Treasure House of Knowledge,* or *Abhidharma Kosha,* written by the Indian master Vasubandhu about 17 centuries ago.

"Here we read that—although the things we do and say certainly do plant karmic seeds—it is our own inner thoughts which are the most powerful. And so it's one thing to try to express to someone how much we value them, and it's another thing to actually *value* them, mentally.

"What I mean is, you'll be collecting a lot of seeds in Step Three, as you sit with your friend in the coffee shop and make sure they feel more valued by yourself and others. But then before you reach the coffee shop, and when you get home afterwards, it's very important that you take some time to think about how much you really do value them, and the reasons why you could value them even more.

"This makes the time that you spend with them, pumping up their feeling of being valued, a lot more credible and powerful—because there probably really are a dozen reasons why everyone could be valuing them more. But all the moments that you set aside to appreciate them just inside your own mind are even more powerful, because the seeds are being planted very close to the inner core of your mind: the place where the seeds are stored.

"And so it's not just important to make your friend *feel* valued; it's crucial that you *do* value them. If you create the seeds for Stephen to realize how much he really does appreciate you, then he'll express that appreciation… very *straight,* if you know what I mean."

Nancy smiles, and we turn back to the performance. I can sell her on the Coffee Meditation afterwards, while we're all hanging out over dessert across the street.

HABITUAL PATTERNS

Question 83

Over the years, it seems like our relationship has evolved into a whole network of habitual patterns—we eat the same foods, we repeat the same stories to each other, we get into the same arguments—year after year. What's the karma to break out of this rut?

I got this question from an Indian couple who live in a suburb of New Delhi; at one point I was spending a lot of time renting rooms from them, while I did grunt work for our refugee project. I met them not long after they got together; early on, they were quite lovey-dovey, and then as the years passed I could feel in their home how yes, habitual patterns did seem to take over. Some were cultural, but a lot more of them were universal, and I have seen them repeated all over the world.

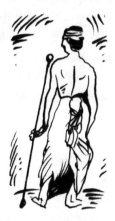

Back in Question 47, we went over some ways to get excitement back into a relationship, and if the present question relates to you, you might want to go take a look at that one once more.

So anyway, Kumar has just come back from sharing a cup of yogurt at the front door with the night watchman for the neighborhood. This fellow walks back and forth among the apartment buildings all night, smashing a huge staff down on the sidewalk every few yards, which I guess is supposed to deter thieves and also assure the residents that he hasn't fallen asleep. After a few weeks you get used to the noise and it doesn't wake you up every half hour as he passes by your door. Kumar's wife Meena is watching the news on the TV, but listening to us with half an ear.

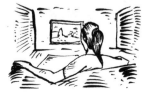

"I mean," I start, "it's really like The Pen Thing…everything is. Some people would find habitual patterns in a marriage to be a very comforting thing: predictable and grounding."

"But we don't!" yells Meena over her shoulder.

"Well that's what I mean. It's not that the patterns in themselves are boring…it's just that the two of you find them boring."

"So are you saying we should find a way to *like* all this repetition?" spouts Kumar.

"No, not at all. I'm just pointing out that the boredom is definitely coming from you. If it were coming from the habitual patterns, then everyone would find them boring. But since some people find them comforting, then how the patterns seem is something that's coming from each person's own mind, individually. And if it's coming from you, then it's something you can easily change.

"And so it's a good thing that everyone sees these patterns differently; if they didn't, then they'd be unchangeable."

"So how *do* we change them?" asks Meena, a little more softly. She's mostly with us now; or it might just be that an endless Indian commercial has just come on.

"Well, anything that the two of you are experiencing together—in this case, a frustration with habitual patterns which have developed in your marriage—ultimately traces back to something similar that together you have done to other people. And there are still seeds in you for that kind of behavior. So we just need to identify that behavior and let it go."

Kumar nods. "Understood. So what do you think we're doing to other people, that makes us go through these same patterns in our day, over and over?"

"Well, let me ask you. What time do the two of you go to bed?" I know that for Indians this can be quite late, because they value a home-cooked dinner made with super-fresh ingredients—which means that you don't get started on cooking until you get home from a slow walk around the nearest farmer's market after work.

"Well, we always go to bed at exactly 11:30," says Meena, and then blushes a bit. "And I guess that's really habitual as well. But anyway, right after the last nighttime news."

"And what time do your neighbors go to bed?"

"Aruna and Ajit? Different times I think, but mostly earlier. Aruna and I text each other sometimes during the day, and I can't recall her ever sending me one after about 10 at night."

"And on what side is their apartment?"

Meena points over the TV. "To that side, towards the street."

The TV is right up against the wall, and I can just imagine what it sounds like on the other side. "So...do you think they can ever hear your TV? I mean, late at night?"

Meena cocks her head. "Well, I suppose...I suppose they can. You know, I never really thought about it."

"So basically they can't go to sleep until you go to sleep."

"Well, perhaps not."

"And if not, then you're imposing your schedule on them, right?"

"I guess so," admits Kumar.

"So this gets into a whole issue, one which is escalating in the modern world. You see, everybody has their own life-rhythm: everyone likes to do certain things at certain times of the day, and it's different for each of us. You might like to go to bed at a certain time, and it might be different for your friends. Same with the time that you like to eat; or watch your favorite TV show; or wake up in the morning.

"And nowadays we all have more contact, you see. We're texting or emailing other people all day, according to our own schedule—and most often we're just not thinking about whether it fits in with their schedule or not.

"Your favorite time to text your sister might be the time that she prefers being quiet and focusing on cooking dinner for her family. The hour that you usually wake up might be the only hour that your friend really gets some good, deep sleep in the day. And so very often in this era of super-connectivity, we're interrupting other people's plans for their day, all day: we're imposing our habitual schedule, and our habitual interests, upon them."

Meena's eyes light up. "I get it. In a way then I'm sticking other people in a rut, in an habitual pattern, if I text them on my schedule, without any consideration for how it fits into their schedule."

But Kumar's not sold yet. "So really what you're saying is that we need to be more considerate of other people's preferred schedules for doing things. That gives them their own options for how their day flows, without demanding that they follow our schedule. And then just naturally the flow of our own days becomes more creative, because we've allowed them to be more creative."

"Right."

"But there's a problem there," he continues. "You're saying that we have to respect the schedules of our friends and family; but that means that we'll have to *learn* and *remember* every other person's preferred meal times, bedtime, and so on and so on."

I nod. "But that's exactly what consideration is all about: thinking of others' needs, which means first learning what their needs are. Consideration of others' needs—says Master Vasubandhu in that same ancient book—is really the root of every good seed you can ever create. The more effort you put into being sensitive to others' daily flows—starting with learning their own daily schedules—then the sweeter your own life will flow. It's one way to break out of those deadly boring cycles that begin to bog down every relationship.

"And again, understand that—as the ruts disappear—it will be organic and natural: effortless. As seeds ripen from being considerate not to impose your patterns on others, then those rigid patterns will automatically drop away. Perhaps you won't even notice it. But one thing's for sure—your own relationship will become fresh and spontaneous."

Meena shuts off the TV and walks over and puts her arm around Kumar's shoulders. "Fun!" she chirps. As usual, just talking about the right way to make a change in a marriage already seems to be changing it.

BREAKUPS

Question 84

I've had a lot of trouble getting over my last close relationship, which ended painfully. What seeds can I plant to help me let this go?

"Well, I can think of two things you can do," I reply. I'm sitting in a conference room at a nice hotel in Jakarta, the capital of Indonesia. The place has been set up to film an hour-long segment on Diamond Cutter business strategies for a popular local TV program. Some of the audience has already come in, and I'm sur-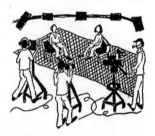rounded by an exotic mixture of Indonesian Muslims and Buddhists; French businessmen; and awesome Sindhi entrepreneurs.

Setiawan is slumped over with his head in his hands, so miserable that he doesn't care if there are a dozen people listening. "Okay then," he sighs. "What's the first?"

"I mean obviously you can go at it with the Four Starbuck Steps." We had discussed those on the plane the day before, during a visit to the exotic Buddhist carvings of Borobudur; but I know it's new to him, so it's better to spell it out.

"Step One: Briefly put, what is it that you want?"

"I want to be able to let my old relationship go: let go of all the hurt, the constant thinking about what happened; let go of Lia, and move on with my life."

"And Step Two?"

Setiawan thinks for a moment. "Well, I guess I'd have to find someone with a similar challenge, and help them get through it." He smiles wryly. "Not too hard to do that; it seems like half my friends have the very same problem."

"Breakup blues do seem to be universal," I agree. "It's so hard to let go of the pain and memories of a failed relationship. Okay. So remember, Step

Two has two parts: Choose, then Plan. Choose a person who has a similar need, and then Plan how you're going to help them. Now what about Step Three?"

"Oh, that's easy to remember. The coffee shop thing. Take them out to a neutral place, share suggestions with them about how to move on from the pain they're in."

"Right," I nod. "And very importantly, remember to mix it all with compassion, a universal compassion. A feeling that—if you test the Diamond Cutter Principles on yourself first, and they work—then you will become a living example for everyone else who has this problem, of moving on from a painful breakup. You could brighten up the lives of hundreds of people, in a big chain reaction, just by succeeding yourself. Step Four?"

"Coffee Meditation: As I close my eyes and fall off to sleep at night, I review the details of all the efforts I've made to help someone else work out the same problem. This is the heavy-duty fertilizer which makes my seeds open fast."

"Well," I say, "you seem to have all that down pat. I don't see where it's going to be any big problem for you to get over this thing really quickly, and move on. But *where* you move on to is also something we have to work on."

"Well I can certainly see that. I do want to find a new relationship, but I certainly don't want it to be the same as the disaster that I just went through with Lia."

"And that gets us into the second suggestion that I wanted to offer. Let me ask you: Do you ever feel like there's some grand plan behind all of this, behind your whole life? Something you can't see, but something that's been there since the day you were born?"

Setiawan nods. The Sindhi and French businesspeople are all clustered around in a knot now, as the sound and camera crews bustle with last-minute adjustments.

"I've always had that feeling," he says. "As if there's some special being near me, my entire life, invisible but certainly there. Like they're trying to direct me, towards something important, something that has to do with the meaning of my whole life."

"Right. I mean, to put it in terms of seeds, the ancient books say that it takes millions upon millions of very good and powerful seeds just to see ourselves walking around in a human body. I mean, there are thousands of different components and systems that make up our body, working together in some kind of impossible harmony.

"According to Tibetan thinking, we must have been *very, very* good people in our last life, just to be blessed with a working body and mind like those that we have now. And according to the same thinking, it's very unlikely that we could have been that good on our own. We must have been under the guidance of a dear and devoted teacher.

"The idea then is that we created a habit—that would be the Second Flower, by the way—of seeing a close teacher, of being in their personal care. So a Buddhist would believe that almost everybody who gets to be a human on this entire planet has seeds to be in the close care of a special, personal teacher. And those seeds might go off in your life as someone invisibly guiding you through each day of that life, and even taking on different roles in your life to do so."

"Sounds like sort of an invisible guardian angel," smiles Setiawan. "We have a very similar idea in the Muslim tradition, here in our country. As you go through your five daily prayers facing Mecca, there's a custom to turn your head both 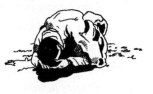 left and right, and whisper something to your guardian angel."

Whisper sometimes to your Guardian Angel

"Exactly the same thing. And if you possess the seeds to have that angel in your life, then they're also going to show themselves, anonymously, as different people around you. Naturally they would choose to appear to you as someone very close to you—someone whose words and actions provide you direction, day by day. And so it's very possible that your guardian angel would choose to appear as your partner."

Setiawan looks confused. "As my partner? You're telling me that Lia was my guardian angel? Then why did she dump me?"

"Ah, now that's the question. Let's say, just hypothetically, that she *was* your guardian angel, in disguise. If that's true, then why would she let you go?"

Setiawan frowns hard—the pain is still so fresh—as he thinks it out.

"Well, if she was some kind of guardian angel, then everything she ever did when she was with me must have had some big purpose—it must have been part of some Grand Plan for my life."

"Even breaking up with you?"

"Well, I suppose so." He pauses and considers for a moment more. "Well, then that would mean that she had some kind of plan for me all along, and that the breakup was part of the plan too. And if that's the case, then it must be that she was…like…sending me somewhere. She saw something up ahead, in the future, and she was sending me on to it."

"Like, maybe, another partner? The next person that your guardian angel will appear to you as, in order to guide you through the next chapter of your life?"

"Well, I guess so," says Setiawan.

"So let's get going," I say, as the cameras roll and the announcer for the TV show starts introducing me. "Stop moping around. The angel has released you so that you can meet the next version of the angel, who will accompany you on the next part of your life's journey. You just have to go find her!"

"You mean *plant* her," Setiawan corrects me.

Question 85

My husband and I have been married for ten years, and it has always been okay. But now I've met somebody who I feel is my real soulmate. What should I do?

"Well, what kind of commitment did you make to each other, in the beginning?" I ask. I'm sitting on the balcony of a really nice house on the edge of the beach in Punte del Este, in southeast Uruguay. Over a hundred thousand of the rich & famous of South America flock here in the summer, and about 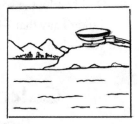 60 of them have been invited to dinner and a business talk.

My assistants and I are feeling distinctly out of place, especially during the photo shoot on the beach by the local fashion magazine; but the event has turned out to be wonderful and warm. It's way past midnight and everyone is still clustered around in little groups, talking intensely about the Diamond Cutter. One of the guests has cornered me over near the reflecting pool, which another over-jolly guest fell into earlier in the evening.

Lucia frowns a bit. "Well, you know, the normal Catholic marriage in Latin America. Ignacio and I made a commitment for life."

"And how does he view this commitment? I mean, how does he see it, now?"

"Well, I mean, we're not madly happy, but we're okay...just okay. I'd say that he still considers it a commitment for life."

"And so if you go for this person you've found...if you go for the soulmate now...then you'd be breaking a lifetime commitment that you made of your own free accord."

"Well yes," Lucia says softly. "I know that. And I'm not happy about it."

"So from what we said at the talk in the living room tonight...what kind of seed would you be planting? I mean, for your new relationship, with your new soulmate."

"I understand," she says. "I understand what you're saying. If I break a very serious commitment to my old partner so that I can be with my new partner—even if he's my soulmate—then it's not just going to hurt Ignacio and the children. It will plant a seed and, according to the First Flower, my soul mate will also leave me, when that seed opens."

"Exactly," I agree, and I'm proud of this person I never met before, that she sees it so clearly after only an hour of Diamond Cutter. I'm constantly surprised this way, that the Diamond Cutter Principles seem so immediately logical to people all around the world, in very different countries with very different cultures. For me it's another confirmation of the universal truth of these principles.

"So I just let the soulmate go?" Lucia is almost crying.

"I didn't say that," I reply. "If you think you need to let the soulmate go, then you didn't understand what I was saying in the talk tonight."

Cakes are made to be both had & eaten

"Well if I don't leave Ignacio, I can't see how I'm going to be with my soulmate," she says, truly believing the logic of what she says. And this particular logic is so completely illogical, and the cause of so much pain and frustration in the world. I mean, what if things weren't like that at all?

"That would be true," I say, "if this situation existed out there, from its own side." I dig a pen out of my pocket—I almost always have one there, just for this purpose—and wave it in front of Lucia. "But in truth the situation is coming from you, from the seeds in your mind. That's especially true of the apparent contradiction between the two things: the perception that you must either stay with Ignacio, or go with your soulmate."

"What are you saying?" says Lucia. "Are you suggesting that I try to set it up so that I can live with both of them at the same time?" She looks strangely outraged at the suggestion.

"No no, I'm not saying that at all. I'm not saying that you should be with both of them; and I'm also not saying that you should be only with one or the other.

"What I am saying is that the apparent dilemma is coming from you, from your seeds. And since it's coming from your seeds, it's something you can change. Just change the seeds, and you can have everything you want, with-out hurting anyone, and without having to choose one or the other."

"So…what will that look like, exactly?" she says, a bit confused.

"What did it look like to stay with Ignacio all these years? And what do you have in mind with your soulmate? I mean, it will look…real. It will be your life."

"No, you don't understand," Lucia persists. "You say that there could be a situation where I have everything I want, and everyone else has everything they want to. I just want to know exactly how that could be."

"No," I persist back. "You don't understand. The point is that you don't have the seeds now even to imagine how it could work out, because you're not even close to having enough seeds for it to work out. When you do have enough seeds, you *will* be able to imagine how it could work out between everyone; and that comes just before it *does* work out.

Don't get stuck trying to figure out how it will be

"Don't get stuck trying to imagine how it could be. You don't have enough seeds for that. Just plant the seeds, and it will come: it has to come. Call it a miracle—call it the impossible coming to give all three of you what your heart desires. But actually it's no more of a miracle than your life is right now. It will be just…the way it is, no more and no less. You will have your soulmate, and you will honor your commitment to Ignacio, all at the same time, as impossibly as you sit on this balcony right now."

There's a long moment of silence, and then Lucia sighs. "Okay; I have a feeling you know what you're talking about, I just feel that's true. But I don't 100% understand how it's going to happen. Anyway, let's say I trust you enough to try to plant the seed that will make it happen; I mean, from what I've heard you say so far, it seems like this seed planting thing always involves helping or serving someone else. And so it can't hurt anything to try; the worst thing that can happen is that I make someone else happy. Tell me what kind of seed I need to plant."

"Well, let's do the Four Starbucks Steps, real fast," I say.

"Okay," says Lucia. "Step One, say what I want: I want a resolution to an apparently impossible situation—a resolution that makes everybody happy, at the same time. Step Two: I choose someone else who's in a situation which they perceive as impossible, and plan how I'm going to give them some advice and support.

"Step Three: I take them out to a coffee shop—or some other neutral space—and just give them the best advice I can, even if it's not perfect, and even if it doesn't solve their problem completely; regardless, the seed will grow. And then, Step Four, I do Coffee Meditation on how nice it was to complete the second and third steps." I nod my approval.

"And you're telling me that's all I have to do? To see a miracle happen?" she asks.

I nod again. "It's no more of a miracle than sitting here right now. Because it will happen, just as this is happening. Both are coming from your mind, from the seeds in your mind. And that means they are real, they both happen. You will have your soul mate, and you will keep your old commitment.

"Nothing is impossible, with seeds. Just try it and see."

PEACE

Question 86

Once in a while, almost by accident, my boyfriend and I fall into a quiet space or moment together that nearly feels like prayer, or meditation. Is there some karma we can do that would make these spontaneous moments happen more often?

We're doing a weekend DCI "success retreat" in a place called Tepoztlan, which is about an hour south of Mexico City. It's an ancient seat of the Toltec people, and the feathered serpent-god, Quetzalcoatl, is said to have been born here. There's an awe-inspiring pyramid perched high on the mountain that looms high over the small retreat center where we're

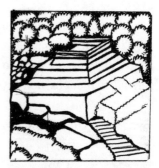

staying. Valeria is asking the question; she and Pablo are leaning back against a tree, looking almost as though they are having one of those moments right now.

"Let me ask you something," I reply. "Is there anything *else* you guys want in your life right now?"

Pablo looks a little surprised by the question. "I don't know," he shrugs, and looks over at Valeria. "I suppose a little more money would be nice; I mean, we don't need much, and we don't actually want much, but struggling for the rent money every month is just stressful."

"Good," I say. "So have you been using the Four Steps on it?"

"Not really," admits Valeria. "I mean, it causes us stress almost all the time, but I guess we've just been lazy about taking care of it—it's just become a regular part of our life."

"Okay," I say. "Well I can see a way here that you can take care of two problems at the same time: you can solve the monthly rent-money anxiety, and plant the seeds for those spontaneous moments of deep peace with your partner."

"How's that?" asks Pablo.

"Well, tell me something. In the old days, before you heard about the Diamond Cutter, how would you deal with a money problem such as coming up with the rent every month?"

Valeria smiles. "We went and scrounged around for money," she says. "Just like everybody else: like cavemen wandering around the forest, hoping to come across some wild berries. Maybe we tried to find something in the house that we really never used, and could sell; or we went and bugged Pablo's mom for some help; or I begged my boss at work for some overtime."

"And now?"

Pablo nods. "And now; well, we know how things really work. And so we understand that we need to plant the seeds for seeing more money in our lives."

"And how do you plant those seeds?"

"I mean, we may have been too lazy to get on it, but we know how to plant the seeds: we need to find maybe another couple who's having some financial challenges, and give them some support on getting out of their hole."

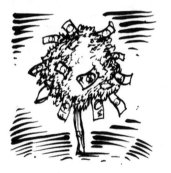

"That's right. Instead of making money the old way, you really *make* money: you create it, you plant it. And you do that by helping someone else make money. And that brings them unexpected relief, comfort."

Valeria's eyes light up. "Oh! I get it! What you're saying is that those 'spontaneous' moments of magic in our relationship aren't really spontaneous at all: we can create them quite consciously. As a couple, we just keep trying to set up moments of comfort or relief for other couples."

Pablo gets excited too. "And what you're saying is that those moments are just the natural result of applying the Four Starbucks Steps to get something that the two of us need anyway. *Just doing the right thing* to get something we already want *always* brings moments of comfort to others; and then we get back both the thing that we ourselves needed, and also those spontaneous moments of deep happiness together."

Valeria nods happily. "We'll have more and more of those magical moments together just by using the Diamond Cutter Principles whenever we can, for whatever we want."

"So get on it," I grump. "There's no reason to be stressing out over the rent money. And you could be having magical moments…"

"…All the time!" smiles Pablo, gazing into Valeria's eyes. It's working already.

"One more suggestion," I say.

"What's that?" says Pablo.

"If it were me, I'd crank up the seed planting here. I mean, in some countries that we visit, people have created little Four Steps Clubs. They get together once a week and help each other track their progress on using the Four Steps for some goal that they have in their life. The people who organize any particular club then are not only planting their own seeds, but they're facilitating other people planting *their* seeds."

Valeria nods. "And I'd guess that there are big buckets of extra seeds being planted when you help a whole group of people plant their seeds."

"You got it," I nod. "So that would be a great way to plant lots more magic moments than you two could ever do just working on your own."

I realize I'm having my own magical moment, right there. I realize how much I crave those moments too, and promise myself to help get more people started on planting.

Question 87

There are two other executives at work that my husband is competing with for promotions and so on—it seems like half our time together is spent with me listening to why these two guys are bad people. I've met them both a couple of times, and they seem pretty nice to me. How do I stop this karma of having to listen to my husband talk bad about someone all the time?

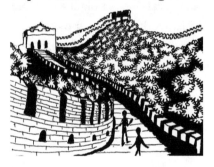

Guangmin asked me this question as we stood on top the Great Wall near Tianjian, China, which is not far from Beijing. Her husband Baochang waves from the balcony of a turret perched above the wall just up ahead; I'm sort of glad to have an excuse not to try climbing up the incredibly steep steps to that one. We lean over a battlement and take in the cliffs and greenery of some of the most dangerous-looking mountains I've ever seen. How they pulled hundreds of thousands of huge stone blocks up these ridges 15 centuries ago boggles the imagination.

"I'll give you sort of a mystical answer," I reply. "Is that okay?"

Guangmin nods. "As long as I can apply it to real life."

"I totally agree with that. So you know about the Dao, right?" I use the traditional Chinese pronunciation, for what a lot of westerners refer to as Tao; we talked about it back in Question 58.

"I know about the *Dao De Jing*," she replies—the text that foreigners have also called the *Tao Te Ching*. "That's the most famous book about the Dao. We had to learn some of it in high school here in China. *Dao* means *the way*, and *de* means *virtue*. *Jing* means *an ancient book*."

"And what is the Dao? What is the Way?"

Guangmin thinks on that for a moment, and then a light goes off in her head. "Well, I never really thought about it this way, but I suppose if you consider it from the point of view of the Diamond Cutter system, you can just say that virtue *is* the Way."

"How so?"

"I mean, it's the way to live your life, the way to make things happen in your life that you want to happen. If someone wants to find a boyfriend, for example, then they have to plant the seed for him, by helping a lonely person. And that's a virtue: a goodness."

"Good. Now people often talk about 'flowing with the Dao.' How would that fit in?"

Guangmin thinks for a moment more, and then snaps her fingers. "I think I get it. There's a wrong way to make things happen in your life—which is 'wrong' only because *it doesn't work*—and there's a right way.

"I mean, in the example of trying to find a boyfriend, you could exhaust yourself searching around the internet; or you could try to endure a week of nightclubs filled with cigarette smoke. That would be the wrong way. Or rather, it would not be the Way: the Dao."

"And what would be the Way? What would be the *right* way?"

"That would be keeping the older person company: planting seeds to have a boyfriend just walk right into your life. And as far as the 'flow' thing, if you tried *this* way to get a boyfriend, you'd be *flowing* with the Dao. You'd be going with the grain of things—with the grain of the entire universe, really—instead of going against it, in a nightclub or on the internet."

Being good to others is a lot more relaxing

"Exactly. And when you're moving with the natural flow of the universe—making things happen by being good or virtuous to others—then life is just a whole lot more relaxing and enjoyable. A lot easier too, and a constant joy. Going against the flow of the Dao is simply exhausting, in part because of the terrible uncertainty involved with trying to get things the wrong way. You *might* find a partner on the internet, or you *might not*. But with seeds, you always know what you're going to get.

"Now how does all this apply to getting Baochang to say nicer things about people, day to day?"

Guangmin's on it. "Considering what you just said, I think I can see how all of this relates to the Dao. If I think about this situation with Baochang—about how he's always criticizing the other two managers at his office—then I get upset, and tired of it. And I guess what you're trying to tell me is that when I *do* get upset or tired of this situation, then that's a pretty definite sign that I'm dealing with it the wrong way: that I'm not flowing with the Dao. Because if I were flowing with the Dao to find a solution, then it could only make me feel light and joyful."

"Right again. Trying to talk Baochang into saying nice things about others is uncertain to have the result you want, and that's going to upset you. But maintaining an unhappy silence with him is just as bad. You can feel how both options work against the grain of the Dao.

"So how would you flow with the Dao instead? Especially if *dao* means *virtue,* or *good deeds?*"

Guangmin nods knowingly. "I would have to plant some good seeds to see Baochang speak more positively. Which means I myself would have to do some virtuous deeds, good deeds. I'd have to work hard—say at work, or with our daughter—to speak more positively about other people." She pauses for a moment.

"I can already think of a real example. I have a women's group that meets together for tai chi exercises three times a week in the park, and usually my daughter Mei comes with us. Afterwards we often stand around under the trees and talk about things that are happening in 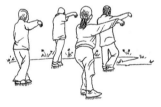 our lives, and I suppose sometimes we do say some mean things about some of the other ladies we know. And Mei is there; I guess she hears all of it, and it probably disturbs her as much Baochang's grousing disturbs me.

"Dealing with Baochang's complaining by cutting down on my own complaining would be flowing with the Dao," Guangmin says decisively. "It's just a very comforting and pleasant way to deal with the problem."

Baochang is crawling his way down the last of the steep steps of the turret, and as always when we begin flowing with the Dao, his face already has a pleasant smile on it.

Question 88

We have a really good relationship, except for one thing. My partner is just really noisy! Whether I'm taking a nap or reading a book or listening to music, there's this constant barrage of slamming doors, clanging dishes, and chair legs screeching across the floor. What's the karma for her to be a little more sensitive to the beauty of quietness?

I'm staying at the home of David and Janet, two old friends and students of mine, in Houston, Texas, where I'm taking a few days of music lessons from a well-known singer who hails from Varanasi, in the east of India. I'm sort of following David around the house, from room to room, while we talk. So far he's checked the email on the computer in his office for messages from his job; walked outside to pick up the daily paper, scanned it for a few minutes and thrown it on the kitchen counter; run through some music on his iPod; and grabbed a handful of grapes out of the fridge.

And now I grab his arm and pull him down on a chair at the kitchen table.

"You know about seeds, right?" I ask.

"Sure," he says. "You covered them in a lot of detail, when you visited last year and gave the talk at the church."

"Okay. So I have a question for you. If you want to plant a seed, for anything—a partner, a credit card that's all paid off, a bad back that doesn't hurt any more—do you need another person?"

"Well sure, that's what you always say."

"But what do you think? Can you ever plant a seed with *yourself?* Just yourself alone?"

David thinks on that one for a moment. "I don't really know. I mean, seeds are good or bad according to whether you hurt somebody or help somebody. And somehow it seems important that it's somebody *else*. I mean, I'm not quite clear on exactly why it's the case, but my gut feeling is that karma is like an echo: that you have to bounce it off somebody else, to have it come back to you."

"I think you're right," I agree. "And it's something I've thought about for a long time. Why is it that you need someone else to bounce your karma off of?"

We sit in silence for a moment, which I can see is already difficult for David. His eyes have settled down on the remote control for the TV, and I'm afraid I'm going to lose him again.

"I mean," I say, "what is it that makes someone else someone else, in the first place?"

"Well, I'm me and you're you," he answers simply.

"Yeah, but *why?*"

"Well, we're separate," he says.

"What makes us separate?" David pops another grape into his mouth and chews and looks over at the TV even as he's talking to me.

"Well, like, when I bite down on this grape, you don't taste it. Only I do. That proves we're separate. So maybe the only way to plant a seed is when you're doing it for somebody else, and not just for yourself. Like, somehow it has to be unselfish."

I frown. Somehow I always get stuck around here.

"But in the end, everything you ever do to help other people *does* help yourself, because it always comes back to you. And that kind of means that other people aren't really separate from yourself.

"I mean, the only way to get the things you want is to help someone else get what they want. In that case, you're both getting what you want, by doing one thing."

David stops chewing. He's actually focusing now. "Well that would kind of indicate that the two of you are, like, somehow a single person—but just in two bodies. I mean, if it helps me whenever I help you."

He thinks some more. "Huh. Well then maybe it's the other way around. Maybe the reason that karma works at all is that somehow the other person is always me. But in that case, I should also be able to do something just to myself, and plant a seed too. What do the old Tibetan books say about that?" he asks.

"Well it's not all that clear," I admit. "Except I can think of one example. When they talk about really serious bad karma, they do mention suicide. They see the human body as something precious beyond words: as a vehicle that we can ride to reach all our dreams, and the dreams of every other person there is. So they say that the wish to destroy this vehicle purposely is one of the worst seeds you can ever plant. And you plant it just with yourself."

"Huh," he says, and goes back to chewing. He's not even aware of it, but his hand is already fiddling with the remote control for the TV.

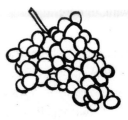

"Well, I was thinking that this might apply to your problem with Janet," I suggest.

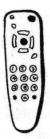

He stops chewing again. "You mean the noise thing?"

"Right."

David shakes his head. "I don't know. I mean, this problem isn't something new. She's been making rackets around her, all the time, ever since we were in high school."

I shake my head too. "When you work on things with the Diamond Cutter Principles, it doesn't matter at all how old the problem is. When you go at something through the seeds, you are working at the real causes, for the first time ever. And then the thing will change."

"So, what? I'm committing some kind of noise suicide? I'm doing something to myself, that makes her pull the same kitchen chair slowly across the floor every morning, screeching like somebody pulling their nails across a chalkboard?"

"I think so. I think this might be one of those cases where—yes—you're planting the seed with yourself, rather than with somebody else."

"How so?"

"I mean, what is it that irritates you the most about what she's doing?"

"It's the noise."

"So what you want is some quiet out of her. You want her to go through a single hour of the day without banging or clanging or slamming something."

"You got it."

"But you don't even do that with *yourself,* you see. You can't sit still, even for a minute. I mean, I've been running around after you all morning, trying to get you quiet enough to talk about this problem with Janet. Maybe being noisy with *yourself* is what plants the seeds for Janet to be noisy all day!"

"So...how do I fix that?" he says.

"Stand up," I answer. "Stand up right now."

David stands.

"Walk over to the fridge," I say. "Close the door to the fridge."

He starts to walk towards the fridge.

"Wait," I say. "Stop chewing. I mean, finish chewing the grape first, then walk to the fridge."

David rolls his eyes and stands still and chews and swallows. The he steps towards the fridge.

"Wait," I say again. "Put down the remote control. You don't need the remote control to walk to the fridge."

David sets it down and shuffles over to the fridge; but his eyes wander off to the newspaper that he left on the kitchen counter. He's moving towards the fridge, but his eyes are trying to read the headlines.

"Wait," I say one more time. "You're walking from the kitchen table to the kitchen fridge. Look at the fridge and focus on the fridge and walk to the fridge. Walk with focus, let your mind be quiet just from here to the fridge. Feel how it feels to walk to the fridge, and close the fridge door, without the mental noise of thinking about three other things on the way."

David focuses on the fridge door and walks towards it with quiet purpose. It's almost like a dance, and I swear that for a moment he looks as graceful as a ballerina. He takes the refrigerator handle in his hand, purposefully; and closes the door, purposefully; and then walks purposefully back to the kitchen table.

"Hey, that felt pretty cool," he says.

"What's cool is that you just made Janet a little more quiet," I smile.

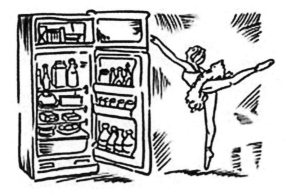

Question 89

What's the karma to have more of those special quiet, peaceful moments in each other's arms?

This question came on a trip to the annual Muslim music festival in Fez, one of the oldest cities in Morocco. Groups come from all over the Islamic world to play, and we are here because we might be invited for next year's festival, to represent Buddhist musicians. We've been out watching amazing performances by groups from Iraq to 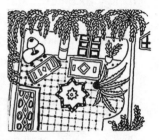 West Africa, and now we're sitting with friends in a *riad,* or open courtyard in the middle of a sprawling townhouse in the old walled quarter. Across the table, Mustapha and Meryem are smiling at each other shyly.

"You know now about the Four Starbucks Steps," I begin, as so often I do.

"Well yes," says Mustapha, "except that here in Fez it is more likely to be a coffee shop serving Moroccan whiskey."

"Whiskey?" I exclaim. "I thought that Muslims were prohibited from drinking alcohol! And you told me that even young Moroccans enjoy keeping the old customs!"

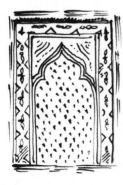 Meryem reaches out for the teapot and pours me another tiny cup of the super-sweet mint tea that most Moroccans drink all day long. "Not to worry—it's just a joke. This is our version of whiskey."

Mustapha laughs and slaps me on the shoulder. Just this afternoon I was asking about the prayers they were doing, and afterwards he came to my room and *gave* me his precious prayer rug—the one he carries around with him every day. And so somehow now we have bonded like family.

"Well, okay. Then tell me what Step Four is."

"Step Four is Coffee Meditation: the one that you do at the end of the day, as you lay down to sleep. You just think about all the good things you've done that day, planting the seeds for something you want to happen. You try to feel happy about the good seeds you've planted, and that makes them stronger, even while you're sleeping."

"Right. But suppose that what you want to happen has *already* happened. Like the moments that the two of you have spent quietly, each in the arms of the other."

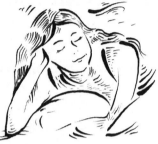

Meryem gives a bit of a puzzled look. "To tell you the truth, we've talked about it, and neither one of us can remember anything in particular that we ever did to plant the seeds for these moments in each other's arms. And anyway, by the time you've had a hug, the seed for that particular hug has already disappeared—like the seed for a tree after the tree has grown. What's the use of doing Coffee Meditation on a seed that you can't remember; and which is gone already anyway?"

I nod. It's a great question. "Let me ask you another question first. You may not remember the original incident that planted one of those gentle hugs from Mustapha, but is there any way to figure out what it probably was?"

"Well yes," says Meryem. "The First Law of Karma says that it must have been something similar to a hug: I mean, something loving and sincere. And the Second Law says that it was smaller than the hug, and then grew up into a hug."

"Okay. So what's smaller than a hug but just as loving?"

Meryem gives that loving look to Mustapha one more time, and we can all see the answer.

"Right. It must have been some small gesture of love—perhaps an affectionate glance at your mother after she put something on your dinner plate, something she'd spent all afternoon cooking.

"So here's a question: Can you lie down at night and figure out roughly what you must have done to create these gentle hugs from Mustapha, and then be happy about a seed that you *must* have planted, even if you don't remember exactly what you did?"

Mustapha nods. "I think you could lay down and take joy in something that you must have done, even if you don't know exactly what it was. I mean, you can just think to yourself that—whatever it was that you did—it must have been something kind, and loving. You could even write a little story about it in your mind, and be happy for it."

"But would that do what Step Four is supposed to do? I mean, would it enhance the power of the seed—make it strong enough to ripen faster?"

Meryem shakes her head. "No, of course not. The seeds that created those hugs are already gone by then. There aren't any seeds left to enhance, or speed up."

But then Mustapha looks at her with even more love. "That's true, beautiful, but I have to think that feeling joy about a seed that you planted before—even if that seed has already been used up—would just by itself create some new seeds of the very same kind. Am I right, Michael?"

"That's exactly the idea," I nod. "We can be happy about things that we *must* have done in the past, just judging from something very sweet that's happening to us now. And even if those seeds are already gone, that Coffee Meditation itself will create more. There's no limit: you can be happy about something you did many years ago; and about a seed that created some beautiful moment in your life which also ended years ago; and still you are planting new seeds, to see that moment be repeated, again and again."

"Never-ending, gentle hugs from my husband," smiles Meryem. "Just by going to sleep thinking about how well I planted the hugs he gave me last year. I like it!"

"I like it too," says Mustapha.

Coffee Meditation has no expiration date

HAPPINESS

Question 90

My marriage with my husband is generally a good one—no special complaints—but even so I sometimes go through long periods when I feel lonely or sad, for no special reason. How can I plant the karmic seeds to feel happy and contented instead?

"This gets into Number Nine," I tell Linda. She and her husband Alvin and I are sitting in the lobby of a beautiful hotel in Zhuhai, a Chinese city on the eastern seaboard not far from Macau. Linda and Alvin, of course, are not their real names: Chinese people who 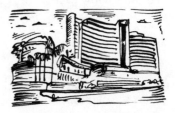 have been studying English will often select an extra, English name, putting a lot of thought into it. As I do so often, I think of how many millions of Chinese people are making a heartfelt effort to learn my language, while almost nobody in my own country shows any interest in learning theirs. It seems to me that we are mostly bogged down wasting our time watching TV and videos instead.

"Number Nine!" exclaims Alvin. "Let's see: Four Laws of Karma; Four Flowers for how these seeds open; Four Steps for speeding them up; and Four Powers for stopping an old bad seed. I don't recall any nines at all."

"No, that's right," I agree. "But this goes back to an idea called the Top Ten."

By the way, this is different from the Top Ten that we talked about back in Question 17. Those were the Top Ten negative seeds: the ones that most of us are planting many times every day. Flip those around, and you get the Top Ten positive seeds.

"These are the ten best things that a person can do to plant seeds. Number Nine is very simple: we just spend time thinking about the good seeds that we see other people planting. You can think of it as a kind of Coffee Meditation, except that instead of being happy about good seeds that we've planted ourselves, we take the time to be happy about other people's good seeds."

"And that's enough to stop those little interludes of sadness that I go through?" asks Linda.

"Exactly," I say. "It's that simple. But it takes some practice. Most of us have trouble just being happy about the good things we're doing ourselves: we have some strange resistance to the whole concept of Coffee Meditation. Being happy about the good seeds we see others planting is even more difficult.

"But think of how satisfying it must be. Rather than noticing what people around us do which is irritating or spiteful to others, we make a special effort—all day long—to pay careful attention to the small kindnesses, the small thoughtful acts, which people offer to each other constantly. When we go to bed, we review each of the ones we've witnessed today, or this week.

"In the beginning, we can't remember a lot of nice things that we've seen others do for each other; but as we continue to practice, these scenes begin to flood our mind as soon as we lay down to sleep. And being *happy* for the happiness that others are planting for themselves is one of the most powerful seeds for witnessing happiness within our own mind.

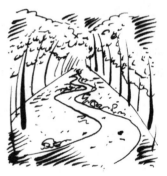

"It is, as the Tibetans call it, 'A happy path to happiness.' And it really works—just try it. Please, just try it."

"I will," says Linda. "I really will."

Question 91

I have this pattern in my life where no matter how wonderful things are going—especially in a relationship—I always start to feel discontented: I'm unable to enjoy the moment, because I'm stuck in thinking about the next thing I want to happen. What seed do I need to plant to find joy in the great things I already have?

This question came on a little motorboat that you have to ride across a bay to get to a popular yoga retreat center near Nassau, in the Bahamas. For years I've been coming here every spring to give small talks about the ancient philosophy of yoga. I understand what Timothy is getting at; here we are, gliding 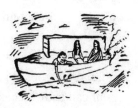 across the bluest ocean water in the world, surrounded by a fragrant ocean breeze punctuated by warm droplets of spray—but all I can think about is how good the dinner's going to be when we get there.

"Well let's go to Step One," I yell over the noise of the engine.

"The essence of what I want," yells back Timothy. Sharon unfortunately is sitting between us, and she ducks her head a bit to avoid the crossfire. "I want to feel content, I want to feel satisfied. I want to be able to enjoy the moment I'm in right now."

I enjoy the sun, and the seagulls following the boat, and think for a moment.

"Look, Tim, you know what a mantra is, right?"

"Some kind of short Sanskrit thing that you say over and over again, counting them on prayer beads," he says.

"Right. So a while back, I was in Asia, speaking to a pretty large audience. One person raised their hand and asked me if there was any mantra I could teach them."

"So which one did you choose?"

"I taught them this one:

Whatever I want,
I will help someone else to get it first.

Whatever I don't want,
I will stop doing it to others first."

"So what's that got to do with being able to enjoy the moment I'm in?"

"You want to learn to enjoy what's right here, right now. So you have to help someone else learn to enjoy the same thing. And that's just very simple. It's learning to be grateful.

"Encourage others to be grateful, and to express that gratitude to the people around them. I mean, it's very common that when we're sitting talking to another person, they might start to complain about things in their life. They don't get paid enough at work; their partner doesn't appreciate them; their bad back is bothering them again today.

"Try to listen, with empathy; and then, if you can, turn the conversation around to the good things that are happening in their life. If it seems like the person can hear it, speak a bit about how it's much more pleasant for them, and for others, if they talk about all the beautiful things that are going on with them—the things they have to be grateful for.

"Your own present state of mind of course isn't something you can decide to have, whether it's good or bad. It will pop up out of the seeds that you've planted, say, the week before. When you encourage others to be grateful, then you plant seeds in your own mind to experience contentment.

"Those seeds will open, and suddenly you'll be able to be here, in the present moment, fully aware and appreciative of the beauty that's happening to you right now."

And again, as so often happens, it seems that just talking about the right way of making things happen starts to work its magic immediately. We all three settle back in a comfortable silence. Timothy's hand drops over the side of the boat, trailing in the warm water of the sea, as if nothing else matters.

Question 92

Sometimes it just seems like relationships never work out—I get tired of trying, and feel like I would rather stay alone, be like a monk or a nun or something. Do you think this will make me happy?

Being a monk, I get this question fairly often. People are having a rough relationship—or they've just ended a rough relationship—and somehow they expect me to confirm for them the "truth," that it really is impossible for any relationship to be successful. They assume that this is the reason why people become monks or nuns, and that somehow people who are running away from relationships are going to find some kind of peace.

"Well," I say to Catherine, "I've known a lot of monks and nuns, and I would say there are two kinds."

"How's that?"

"Well, there's one kind that's been hurt in relationships. Having a partner can obviously be one of
the greatest joys that anyone experiences in their entire life. But we all know that it can also end in the
deepest pain we've ever felt. And so some people
take robes because they've been hurt, and they've
given up on relationships.

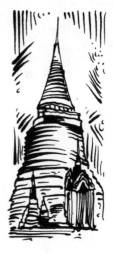

"In my own experience, these people often become incapable of enjoying other kinds of relationships as well: the warmth between good friends; the
camaraderie of people who work at the same job.
They begin to mistrust all forms of closeness.

"But what I've observed is that this often descends into a kind of bitterness about life, rather than the peaceful contentment that we like to imagine
fills the mind of a monk or nun. There do exist monastics who have found
this contentment—they are the second kind I was talking about—but in my
belief it's not *because* they have run away from life.

"Rather, they embrace that life, and they embrace the lives of others. They enjoy close relationships on many levels, because they've learned how to have a successful relationship. That is, they have actually followed the teachings for monks and nuns: teachings which say that we can plant any beautiful thing which our heart desires.

"Reach out to lonely people, wherever they might be, whatever age they might be. Plant the seeds for true companionship. Those seeds might ripen as a lifelong partner in the flesh, or they might ripen as a lifelong partnership with some divine presence—or even as a combination of the two.

"Become a nun if it calls to you, but only because you seek beauty, and not because you are running from your own failure to learn how to plant a seed. All things are possible, with seeds."

GETTING OLD
TOGETHER

Question 93

I'm getting older—I take good care of myself, but I can feel the sags and wrinkles, and I worry that my husband will find me unattractive. Is there any way karmically for me to stay looking young?

This is one of those questions that many people *want* to ask me, but for some reason they seem to hesitate. I think sometimes they're afraid to sound vain, because that wouldn't seem spiritual, and then somehow that would turn me off.

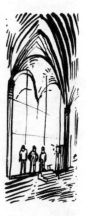

But more often, I'm sorry to say, I think that people believe that aging is inevitable, and that it's hopeless even to ask the question. It's not.

Clara and her husband Felipe and I are out for a late-night walk in Barcelona, where I've just finished delivering an evening business talk. We're standing in front of a bookstore admiring hand-bound editions of Cervantes' *Don Quixote,* an *Hidalgo Ingenioso.* But I can see that Clara isn't looking *through* the large plate-glass window; she's gazing at her own reflection in the glass, with a look of sadness and uncertainty.

I take a pen out of my pocket and wave it in her face.

"Why do you see a pen?"

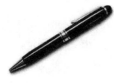

"Not because it *is* a pen," she answers confidently. "I see a pen because there are pen-seeds opening up in my mind. Seeds that I planted in the past, when perhaps I helped someone else communicate something they needed to communicate."

"And so why do you see your hand this way?" I ask, touching her hand. It's crisscrossed with wrinkles, and it's clear that some arthritis is setting in.

"Seeds?" she asks simply.

"Yes and no," I reply. "Was your hand always this way?"

"No, of course not," answers Felipe, with a touch of indignation. "Clara had the most beautiful skin of anyone in the university; and the most delicate hands."

"Why?" I ask simply.

"Well according to what we've said," she answers, "I must have had the seeds to see my hands that way, and to see others see my hands that way too. I was young, I was full of the energy of life."

"And what happened to that energy? Where did the seeds go?"

Life is a debit card

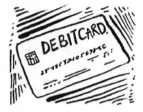

Felipe is ready. "It's what you were talking about tonight. It's as if we start our life with a debit card; and then every hour of our life that goes by, that hour burns up some of the credit left on that card, and finally the seeds are almost all gone. We still have enough seeds to see a hand—

we haven't died yet—but we don't have enough seeds remaining to see that hand be beautiful."

"Is that it then? We start out with a certain number of life-seeds, and we use them up? Can't we get new ones?"

"Well yes, in theory, we could," says Carla. "We know that nothing happens from nothing: and so we must have done something, somewhere, to plant the seeds we've used so far in our life. And if we planted those old ones, we must be able to plant new ones too."

"What kinds of things would we have to do, to plant those kinds of seeds?"

"To *get* life, we would have to *give* life," Felipe says with conviction.

"And what are some ways to *give* life?" I ask. "Give me three ways, each of you."

Carla nods. "Well I guess you could protect life. Help older people get around safely. Be super-careful when you drive. Try not to eat things that have to be killed—the bodies of animals."

Felipe pauses, and then adds: "Refuse to support war; work against it, but *peacefully.* Visit the sick."

He thinks a bit more. "And, I guess…be kind to your own body too. I mean, recognize that you need a body to help others, and be responsible about feeding it in a healthy way; exercising it regularly; and watching your emotions, which seem to have a powerful effect on the aging of the body. I think that taking care of yourself in general is probably a really good karma; but I suspect it's even more powerful if the *reason* you take care of yourself is so that you can help more people, longer."

"Good," I say. "Now I have a few questions more. Do you think that this process could go on indefinitely? I mean—in theory—could you plant enough new seeds for life to keep up with the old seeds wearing out? Could a person stay young forever?"

Carla nods. "In theory, I would say yes. I mean, if it's true that the seeds which you already possess inside of you double in power every 24 hours, then it's obviously *possible* to plant more new life-seeds than you are using up."

"But there's a problem," interjects Felipe. "It may be possible *in theory,* but in actual life we just don't see people walking around who are immortal."

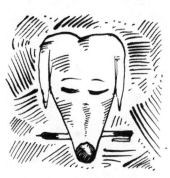

I wave the pen again. "A dog doesn't have the seeds to see it as a pen. Does that mean that pens don't exist?"

"Well maybe not, for dogs."

"But what about for people?"

"For people, pens do exist."

"Then, *in theory,* could it possible that some people *do* see a certain number of immortal people walking around, even while their neighbors *don't* see immortal people walking around?"

"Well yes," agrees Carla; and then she pauses. "Why, I guess you'd have to say that none of us ever sees anyone else in exactly the same way that another person does. I can't really know how either one of you is seeing the same people that I'm looking at."

"Right," I agree. "As my own dear teacher used to say, 'There are *lots* of things you haven't seen, boy!'" Both Carla and Felipe laugh, a laugh with the sound of new hope in it.

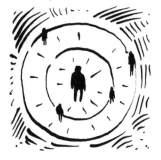

"Last question," I say. "If you *did* manage to collect enough new life-seeds that you *didn't* grow old; and if there were people who had good enough seeds to *see* you not growing old; what would happen then?"

"Well," says Carla, "I imagine that they would ask you how you did it. And then they would copy what you had done, if they could."

"And if *they* planted enough seeds to stay forever young?"

"Then *their* friends would copy *them*. And it would keep spreading."

"In theory," Felipe repeats the phrase, "it would spread almost infinitely."

"Just so," I agree. "And how many seeds would *that* plant?"

"I suppose," says Carla, "that a person who was responsible for triggering a chain reaction that big would plant an almost infinite number of seeds."

"Exactly. If we succeed for example in staying young, because we have learned how to plant the seeds to do so, then other people will copy us. We become a living example for others to follow, and that in itself keeps us living and young.

Question 94

My husband and I are both getting on in years. Can you give us some karmic advice for aging gracefully together, as a couple?

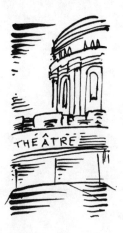

"I don't like the question," I scowl at Irina. She and her husband Maxim have travelled from Krasnodar, an historic city in southern Russia, to attend a talk at a theater in Paris. We're walking back to our hotel together, through the Montmartre section.

"I call it the 'coping question,'" I grumble.

"Meaning what?" asks Irina.

"Meaning don't ask me for advice on how to *cope* with bad situations. Ask me how to *stop* bad situations. And then you don't have to stress over figuring out how to *cope* with them.

"If everything that happens in our life is coming from seeds in our mind, then we can forget about trying to cope with things like getting old with our partner. We just stop it from happening in the first place."

And then I went over Question 93 with them, and that was that. Please stop coping, everybody.

Stop coping

DEATH

Question 95

I love my husband very much; our journey together has been long and sweet. But I have terrible worries about what I would do if he died. What can help with this?

This question came to me on a visit to the town of Princeton, at the home of a dear friend not far from the university. He had taught me as a college student, and was now living in retirement with his wife, also a dear friend. She is asking me the question as he rummages upstairs through a box of books that he wants me to have.

"For me," I reply, "it's a question about the entire course of a human life."

"How so?" replies Ann.

"There is a truth about life: a truth about where life comes from, and what life is for."

"And how do you think about that?"

I shift forward in my seat, and try to find the words.

"Imagine that you are a painter. A friend comes and says that she is organizing an exhibition, to celebrate the colors of autumn. She commissions a series of paintings depicting the forest in fall.

"You work for months and finish your paintings on time. You deliver them to the gallery, and they go up on the walls. Visitors will be walking down a line of three connecting rooms, laid out one after the other, showing the brilliant colors of nature as they progress from emerald to gold to crimson. And in the back room hangs the final painting: the first shoot of spring green emerging from a barren branch.

"Your friend sends out invitations to the exhibition; refreshments are ordered; cars for the guests are confirmed.

"And then the long-awaited night arrives. People file in, one by one, dressed in their evening finery.

"Except that every one of them is blind. Completely blind."

Ann frowns. "What are you saying?"

"I'm saying that this is how almost every person on this planet spends

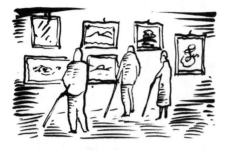

their entire life. They walk from the front door, oblivious, through the colors, on back to the final master-piece: they pass from birth to death, and nothing has happened. They have experienced nothing; they have missed the entire purpose of their time here."

"And how would you describe that purpose?" she asks.

"It is simply to *know,* and to share that knowledge; to help others see the ultimate beauty."

"And then it's alright to die? We learn something that makes us unafraid of death?"

I shake my head slowly. "Imagine another place. An entire world. Imagine that all the people of that world speak the same language.

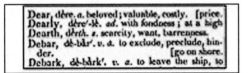

"And in that language, there is no word for death.

"Because the thing that the word is used for simply doesn't exist there.

"If everything is coming from seeds, then death is coming from seeds too. Learn about the seeds, how the seeds work: learn the seeds for life, and teach them to others. *Use* your life, to give life to others.

"And then you not only continue to live, you continue to live a life that has meaning, the highest meaning of all. It's as if all the life you lived before, you were already dead, and now you've woken up. You were blind, and now you see the colors.

"Learn about the seeds, master them, and most importantly, teach them to others. You have a whole new life to look forward to."

Question 96

I lost my wife several years ago; I miss her terribly and still love her. Is there any karma that I could do that would let me talk to her sometimes, to know where she is, and if she is okay?

I first got this question before a talk at a small yoga studio in a suburb of Buenos Aires, quite near the bank of the Rio de la Plata. Since then I have heard it, or some variation of it, in countries all over the world. It is sad how many relationships fail; and it is infinitely sad that—when a relationship doesn't fail—one partner always leaves the other behind, in loneliness. Karl's face told me that something like this was going on, even before he began to speak.

"This gets into miracles," I begin.

"I understand," says Karl. "And that must take a lot more seeds than normal events."

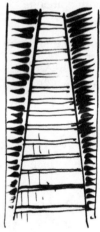

"Yes and no. Look, we're sitting here right now, in the waiting room on the second floor of the yoga studio. In five or ten minutes, somebody's going to come up and tell me they're ready for me downstairs. Tens of thousands of new seeds are going to rise up to the conscious part of my mind and break open; and they're going to create the stairs that I walk down, and the ground floor that I walk across, and all the people that I see on the way.

"That's the same every day, all day, and everywhere I ever go. It will be the same even if I sit here, and no one ever comes and asks me to go start the talk. In that case, tens of thousands of new seeds will open up to sustain these same four walls that we see around us right now.

Karl thinks for a moment, and then nods. "It makes sense," he says. "But how does that relate to my making contact with Ellen?"

"It has to do with the miracle. I mean, it takes the same number of seeds to make a miracle happen for the next five minutes that it takes to make normal life go on for the next five minutes. It's just different seeds. And from that point of view, normal life *is* a miracle."

Karl's face softens. "So it sounds like it *would* be possible to speak to Ellen. I just need to find out what the seeds are, and plant them." He looks to me expectantly.

"It's the same as always; let's go through the Four Starbucks Steps," I say. "What is the essence of what you want, in a single sentence?"

"I want to make contact with my wife, who died three years ago."

"And Step Two?"

Karl thinks for another moment. "That's the hard part, it seems to me. I guess I have to find someone who needs to overcome some extraordinary obstacle to communicating with someone else."

"I think you're right," I agree. "I had a case like this with a woman from Galway, in Ireland; and I think it might help here. She came and told me she'd had a falling out with her mother, and that they hadn't spoken to each other in more than ten years.

"She asked me what seeds to plant, and I asked her to do the Four Steps with someone else who was having a serious problem in their family. And her mother called *her,* out of the blue, the very next day. It really gave even me more belief in the whole Diamond Cutter system."

Karl is quiet, and I can tell his mind is already in Step Two. "Okay," he says. "I've got one. It's really the same situation as the one you just described: a family I know, where one of the daughters decided to come out as a lesbian. She brought her partner home, hoping that things would be better if she were just very open about her feelings, but her parents have refused to see her since that day. Perhaps I start there, work on opening up the lines of communication."

"Any more on Step Two?"

"Well yes, I choose the father; and for our first talk I'll take him out to the Starbucks in the town down the highway from our home."

"Step Three, then."

"That's easy, just actually do it, take him to the Starbucks. Talk to him about his daughter. Keep my heart in the right place: try to help, and understand that my intention to help is planting the seeds, whatever the outcome of the meeting."

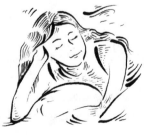

"And the most important step of all?"

Karl nods. "Step Four, the Coffee Meditation. When I lay down to go to sleep at night, work really hard to pull my mind out the usual hopes and fears: push it over to thinking about the dad, sitting in the coffee shop, at least imagining what it would be like to speak to his daughter again.

"But what will it be like?" he asks then. "How will Ellen contact me; how clear will it be; what to expect?"

I smile. "That goes back to the miracle, the miracle of every day that we live our life. We don't know exactly what will happen when we go downstairs, right now. We simply plant the most beautiful seeds we can. And then we can trust, completely, that something even more beautiful will come to us, will become the next part of our life.

"You can spend some quiet hours imagining what it will be like to talk to Ellen—how it will feel, how it will happen. But the reality of it, when the seeds ripen, will be more beautiful than you could ever imagine beforehand.

The Four
Starbucks Steps,

one last time!

1) Say what it is you want in your life, <u>in a single short sentence.</u>

2) <u>Plan</u> who it is you're going to help get the same thing, and which Starbucks you're going to take them to, to talk about it.

3) <u>Actually do something</u> to help them.

4) Do your <u>Coffee Meditation</u>: as you go to sleep, think of the good things you're doing to help them.

HIGHER THINGS

Question 97

Sometimes when I look at the state of the world I feel like all this relationship stuff—and especially the intimacy—isn't really helping anybody, and is just sort of a selfish indulgence. Do you think that I should follow this train of thought, and maybe just become celibate?

We had a similar thought back in Question 92, where a friend was ready to give up relationships forever, because they had gone through so many heartbreaking failures in the past. This though is a different question—The world is for many people a place of great pain: starvation, poverty, and war. Is it irresponsible for us, especially if we are trying to follow a spiritual path, to even spend time discussing relationships—especially intimacy—while others around us are suffering and dying?

A friend from Shanghai, Chuhua, is asking me this question as we walk down the panorama of the Bund, on the Huangpu River, downtown. Her husband Jianmin walks with us, on her other side, holding their baby son Rusong in his arms. I know 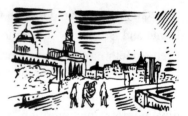 that they care deeply about their family, especially their child, and I also know the depths of their belief in humanity, their overwhelming desire to help make the world a better place for everyone's children. And I know that they will take my answer seriously, even if it means—in essence—giving up the physical side of their relationship.

"Our minds have a certain tendency," I begin, "an habitual way of seeing things. I don't know exactly why, or precisely what the seeds for it are. But I do know that—for all of us—the mind tends to put things into *this* or *that*. Either intimacy is something meaningful, or it's a waste of time.

"And as usual, intimacy is neither *this* or *that*, at least from its own side. It is whatever our seeds make it.

"There is perhaps no more powerful force in the human psyche than the sexual urge. What you're asking then is just this: Is there any way to use this force in the service of humankind, or is it simply something base, like the urge to eat donuts, or to have a drink?"

Chuhua nods. "That's the question; exactly." Jianmin chimes in, "And there's this feeling which we have, both of us, that there may be some good use for this powerful force—that the relationship between the two of us has some higher meaning."

I think for a moment and start working my way. "Obviously the compulsion to mate can be a low thing: we see every day how it can make a fool of people—men and women spending money they don't have to attract someone; hopes that are never fulfilled, as people pine their whole lives for someone who never reciprocates; the tremendous pain which is caused as people become dissatisfied, and break off one relationship to seek another."

We are each quiet for a moment, walking, remembering, agreeing silently about the suffering that love can bring. Rusong is quiet, almost asleep, and Jianmin shifts him to his other shoulder.

Dante had Beatrice

"On the other hand though we hear of epic relationships: Jesus and Mary, Dante and Beatrice—and somehow deep inside we feel that there must have been something important there, even world-saving. We have the same instinct about our own relationship.

"The question then is only: How does it work? How do we turn our intimacy into something high, and not just an indulgence, or even something degrading to the both of us?"

I point vaguely toward the high-rises of downtown Shanghai. "Do you remember the yoga class we did earlier this week? The stuff we talked about, the inner body?"

Jianmin nods. "The main thing I remember is that the whole purpose of yoga is to loosen the knots of the inner body. The movements help us do that: twisting at the chest, for example, helps loosen the knot behind the heart."

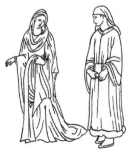

"And what put the knot there in the first place?"

"You said we've had the knots in our body

since before we were born: that they begin forming even in the womb, during the first month of pregnancy."

"And how do they form?"

Chuhua draws three fingers down her forehead. "The knots tie up the three main channels in the body: little straws of light that stretch from the tip of the head down to the groin, between the legs. Inside the channels flows an energy, something like a spiritual electricity—something they call *prana* in India, or *chi* in Chinese. The Tibetans call it *lung,* meaning *the inner winds.*"

"And what is the use of this energy?"

"One of the uses of prana is simply to run the body: when you need to swallow some food, these inner winds gather near the throat and supply the impetus for the muscles to move; when your body eliminates waste, the inner winds gather in a different configuration, and trigger the different muscles which allow that to happen."

"But prana has another crucial function," adds Jianmin. "It acts as a carrier. It is something physical, although extremely subtle, as fine as light. As the inner wind flows, it carries the thoughts upon it, as a horse carries a rider. In fact, this is the place where the body meets the mind: the mysterious interface between the physical—which is all about things which are touch-able—and the mental, which cannot be touched."

"Now connect it to your emotions," I prompt Chuhua. "Somewhere here we have an answer to making a higher force of the physical love between two people."

She nods. "They say that our body, inside, is covered by a network of 72,000 different channels—some bigger, some smaller, all with their own functions. But these main three," she draws the three fingers down her fore-head again, "are by far the most important."

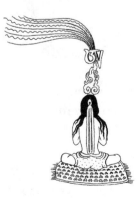

I nod, and Chuhua continues. "When prana, the inner winds, are flowing down the middle channel, we feel happy, and clear. Our creative juices flow; love for others comes easily; prob-lems at work or at home are easily solved."

"And when the middle channel flows," adds Jianmin, "our mind is in a mood to think the highest thoughts of all: to look deep into the very roots of reality and comprehend that it is all coming from us, from the seeds in our own mind—seeds that we have planted by being good or bad to others around us."

I turn to Chuhua. "And what happens when prana flows down the left-hand channel?"

She makes a face. "Problems. Like I'm sitting in a coffee shop, and I've already had a nice pastry, and now I'm not hungry at all, but suddenly I get this unreasonable urge to have a second pastry. I guess you could call it just mindless desire."

Jianmin nods. "And that's what we were talking about with the sex, you see. Is it all just left-channel stuff? I mean—aside from creating beautiful children like our little gem Rusong here—is there really any point to it, any real purpose that can help all other people?"

"It's a beautiful question, an important question," I agree. "Let's get at it through the right-hand channel. What happens when inner wind flows down that side?"

"I get angry, I get upset," says Chuhua.

"And how could that relate to sex?"

"Like Jianmin might have prana flowing down the left, and he feels like being intimate tonight; but maybe I'm exhausted from dealing with Rusong all day," she raises a significant eyebrow at her husband, "and I ask him if we could maybe wait until tomorrow. And then possibly he gets upset, and prana shifts from his left channel to his right."

"Exactly," I agree. "And there's another problem—the thing about the knots. How does that work?"

Jianmin crosses two fingers across his forehead. "There are places in the body where the three channels cross over each other, and create a knot. Let's say I'm sitting at home thinking clearly about how to solve a problem at work—I have prana running down the middle—and then suddenly all I can think about is taking my wife to bed.

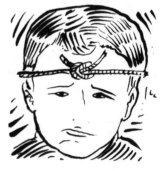

"The inner winds begin running to the left, and the left-hand channel gets fat and full, and it chokes the middle channel where they overlap. And so when my mind's obsessed on sex, I'm actually incapable of thinking straight." He smiles at Chuhua, who gives him a playful smile back, as if to say that's not always so bad.

"But deeper," I urge them. "You said that the knots start even in the womb. Aside from stopping Jianmin from solving his challenges at the office, do the knots cause any other problems?"

Chuhua nods, and now she looks sad. "I heard what you said about that, and I can feel the truth of it, when I look sometimes at Ru. In the first months after conception the body is no more than a tiny tube, less than an inch long. But inside that tube the three major channels are already formed, and prana is already running through them.

"And where the inner winds are running, thoughts are being carried upon these winds. The baby at this point may not be working out math problems, but he does have rudimentary thoughts. 'It's hot in here, uncomfortably hot' is already flowing through the right channel. 'I want to get out of here, away from the suffocating heat' is already flowing through the left channel. And so the middle channel, of reason, and of love, is already being choked off, even in the first weeks of pregnancy. And that choking creates the knots."

"What happens then?"

Jianmin picks it up. "The prana in the middle is blocked, like water pressure building up in a garden hose that has a kink in it. Eventually it reaches a point where the middle channel splits open, and more channels flow out sideways, towards the sides of the body. Soon you have a pattern of smaller channels radiating out from each of the knots, like the spokes of a bicycle wheel."

"Which is why they call that pattern…"

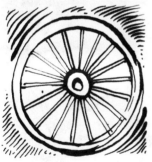

"A *chakra,* which is the ancient Indian word for *wheel.*"

"Oh I've seen pictures of those," I smile. "Pretty little flowers of all different colors, with Sanskrit letters in the middle."

Jianmin shakes his head bitterly. "Not pretty, but death."

"Death? How so?"

"Prana accumulates in the areas where it's choked off, around the knots, around the chakras. In time it congeals into a substance like jelly, and there inside the womb, it causes the formation of the child's body: the flesh and the blood and the bone.

"You can point to the seven main knots—the seven biggest chakras—and trace the formation of the principal structures of the child's skeleton, for example. The pocket of the skull forms around the chakras of the forehead and the tip of the head; the crucial bones of the neck and upper spine form around the chakra behind the throat.

"The chakra at the back of the body behind the heart has the worst knot—

three turns of the three main channels—and from it form all the ribs, and the middle part of the spine. Behind the navel is another knot, and around it accretes the lower part of the backbone. At the very bottom of the spine is another knot, and a final one between the legs, and these create one of the largest bones of the body, the pelvis. The entire skeleton—my son Ru's entire tiny skeleton—formed around his chakras, during his time inside my womb."

"So what's so bad about that?" I ask.

Jianmin says it all. "Think about it. Negative thoughts tie up the channels, even inside the womb. The knots in the channels—the chakras—create our physical body, the body which we then come out of the womb with. And in the moment we leave the womb, we begin to die. Anyone who has a physical body must die; our son Rusong must die, simply because he was born." As he speaks he clutches Rusong ever more tightly, trying to protect him from something which seems inevitable.

"And so you can say," concludes Chuhua, "that it is our desire, and our anger, which make us mortal."

We are quiet for another moment, walking through a rare patch of sunlight in the perpetual grey of the fog rising from the river to our right.

"And what then?" asks Jianmin. "How does all this relate to our question: Is there any higher meaning to physical love, between a man and a woman?"

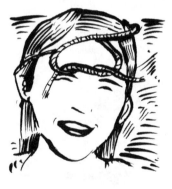

"It can be reversed," I say simply.

"What?" asks Chuhua.

"The process can be reversed. Left in our original condition—in our raw condition, before the left and right channels ever started—we would have had no knots. We would have been angels, in bodies of light, pure energy flowing up and down the middle channel."

"And you're saying we can go back to that?" whispers Jianmin.

"Can, and must, each one of us. The only question is whether we can untie those knots; and unmake those chakras; and melt the flesh and bone back into the light they were meant to be."

I look at Chuhua's face and I can see a bit of tension there. "Oh don't worry," I laugh. "Your little son Rusong won't turn into a light bulb. The basic shape of the body—head, arms, legs—remains the same, only it is perfectly exquisite, and beautiful, and deathless, and compassionate."

"And how does this transformation take place? How do we untie the knots?" demands Jianmin.

"The answer is quite famous; in the ancient books, they call it *Chi nang tab la tsowor bey.* It means *To untie the knots, work from the inside, and work from the outside too.*

"Working from the inside is pretty much what you might expect: meditation, contemplation, and prayer—to develop wisdom and love. Here a change in the person who rides on the horse changes the horse itself: if our thoughts are gentle, this causes the inner winds to move gently, and to move where we want them to go, into the middle—all because of that link between the windflow and our thoughts."

"And working from the outside?" asks Chuhua.

"Jianmin has already said it. The original purpose of yoga, and of many similar forms of exercise from Asia, was simply to untwist the knots, and return all of our winds to the middle channel.

"And there is one more very profound, very powerful way to move this prana…"

Chuhua can see it. "The intimacy that Jianmin and I share, right? I mean, in those moments it does almost seem as though our middle channels are connected, as though they literally become a single channel."

Jianmin nods. "And of course there is this intense release of a very powerful energy, jolting through the body."

I nod in turn. "That's right—in the right circumstances, the physical union between the two of you can become a very high thing, an even higher act of creation. It could help you move all the prana to the middle; it could help you become an angel of light, with a body that can appear on many worlds at the same time, and bring countless people out of their own pain."

Chuhua's face takes on a look of certainty. "I mean, it's something I think that we all feel, somewhere inside, about human intimacy: that somehow, it can be a very sacred thing, the giver of life, higher life…" Her words leave us all quiet, as we look out across the water.

After long minutes, Jianmin breaks the reverie. "But what did you mean when you said 'in the right circumstances'? I'm guessing that these circumstances are what make the difference between sex as an indulgence of little importance, and as a higher act of creation."

"I think you're right," I agree, "and that's exactly how the ancient scriptures put it too. It all has to do with that idea of the interaction between our thoughts and our inner winds, the prana. If the prana flows smoothly, our thoughts are kind, and gentle, and wise. And if we want to move the kind of prana that will change us back into light, then we can do so by working on our thoughts.

"The combination then is what we're looking for: using intimacy to move the winds, and developing the noble kinds of thinking that would move them to the right place, to the middle."

"And what are those thoughts?" asks Chuhua.

"Just about what you would expect," I an-swer. "I mean, first and foremost, the feelings of love and respect between yourself and your husband. It's something anyone can see, as they go through life. Physical intimacy between two people who don't really have any great concern for each other's happiness becomes just more or less of a wrestling match, each partner demand-ing physical sensations from the other, trying only to fulfill their own needs.

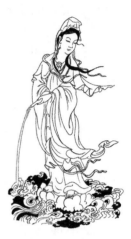

"The deepest of all human emotions is sim-ply to care whether someone else is happy or not. And so ideal partners—partners who are able to make intimacy into this high-est act of creation—are those who truly love each other. They are soul mates, they are lovers for life, they were always meant for each other; and each was heaven-sent for the other. They have spent a good part of their lives serv-ing each other, getting to know each other, respecting and loving each other. Even before the act of physical intimacy they have bonded, into a single be-ing. It is nothing casual; it is as though their union has always been, long before their birth—and perhaps it was."

Another lovely pause of silence, looking out over the waters. Even Ru-song is gazing out in quiet reflection.

"And there should be a sense of purpose," I add. "An intention, a holy in-tention, which by itself brings the winds to their single, ultimate resting point, deep within the heart." I nod at Ru. "It goes back to that idea of changing the world by example. If one of us could pull off what seems to be impossible, then our children would know it was possible, and it would save them too. The purpose of the union has to be a greater union: we need to do it for the world, for the children of the world."

"And is there anything else?" asks Jianmin.

"I think just to understand *why* the impossible is possible. In the end, our bodies are no different than the pen. What one sees as a dog's chew-toy, another sees as a writing instrument; what has always seemed a mortal coil can be equally experienced as a body of light. It all depends on our seeds."

Rusong has this wonderful habit of bursting out with a little "Oooh" of delight every once in a while, for reasons known only to himself. And of course he chooses this moment.

Question 98

Every once in a while I look out of the corner of my eye at my partner and I get this distinct feeling that they are some kind of Angel who was sent to me, to guide me. What's your take on this?

We're nearing the end of this book, and I know you're probably tired of me harping on seeds and pens over and over again. But there's really nowhere else to go. Everything depends on this one idea. The Buddha once said that anytime he ever talked about anything *other* than the seeds and the pen, he wasn't really talking about what he wanted to. And I truly believe the same.

Okay, so Tom and Kaia are not exactly your normal couple. I mean, they've been married almost ten years, and they claim that they've never had a fight. Be that as it may, the answer's the same. I pull out a pen and wave it in front of Kaia's face.

"Is Tom or is Tom not a holy angel sent to guide you?"

Kaia laughs. "Okay, okay, I know. I could be seeing him as a pen, or I could be seeing him as a chew-toy."

I get serious. "That's right—you could see him as just a regular guy that you sat down next to on a plane one day, or you could see him as a

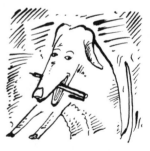

divine angel who maybe slipped into the plane from the top, and either one would be correct; either one would be real. But let me ask you: *Which one is more fun?"*

"The angel!" burst out Tom and Kaia in the same moment, as they so often do.

"So what kind of seeds?" asks Tom. "How can I see her this way all the time, instead of just getting a glimpse at random moments?"

We talked about this back in Question 9; but let's go at it a different way, because it's such a beautiful place to be.

"The ancient Tibetans called it *Takpay Nelnjor,"* I begin. "The Yoga of

Make-Believe. It means that if we want to reach a place where we just naturally see the world in a special way, we can plant the seeds by sort of artificially trying to see the world in that way."

"How's that?"

We touched on this back at Question 20, and you might want to go back and re-read that part. To Tom I say, "I mean, start with the moment that you first met Kaia on the plane, and work through your time together, up to now. Artificially choose certain moments as special, and try to see them that way. That plants the seeds for them to *become* that way, in reality."

"Well, the first moment really was on the plane, when she got assigned the seat next to me."

"Got assigned? Or was it set up? I like to call it *Central Casting.*"

"Meaning what?"

"Meaning you can *make believe* that there are sneaky angels spread all throughout the general population. Kaia is one of them, of course; but so was the ticket agent at the airline counter—she got assigned from Angel Central Casting to work that particular day at that particular counter, so you could meet each other.

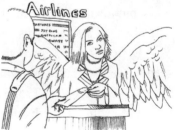

"Kaia comes in and winks at her (angels don't need to talk much), and nods towards you waiting over in the other line. The angelic ticket agent gives a nod and does some angel voodoo on the computer to guarantee that Kaia and you get seats next to each other."

Angels are sneaky

"But that's pretty far-fetched, don't you think?" Tom glances at Kaia. "I mean, a big conspiracy of angels around me my whole life, just trying to… what? Get me enlightened? Make me totally happy? Guarantee that I get to save the world?"

Dead silence.

Question 99

I find this whole idea pretty attractive: That everything which ever happens to me, and everyone I meet, is actually coming from seeds I've planted in my mind, by being good or bad to other people. But my husband doesn't think it makes any sense at all, and so I feel sort of a gap being created between us. What karmic seed do I have to plant to see my husband get the idea of karmic seeds running the show?

We live in a world where people *don't* really believe that seeds are running the show: that the people and the world around us are actually created by how we treat others. We talk about being good, and we all really do try to be good, but it's not like we totally believe that the irritating person at work has actually been created by us yelling at our kids every once in a while.

"Basically then," I say to Elena, "you aren't just asking how to plant a seed to see your husband trying to run his life on seeds. I mean, it could just as well be everybody. That is, what kind of seed does it take to see a whole planet of people living by a single principle: Everything that happens in my life comes directly from how well I take care of other people."

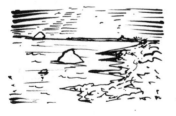 Elena and me are sort of yelling, because we're sitting across the aisle from each other on a noisy Russian bus working its way up the coast of Neva Bay, north of St Petersburg. Next to Elena sits her coworker Svetlana, who is focusing on our conversation in such a way that I'm guessing she has the same issue at home. Behind is a big crew of teachers from our Diamond Cutter Institute, all headed to a business retreat in the beautiful forested countryside outside the city.

"What you mean," she says in that lovely Russian accent, "is that if I figure out how to live in a whole world that runs itself by seeds, then automatically I'll see Aleksandr running himself by seeds."

I nod. "I mean, consider when we were little kids. I grew up in America, in a state called Arizona, in a city called Phoenix. I went to Maryland Elementary School. I felt like Maryland Elementary School was pretty much the 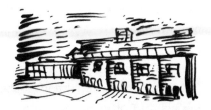 center of the entire universe. And that the chimes that they played over the loudspeaker when we were supposed to walk to our next class were pretty much the standard for classroom chimes all over the world.

"Then we grow up, and slowly we find out that there are other kinds of classroom chimes; and other elementary schools—other states, and other countries. I mean, even in college studying Russian, I thought Russia was impossibly far away, and that I would never be able to go there. And now here I am, sitting on a bus in Russia with a whole busload of Russians who seem like family." I wave my arm off towards the rest of the seats behind us. The family is also getting a little boisterous—too many *ponchik,* Russian pastries, washed down with American coke. Ah, the perfect melding of the two cultures.

"Yes, it is quite nice…" says Elena, obviously trying to get me back to the problem with her husband.

"Well you see, worlds are just the same. I mean, maybe even now, as we are here—as adults—we are thinking not that much differently from the little boy at Maryland Elementary School. How could this be the only world? How could there be that many stars in the sky, billions upon billions, and not another elementary school, somewhere? And do they move by the same classroom chimes that we do?"

"I see what you're saying," and I can feel that Russian intellect rising, one that we've seen in our audiences throughout the trip, as lovely as the accent. "There are certainly other worlds, and there are certainly ones that march to a different beat. Of the infinite worlds that must be there," she looks towards the sky, "there are certainly worlds which have already evolved in their thinking to this one idea, that our world is created by how well we treat other people."

Svetlana pipes up: "So it comes down to, what are the seeds to see a worldful of people who know enough to run their lives by seeds? And that would automatically cover Elena's husband and mine!"

"This is a famous question, and a famous answer. It all comes down to… *zhivoy primyer.*" I sit for a moment, kind of shocked that this Russian expression has suddenly popped into my head, quite clearly, without my having heard it for like over 30 years, since my torture sessions in college Russian class.

"A living example," translates Elena.

"That's the seed," I nod. "The seed to see a whole world of people being good to other people, because they know that's the seed for a perfect life. What plants the seed to see Aleksandr run his life by seeds is simply that you yourself have to keep in mind, constantly, that the seeds you plant are what create your own world. Because then you'll act on that understanding—you'll be a living example, of a person who achieves their goals in life by making very sure that others achieve theirs.

"So see that we're talking about the bigger picture of how you live your life. It's not just that you achieve your own financial independence by helping others achieve theirs; it's not just that you sustain a great relationship with your husband by attending to the needs of those who have no companionship.

"These are specific seeds that you plant to get specific things that you want in your life. On a larger scale, the point is that *you're dealing with everything* by identifying the seeds you need and planting them. No more clumsy attempts to manipulate the outside world: If I'm looking for a partner, do I go on the internet, or go to a nightclub? Which works best, red lipstick or pink?

"You just don't think that way anymore. Whatever you want, big or small—losing 5 pounds this month, or eliminating war in the world—you go at it from the inside, by planting the seeds inside of yourself. And then the outside just automatically changes.

"People see you acting this way, in a different way; maybe they understand the principles behind how you're acting, but more likely they just *feel* how you're acting, the power of a living example. And then they pick it up, and it spreads.

"Bottom line is you'll see Aleksandr start using the seeds, when you are using them for everything in your life yourself."

The driver suddenly pulls over and points to his left; the Gulf of Finland fills the horizon, and there's a small little beach. We all pile out to go touch the water and run right back to the bus, laughing and freezing.

Help others by being a living example of happiness

Question 100

How can we use our relationship to help the world?

I've spent a good part of my life teaching spiritual things around the world, because I love them and they make me very happy. But still it took me a long time to realize what people really want. It mostly boils down to four different things.

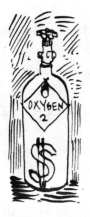

First we would like to be physically comfortable—which for me means financially independent. I like to call it "oxygen money." I don't think that most of us are greedy: that we want to live in a mansion and own twelve expensive cars and wear hats made of gold. But we would like to *have enough money that we don't have to think about money.*

When you decide to go to a movie, you don't call the theater ahead of time to make sure there will be enough oxygen in the room for everybody who attends the show. You just assume that the air will be there; it always is, everywhere we go. Money should be like that, for all of us. We should all have enough, and it should flow in smoothly all the time, so that we can just do all the things we'd like to do with our lives, without worrying about credit card balances and stuff like that.

And so oxygen money is goal #1. You can't meditate, for example, if you don't have a place to meditate which is reasonably comfortable. I tried meditating once in a cave at a place called Sycamore Canyon, in Arizona; but I got chased out by spiders and an especially venomous species of rattlesnake. A reasonably safe and comfortable place to meditate is going to cost, not a lot of money, but some.

Money by itself though doesn't make you happy: there are a heck of a lot of rich people who are terribly lonely. And so I think very naturally the second goal that most of us have is to find our special partner, someone to be our companion as we go through life, someone to have a family with if that's what we want. We'd like to find them, and keep them, and be as crazy in love with them 20 or 30 years later as we were on the first date.

But the comfort of a home and the companionship of a partner aren't completely comforting if we have no energy, or we are in poor health. And so I think that goal #3, for most of us, is to stay young and strong, so that we can really enjoy our life to the fullest.

By now you know how to achieve each of these goals. Plant the seeds, use the Four Steps, especially the last one: Coffee Meditation, wrestling with your mind when you lay down to sleep, forcing it to think about all the good things that you and others have been doing, fertilizing the seeds of goodness that every person already has in their mind.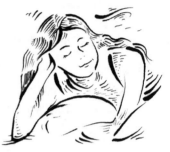

But there is one more goal to reach, one more human need that every one of us craves to fulfill. And that is to take care of others: to help make a world where no one has pain, where no one is sad. The need for shelter, the desire for another's touch, and the pursuit of youth are powerful forces in every human heart; but beneath them, deep in the soul, is the most powerful urge of all, and that is to provide each of these things, to provide happiness, to every *other* living being. We all want to be a superhero, we all want to be everyone else's mother.

So how do we use our relationship to save the world—to bring safety and comfort and happiness to every other person in the world? How do we fulfill our deepest desire of all?

In the Diamond Cutter system we achieve our own needs by planting seeds, and the only way to plant seeds is to fulfill the needs of others. When we work for others, we are working for ourselves; and the only way to work for ourselves is to work for others. It's not just that the two goals overlap; in truth they are the same goal, and deep down we feel it.

And so if you want your relationship to help the world, all you have to do is to make it a *successful* relationship. The best thing you can both do for the world is to be that living example; because in the end people don't care what you say, they only watch what you do. And if they see that what you do works, they will try it for themselves.

In the end then your greatest responsibility, and the best way you can help

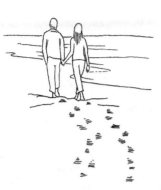

the entire world, is to be a success at that most difficult task in an entire   human life: Become a happy person, become a happy couple. People will watch you, and if the seed thing works for you and your partner, the world will copy you. And in this way we change the world, like a computer virus that spreads quickly, from one person to countless others.

Your only job, if you love the world, is to be happy. And the only way to be happy is to plant the seeds.

**Your only job,
if you love the world,
is to be happy**

ACKNOWLEDGEMENTS

I am very blessed to live my life to in a wonderful network of talented and dedicated friends who have always been willing to devote their time and skills to projects, like this book, which we all hope will help other people. I would like to thank a few of them here by name, and also thank all the many others who are not named here, and have happily given their time and energy for all these years.

Our publishing team was headed by John Cerullo, founder and director of Diamond Cutter Press, and one of those rare and beautiful combinations of humility and high expertise, in this case with decades in the national publishing business. Brooks Singer, DCP's Subsidiary Rights Manager, skillfully and cheerfully juggles dozens of overseas contracts at any given time, including those for the upcoming foreign editions of this book.

Ven Jigme Palmo (Elizabeth van der Pas) coordinated all the teams working on the book, all over the world, working non-stop through many time zones. Alejandro Julien, the ebullient head of ACI and DCI Mexico, brought together many members of his Guadalajara team to get the book finished. Paramjeet Singh, director of Fine Grains India, worked very hard to meet a tight printing deadline, with expertise and care.

The design team included Georgina (Gina) Rivera of Guadalajara, the quiet genius behind many related publishing efforts; as well as Robert Ruisinger, from the USA, and another delightful combination of cheerfulness, dedication, and mastery of the printed word.

Editorial duties were shared by an entire group from the ACI Phoenix team, including Rebecca Vinacour, Nicole Vigna, Ven Jigme Palmo, John Oyzon, Esther Giangrande, Christine Walsh, and Robert Haggerty. Each of these friends has their own special talent—whether it be performing in a Broadway musical or training hundreds of professional psychologists in a single sitting—but together they also share a fine eye and ear that has made the book flow much better, and more accurately.

Our team of illustrators was again asked to meet a nearly impossible deadline, and rose to the challenge—especially Gibran Julian, founder of Studio Gibravo (*www.gibravo.com*) in Guadalajara, who was trained in both Mexico and Europe. Imelda Espinoza—one of the organizers of the ACI and DCI Mexico teams, and also a magazine and book designer, as well as translator—

also contributed. Other illustrations were completed by Ana Maria Velasco of Santa Marta, Colombia, who was trained at the School of the Museum of Fine Arts in Boston and directs the wellness non-profit NEEM (*www.anavelasco. co*). Ori Carin, a highly talented painter from New York and contributor to previous books, completed a number of the illustrations requiring portraiture. Nicole Vigna and Ula Byglewski assisted with the selection of the sample images for the illustrations.

Nicole is also taking charge of the worldwide releases and marketing of the book, with Mark Tripetti and Miriam Parker heading the core marketing effort in New York. As usual, indispensible support has been supplied by several dear members of my personal staff, who between them have logged almost 50 years providing me with all the help and friendship I could ever hope for: Ven Jigme Palmo (Elizabeth van der Pas), concentrating on finance; Mercedes Bahleda, on business development, global operations, and scheduling; and Ven Lobsang Nyingpo (Eric Brinkman), communications and technology. Nick Lashaw also helped immensely with logistics as the book neared completion.

Roy Phay of Singapore, who helps spearhead DCI operations throughout the East and Southeast Asia, and his wife Michslle Phay are the masterminds behind the Karma of Love website (*www.KarmaOfLove.com*) and the online and cell phone Karma of Love apps. I am also grateful for the many hours they have devoted to our charitable work for needy people around the world.

Finally I would like to take this opportunity to thank the friends who have labored for decades to make my books available in countries all over the world. Many of them are producing foreign-language editions of the *Karma of Love,* for which I am also very grateful. In Asia these include Xia Liyang and John Bentham (China); Chiafang Chang of Oaktree and Cite Publishing (Taiwan), with dedicated assistance from Rob Hou and his wife Jessica Sung, as well as Kay Chen; Nguyen Man Hung and his wonderful staff at Thai Ha Books (Vietnam); Leza Lowitz (Japan); Sheshadri and Melissa Mantha (India); and Jaki Fisher (Singapore).

In Europe I am indebted to the publishing efforts of Silvia Engelhardt, Ulla Bettmer, and Beate Ludwig of Edition Blumenau (Germany); the decades of devoted publishing by Isidro and Marta Gordi of Ediciones Amara (Spain); Pavel Belorusskiy of Niguma Publishing House (Russia); Elena Novik and Marina Selitsky of Almaz Publishing (Ukraine & Russia); the superstars of Zhanaua '98 publishing—Jana Ivanova, Kiril Voinov, and Yasen Nikolov (Bulgaria); Per Flood and Peter Mörtl (Sweden); Cecile Roubaud (France);

Gerard van Bussel of Petiet Publishing (Holland); Yelena Zaric (Serbia); Andrei Soeanu (Romania); Niki Lambropoulos (Greece); and newcomers Zoltan Saghy (Hungary); Sergei Mironov (Estonia); Ralitza Nikolaeva (Portugal); and Maxim Shkodin (Krasnodar, Russia).

For Latin America I would like to give thanks to Alejandro Julien and the Mexico publishing team; to Carola Terreni and her husband Tomas Laredo (Argentina); and to Maria Rita Stumpf (Brazil and Peru). For Israel, great thanks to all the publishing efforts of many groups, and the coordination of them headed by Liran Katz. And finally, my grateful thanks to Trace Murphy and Gary Jansen of Doubleday, Crown, and Random House, for having the faith to get me started as an author in the first place. I hope that between all of us we have helped spread the great ideas of the Diamond Cutter, and contributed to the lives and happiness of people we know, and those who are yet to come.

INDEX

Note: The numbers refer to the question number, and not the page number

Karma of Love

The app is coming!

Trouble with your partner? *We're here to help you.* Go in the bathroom, pull out your cell phone, and use your Karma of Love App for instant advice, tailored to your needs. Check the karmic seeds you need to plant, right now! See our website *www.KarmaOfLove.com* for updates on an app that will change you and your partner's life, forever.

The site

Order the app, get copies of the book, see how people around the world are using karmic seeds to deal with exactly the same challenges that you have. And get expert advice from our KOL Counselors. All in many different languages of the world. Go to *www.KarmaOfLove.com.*

The talk

Have a KOL Counselor or Senior Staff Teacher visit your city for one or two evenings of talks, to groups from ten to a thousand people. Let us know what you need at *info@KarmaOfLove.com.* We'll be there!

The training

In conjunction with senior coaches from the Diamond Cutter Institute, we offer teacher training seminars to help you learn to use the principles of the Karma of Love in your own business, school, or wellness practice. See either website for details: *www.KarmaOfLove.com;* or *www. diamondcutterinstitute.com.*

The book

Order copies of this book online at Amazon or other major bookselling sites.

For wholesale or bookstore orders contact
Diamond Cutter Press at:
www.diamondcutterpress.com/contact.html

Other languages

Publishers all over the world are coming out with *The Karma of Love* in different languages. Check our website *www.KarmaOfLove.com* to see what's available and what's upcoming. If you'd like to publish the book in your country, we'd be happy to help; contact *info@KarmaOfLove.com*.